T0372694

Knowledge and the scholarly medical traditions

However much the three great traditions of medicine – Galenic, Chinese and Āyurvedic – differed from each other, they had one thing in common: scholarship. The foundational knowledge of each could be acquired only by careful study under teachers relying on ancient texts. Such knowledge is special, operating as it does in the realm of the most fundamental human experiences – health, disease, suffering, birth and death – and the credibility of healers is of crucial importance. Because of this, scholarly medical knowledge offers a rich field for the study of different cultural practices in the legitimation of knowledge generally. The contributors to this volume are all specialists in the history or anthropology of these traditions, and their essays range from historical investigations to studies of present-day practices.

Knowledge and the scholarly medical traditions

Edited by

Don Bates

McGill University

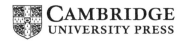

CAMBRIDGE
UNIVERSITY PRESS

University Printing House, Cambridge CB2 8BS, United Kingdom

Cambridge University Press is part of the University of Cambridge.

It furthers the University's mission by disseminating knowledge in the pursuit of education, learning and research at the highest international levels of excellence.

www.cambridge.org
Information on this title: www.cambridge.org/9780521480710

© Cambridge University Press 1995

First published 1995

A catalogue record for this publication is available from the British Library

Library of Congress Cataloguing in Publication data
Knowledge and the scholarly medical traditions / edited by Don Bates.
   p. cm.
Includes index.
ISBN 0 521 48071 X (hardback)
1. Medicine – Philosophy.
2. Medical anthropology.
3. Knowledge and learning.
I. Bates, Donald G. (Donald George), 1933– .
[DNLM: 1. Learning.   2. Philosophy, Medical.   3. History of Medicine.
4. Medicine, Traditional – history.   W 61 K725 1995]
R723.K54   1995
610'.1 – dc20   94–40968   CIP
DNLM/DLC for Library of Congress

ISBN 978-0-521-48071-0 Hardback
ISBN 978-0-521-49975-0 Paperback

To Owsei Temkin and Charles Leslie

Contents

Illustrations

Contributors

DON BATES
Department of Social Studies of Medicine, McGill University, Montreal

FRANCESCA BRAY
Department of Anthropology, University of California, Santa Barbara

LAWRENCE COHEN
Department of Anthropology, University of California, Berkeley

LAWRENCE CONRAD
Wellcome Institute for the History of Medicine, London

LESLEY DEAN-JONES
Department of Classics, University of Texas, Austin

JUDITH FARQUHAR
Department of Anthropology, University of North Carolina, Chapel Hill

AMOS FUNKENSTEIN
Department of History, University of California, Berkeley

LUIS GARCÍA-BALLESTER
CSIC, Historia de la Ciencia, Barcelona, Spain

ROBERT JAMES HANKINSON
Department of Philosophy, University of Texas, Austin

SHIGEHISA KURIYAMA
International Research Center of Japanese Studies, Kyoto

GEOFFREY LLOYD
Darwin College, Cambridge University, Cambridge

NATHAN SIVIN
Department of History and Sociology of Science, University of
Pennsylvania, Philadelphia

MARGARET TRAWICK
Department of Social Anthropology, Massey University, Palmerston North, New Zealand

FAITH WALLIS
Department of Social Studies of Medicine, McGill University, Montreal

ANDREW WEAR
Wellcome Institute for the History of Medicine, London

ALLAN YOUNG
Department of Social Studies of Medicine, McGill University, Montreal

FRANCIS ZIMMERMANN
Laboratoire d'anthropologie sociale, Ecole des hautes études en sciences sociales, Paris

Acknowledgements

The organizing of a workshop followed by the production of a volume inevitably depends upon the time, effort and co-operation of a great many people, only a small number of whom I can mention here. The idea for the workshop 'Epistemology and the Scholarly Medical Traditions' arose out of a number of conversations with my colleague, George Weisz, and had its origins in a course in the history of medicine which we have been teaching together for many years. Moreover, at all stages of the project – from planning the meeting through to editing and introducing this book – I have received many helpful suggestions and advice from George and all my other colleagues – Margaret Lock, Allan Young, Faith Wallis and Alberto Cambrosio. Indeed, although ultimately my responsibility, this volume is in many ways a product of our whole department in which medical history, medical anthropology and medical sociology have worked closely together for almost twenty years.

While contributors to an edited volume are generally assumed to receive their due by virtue of their authorship, only the editor knows how much he has benefited from their participation in the workshop, their co-operation in preparing their papers and their patience with his idiosyncrasies. Moreover, I want to offer a special thanks to Geoffrey Lloyd, Nathan Sivin and Francis Zimmermann for their very early and unwavering support and advice for this project, and for their helpful suggestions on the introductory chapter, and to Judy Farquhar for several useful conversations during her time as a visiting scholar in our department.

No effort of this kind can succeed, however, without a certain amount of luck, and that luck came in the persons of Fern Brunger, Teresa Gray and Fiona Deller. Fern played such a major role in organizing and putting on the workshop that it would not be an exaggeration to say that I was her assistant. Teresa and Fiona very ably performed the highly exacting task of copy-editing and bringing into editorial harmony this very interdisciplinary group of contributions. Meanwhile, Claudine

Houston diligently tracked our finances and Stella Zoccali provided the first-class secretarial assistance for which she is highly reputed. Early on, while Stella was at home making her own contribution to the next generation of humanity, Jane Scribner pitched in cheerfully, enthusiastically and very effectively. I would also like to express my thanks to Jessica Kuper and Virginia Catmur of Cambridge University Press.

Last, and possibly most, I want to thank those who provided the financial support that made the whole thing possible. The Hannah Institute for the History of Medicine in Toronto was not only generous in its funding, but exceptionally flexible and understanding in responding to our requests. The Wenner-Gren Foundation for Anthropological Research was also a major contributor. Additional financial support was provided by the Social Sciences and Humanities Research Council of Canada, the Wellcome Trust in London, and the Dr Joseph Nathanson Center for the History and Culture of Medicine.

1   Scholarly ways of knowing: an introduction

Don Bates

The title for the workshop from which this volume evolved was 'Epistemology and the Scholarly Medical Traditions'. The original idea was to look at the question, 'How did Galenic, Chinese and Āyurvedic doctors use written texts as authorities for their claims to knowledge?' Contributors were left considerable freedom, however, to interpret the original title as they pleased because enforcing any particular orientation would have risked subverting our comparative enterprise before it had begun.

That proved to be a wise decision. In our very first session together, Jim Hankinson defined 'epistemology' as 'a self-conscious theory of knowledge'. A little later, Judith Farquhar observed that, for a Sinologist, every word of that definition would have to be reinterpreted, 'quite possibly including "of"'. As the reader will discover, 'episte-mology' turns up frequently, and it is indeed a troublemaker. It has a decidedly Eurocentric ring to it. In an effort to avoid some of the pitfalls associated with the term, this essay will step back a bit and reflect, historically, anthropologically and meta-epistemologically, on the ways in which these traditions have (or have not) claimed special status for their scholarly medical knowledge at various times in history.[1]

But first, a word or two is needed about the overall strategy of the volume. All the chapters are devoted to the past except for those by anthropologists Judith Farquhar and Lawrence Cohen who talk about present-day events in China and India, respectively. In retrospect, I regret the omission of something about modern Unani medicine so as to

---

[1]   See Ian Hacking, 'Historical Epistemology', an unpublished discussion paper for the Chicago–Paris–Toronto graduate students' workshop, University of Toronto (October, 1993). Hacking sees historical epistemology as dealing with 'organizing concepts that we are stuck with' such as objectivity (p. 24f.). Moreover, 'historical epistemology is ... totally locked into the Western tradition of reason and causality in which philosophy, science, and history arose, and it has no pretension to go beyond that' (p. 29). From Hacking's perspective, this introduction is an exercise in historical meta-epistemology because, on the one hand, it seeks a level that will reach beyond the Western tradition, but on the other hand, addresses a classical epistemological question – how is knowledge, in this case medical knowledge, legitimated?

have touched on living examples of all three traditions. But, in a book such as this, comprehensiveness is just not possible.[2] Also omitted is any extended reference to modern medicine, or 'biomedicine'. This omission was deliberate, not because our medicine represents some sort of culture-free, transcendent truth but because we wanted to compare text-based traditions.

As for what is in the volume, a look at the table of contents will reveal that half of it is devoted to Western medical history, especially Galenism, while the Chinese and Āyurvedic traditions share the remainder.[3] This imbalance was intentional, for a major aim of the exercise was to bring historical Galenism into its rightful place as an obvious subject for comparison with the other great traditions. Several of the scholars who are presently leading the way in this kind of comparison – people such as Geoffrey Lloyd, Nathan Sivin, Shigehisa Kuriyama and Francis Zimmermann – are contributors to this volume.

The central purpose of the book is to offer for comparison some studies on the ways in which healers in the three great scholarly traditions of medicine claimed to know something about the promotion of health and healing. What makes comparison seem promising is that the knowing involved has certain characteristics in common. First, all these scholarly healers (with the exception of the Hippocratics) rest their claims to healing power largely on knowledge which is grounded in the study of written texts. They are not shamans, craftsmen, wise women, bonesetters nor folk healers. For the most part they do not claim to get medical knowledge through direct revelation, mystical experience, simple trial and error, nor even through mere apprenticeship, however much apprenticeship may also be involved. They are all scholars of literate traditions.

Second, such learning is at least partly theoretical, and, as such, operates at the interface between human beings and the universe. Like religion, medical theory (or doctrine) is cosmic in its orientation.[4]

[2]   See 'The Comparative Study of Greco-Islamic Medicine: The Integration of Medical Knowledge into Local Symbolic Contexts', by Byron and Mary-Jo DelVecchio Good, and indeed the whole volume of which it is a part, Charles Leslie and Allan Young (eds.), *Paths to Asian Medical Knowledge* (Berkeley: University of California Press, 1992). The Goods' article is on pp. 257–71. The other classic of comparative studies in this field, of course, and the original inspiration for this volume is Charles Leslie (ed.), *Asian Medical Systems: A Comparative Study* (Berkeley: University of California Press, 1976).

[3]   As this introduction argues, and the rest of this volume attests, there are just as good (and just as dubious) *historical* grounds for speaking of 'Western' as for 'Eastern', 'Chinese', or 'Āyurvedic'. Like all conventions, they have their benefits and their costs.

[4]   For example, the ubiquity of concepts about a correspondence between the microcosm and macrocosm.

Third, however theoretical or abstract, learned medical knowing must confront experience, in fact some of the most profoundly important human experiences – health, illness, disease, pain, suffering, birth, death. Therapy involves interacting with the world.

Having staked out what I see to be the common ground on which a comparison can be made, my aim in this introductory chapter is to mine the contributions to this volume for what they can tell us about knowing in the three traditions.[5] As a preparation for that exercise, though, I want to dwell for a moment on the fundamental issue of knowledge and knowing, because the following chapters suggest basic differences among the traditions, and within individual traditions at different times, with respect to their attitudes towards knowledge and the knowing person.

If, for example, we compare the classical Greek tradition with its Chinese and Āyurvedic counterparts, a difference is already apparent. In the latter two, knowledge gets much of its status from the person who knows it, while, in ancient Greece, the known gets much more of its status from the knower's capacity to justify it in terms of other knowns. And connected with that need to justify is the very Western phenomenon of active epistemology.

In an effort to design some analytical tools that would deal with this difference, two concepts were constructed and given names: 'gnostic' and 'epistemic'.[6] Largely on the basis of the contributions to this volume, I then tried to think through, in idealized terms, what these contrasting concepts could mean. On the one hand, it seemed, gnostic knowing is centred on the knower. Knowledge is certified by the status of the knower. It is acquired through learning and experience. The student is a disciple who is guided by an orthodoxy which is elaborated, corroborated, enriched and embellished by experience. Study is as much a rite of initiation as it is learning. The highest goal is wisdom.

On the other hand, epistemic knowing is centred on the known. The credibility of the known is grounded in how it is known ('methodology'), and attention is focused at least as much on the constitution of knowledge as on the means of its transmission. Rather than as an accompaniment to learning, experience is often set up in opposition to intellectual pursuits of theory making, reasoning and rationality. The relation of student to teacher is problematic because epistemology

---

5 I have richly benefited from the comments of several contributors and colleagues who read earlier drafts of this introduction. Nevertheless, any ideas or interpretations put forward here that do not appear in subsequent chapters or references are entirely my own responsibility.

6 In using 'gnostic' I am not referring to 'Gnostic', though the choice of the term was influenced by some of Gnosticism's ideas about knowledge.

furnishes the final criteria of certification. To the extent that epistemological principles have been established, the role of experience is also defined by those principles. The ultimate goal may be wisdom, but it is often thought of as expertise.

In its idealized form, gnostic knowing cultivates stories of transcendent origins in divine authority or the superior knowers of a golden age, and reveres continuity through genealogies and lineages (of persons and/or texts) that tie the known to those transcendent knowers. More loosely, this value is manifested simply as archaism. Epistemic knowing, on the other hand, depends on the things already known, and concerns itself less with continuity than with justifiability (rational and/or empirical, depending on the epistemology espoused). Moreover, whereas the gnostic reverence for knowers often accommodates multivocal knowing when there is a multiplicity of superior knowers (gods, sages, etc.), the epistemic variety more typically combines its focus on the known with a commitment to univocal truth. And finally, keeping in mind Hankinson's formula for 'epistemology', but backing up to the level of our meta-epistemology, we might think of gnostic scholarship as self-consciously cultivating superior knowers, while epistemic scholarship self-consciously searches for ways to justify knowledge.

Those familiar with the work of Max Weber will no doubt notice that there are some interesting similarities between these two concepts and his three types of 'authority'.[7] Epistemicism makes one think of his 'legal' authority, and gnosticism sounds like some combination of his 'traditional' and 'charismatic' forms of authority.[8] But it would not serve our present purposes to follow up on these resemblances which are by no means straightforward.

On the other hand, the manner in which Weber used his types of authority as 'heterogeneous elements' which are always 'combined in different historical configurations' captures very well the way I intend gnosticism and epistemicism to be understood. As spelled out above, I am not suggesting that they will be found as 'pure types' in history, but am proposing them, rather, as 'clear concepts' for analysing the combinations of ways of knowing that actually turn up in the three scholarly traditions.[9]

Besides emphasizing that the notions of gnosticism and epistemicism are meant more to serve as heuristic devices than to reflect historical

---

[7] I am grateful to Allan Young for drawing this to my attention.

[8] In a preliminary version of his chapter in this volume, Nathan Sivin spoke of 'charismatic scriptures' as sources of Chinese traditional medicine.

[9] With respect to Weber's concepts and how he used them, I am employing the language of Reinhard Bendix in his *Max Weber: An Intellectual Portrait* (Berkeley: University of California Press, 1977), pp. 290–7, esp. p. 296.

realities, there is a second methodological point that I would like to make. A number of constraints oblige me to treat the history of the three traditions, themselves, in superficial, schematic and discontinuous ways. These constraints are first, that this introduction must be brief; second, that I want to focus largely on the richly suggestive material furnished by the succeeding chapters; and third that, despite the generous help of several of the contributors,[10] I can make no claim to the kind of expertise that would be required for an adequate historical overview, even of Western medicine, let alone of the other traditions. Therefore, as the reader proceeds, both the concepts of gnosticism and epistemicism, and the analysis which follows, should be looked upon largely as suggestions for thinking about the history of scholarly ways of knowing in the three traditions.

Perhaps this is also the best place to clarify a third point. Weber treated his three elements as 'types of authority'. In this essay, I am treating gnosticism and epistemicism as types of knowledge legitimation or ways of knowing. When *we* study these types, *we* are engaging in epistemology; we are behaving like the followers of epistemicism insofar as we are studying knowledge legitimation in and of itself. But we are not behaving entirely like classical epistemics in that our disciplinary perspectives are not those of philosophy, nor even cognitive psychology, but rather those of history and anthropology. This socially oriented approach positions us better for our study of gnosticism where the concerns of legitimacy are (in the idealized type) more the *social* concerns of legitimating the knower than the philosophical concerns of legitimating the known.

In addition, this social perspective helps in another way. We are engaged, here, in the study of what people *claimed* to be the basis of their knowledge, i.e., in *the study of their rhetoric and behaviour* insofar as it was aimed to convince themselves and others that they were indeed in possession of the truth, or at least of knowledge of special value. The motives behind that rhetoric and behaviour were undoubtedly many and varied. Those motives may have often included the desire for truth, but not always. Indeed, with respect to scholarly medicine, it is clear that the strongest motives usually had to do with a desire to maintain health and promote healing, on the one hand, and to gain a social purchase over the patient and/or one's rivals, on the other.

Now, keeping these methodological points in mind, let us turn to a contemplation of how gnosticism and epistemicism might have played out in actual historical situations. To begin with, the different values

---

[10] I want particularly to thank Nathan Sivin and Geoffrey Lloyd in this regard.

expressed in gnostic and epistemic ways of knowing no doubt reflect the wider frameworks of meaning and value, the 'cosmologies' as it were, of the societies that subscribed to them. In classical Hindu thought, for example, it is spiritual moral order that dominates, while in classical Chinese thought it is more of a civil moral order. In either case, though, the fundamentals of how the world works are underwritten by the status of transcendent or at least superior knowers who reveal them. Greek thought, on the other hand, seems to have evolved in a somewhat different direction.[11] In particular, with 'the invention of nature'[12] comes a philosophical tradition (chiefly Aristotelian) that does not depend on revelation for its foundational knowledge.[13]

True, Greek nature is divine, and, in view of its divinity, in some sense a knowing other. (For example, nature is a skilled craftsman; nature does nothing without a purpose, etc.) Yet, from the human perspective, it is not knowing in an altogether helpful way. It is as if society were situated, not at the feet of a divine revealer, so much as inside its knowing self, and having to infer that knowing from the state it finds nature to be in. As a result, the Greeks had only their own all-too-human knowers (i.e., natural philosophers), to tell each other about it.

This is a bit fanciful,[14] but what I am trying to suggest is a congruence between the gnostic way of knowing and cosmologies headed up by knowing and revelatory others, on the one hand, and between the epistemic way of knowing and cosmologies dominated by a 'nature' which, if knowing, is nevertheless accessible to humans largely as a non-communicating other.

I do not mean to suggest by this that any of the cosmologies of the three classical societies was unitary or unchanging. They are as historical and pluralistic as the communities which gave them expression. By the same token I do not mean to imply that they were 'mentalities' that necessitated the particular ways of knowing which they reflected.[15] I am

[11]   For a comparison of ancient Chinese and Greek cosmological thinking, see G.E.R. Lloyd, *Demystifying Mentalities* (Cambridge: Cambridge University Press, 1990), ch. 4, pp. 105–34.
[12]   G. E. R. Lloyd, 'The Invention of Nature', in his *Methods and Problems in Greek Science* (Cambridge: Cambridge University Press, 1991), pp. 417–34.
[13]   For earlier Greek thought, see Edward Hussey, 'The Beginnings of Epistemology: From Homer to Philolaus', in Stephen Everson (ed.), *Epistemology* (Cambridge: Cambridge University Press, 1990), pp. 11–38.
[14]   And greatly oversimplified. For a detailed discussion see Owsei Temkin, *Hippocrates in a World of Pagans and Christians* (Baltimore: The Johns Hopkins University Press, 1991), esp. ch. 15, pp. 197–208. However, no ancient Greek healing gods (and particularly Asclepius) gave rise to a *scholarly* medicine based on revealed knowledge conveyed by teachers and texts. Asclepius, for instance, *was* the healer.
[15]   See Lloyd (note 11). Later in this essay, I shall return to the issue of cultures and cosmologies.

only saying that these different cosmological outlooks came with different potentialities for ways of knowing just as they did for what was known. In short, a cosmology offers its own ways of legitimating knowledge.

But I have a reason for taking such a broad and roomy perspective. It helps us when we shift our focus from the last five hundred years BC, i.e., roughly the classical period in which each of the traditions was born, and begin to roll the camera of history forward over the next fifteen hundred years. For it allows us to take notice of another difference between the Greek medical tradition and those of the East – the successive transplantation of the former into a series of other cosmologies not only different from the one in which it was born, but cosmologies that fostered different ways of legitimating knowledge.

Our knowledge of the history of Chinese and Āyurvedic medicine is limited, particularly from a comparative perspective of the kind that would help us here. Nevertheless, it is clear that we tell their stories very differently. For there is no counterpart to our Western account of a corpus of ancient texts migrating for over eight hundred years (and some parts for more than fourteen hundred years), starting eastward from the Aegean, then circling clockwise around the Mediterranean basin via North Africa, and ending up in Western Europe after 1000 AD. In their journey, these texts passed through early Christianity, Judaism and Islam, and then into medieval Christian Europe, writings that were translated, often serially, into Persian, Syriac, Hebrew, Arabic and Latin. Once more, at the end of the Middle Ages, they received a new infusion of texts translated from the Greek. Indeed, the very existence of this narrative is testimony to our Western proclivity for focusing on an ontologized 'knowledge' rather than on the knowing society.[16]

In the course of its remarkable journey, this body of literature was itself subject to much variation in its constituent parts by virtue of the ever-changing amounts of omission and addition. Of more importance here though is the fact that very different societies, with different languages, religions and cosmologies, constantly transformed and retransformed this legacy from ancient Greece. Admittedly, the Chinese and Āyurvedic texts were not static either, but the central theme of our stories about them is much more one of continuity and return to traditionalism than of geographical migration and profound linguistic and societal transformation.

---

[16] Apart from providing a rich body of literature for historians to work on, the story of 'Galenism' has undoubtedly been shaped by longstanding values that privilege scholarship and cultivate the central narrative of 'Western' history – the roots of modern European and North and South American society in Greek and Roman antiquity.

Scholarly texts

Perhaps this difference will become sharper if we look more closely at that Western migration of texts in the context of gnostic and epistemic knowing. The period from before the time of Hippocrates in 400 BC to that of Galen six hundred years later seems to offer the purest instance of what I am calling the epistemic approach to knowing (at least before the modern era, which is not being considered here). In Geoffrey Lloyd's exploration of epistemological issues in early Greek medicine, and Jim Hankinson's description of the growth of medical empiricism in later antiquity, we get a detailed introduction to this story and to its strong epistemic character.[17] Consistent with this, texts served throughout only as vehicles for discourse and communication. In terms of Faith Wallis' typology (p. 125), they were not 'sacred' nor 'classic', but just 'plain' texts.

This situation may have been changing, however, even during Galen's own lifetime. Certainly for him, and for many of his contemporaries, Hippocrates had taken on god-like qualities. Moreover, by the fourth century, i.e., well before the rise of Islam, the text had definitely become invested with a significance consistent with gnostic knowing: Galen's own works were beginning to enjoy a privileged status and Galen, both as the source of Hippocratic knowledge and in his own right, was becoming a superior knower, even though both were pagans in a now predominantly Christian cosmology. By the time of the rise of Islam in the seventh century, there was a fairly strong gnostic tradition of medical knowing centred on the Galenic texts.[18]

As with Christianity, in the Muslim religion itself we have an example of a very strong gnostic tradition of knowing in which the Koran is the epitome of a sacred text. Yet, just because the lineage of the Koran was so clear and so exclusive, the ancient Greek knowledge of nature and medicine lay outside this main trunk of relatively pure gnostic knowing.

With regard to Arab-Islamic medicine, then, the ancient Greek legacy of natural and methodological philosophy and medicine was assimilated into early ninth-century Islam. But, even though the ancient texts were privileged, those privileges were not generally on a plane with the gnostic knowing that society bestowed upon its indigenous, religious verities. Not surprisingly, Arabic scholar-practitioners eventually began to add to

---

[17]   Indeed, the empiricists were explicitly anti-gnostic. (See Hankinson, p. 68).
[18]   Owsei Temkin, *Galenism: Rise and Decline of a Medical Philosophy* (Ithaca: Cornell University Press, 1973), esp. ch. 2, pp. 51–94; also, Temkin (note 14), esp. ch. 5, pp. 47–50.

the Greek inheritance on the authority of their own experience and understanding.

Even in this greatly simplified account, it is clear that both epistemic and gnostic elements are present and our sharp distinction between their idealized types has been blurred. Over the centuries, the cumulative impression one gets from the early Christian and Arabic handling of the ancient corpus is that of archaism and learnedness. This is gnostic to the extent that the ancient texts are revered because they are ancient. It is also gnostic in its cultivation of learnedness. But ultimately the degree of gnosticism involved must be measured by the degree to which those texts serve as a framework that constrains meaning and the possibilities for new knowledge by virtue of their authors' transcendent authority.

If the Arabic regard for these medical texts wasn't thoroughly gnostic, neither was it as actively epistemic as it was among the ancient Greek authors whom Lloyd and Hankinson tell us about. Compared to the Greeks' self-conscious and unresolved struggle and competition over theories of knowledge, the Arabic approach was epistemologically more passive. Its epistemological activity resided in the fact that it applied the methodologies of ancient philosophy (most particularly Aristotle, but also Galen and others) to the medical knowledge of antiquity in order to make it more 'rational', more consistent, systematic and coherent, i.e., in true epistemic spirit it tried to make that knowledge more or less self-consistent, quite apart from its being ancient. But it was a passive, i.e., traditionalized, epistemology insofar as it privileged and took for granted both those methodologies and that knowledge *because* they were ancient.

When we compare this with Faith Wallis' chapter on the composition of texts and manuscripts in early medieval medicine, these epistemic differences become even more apparent. On the one hand, the early medieval, Christian, European society that Wallis is talking about was, like its Islamic contemporaries, observing a religious brand of gnostic knowing.[19] On the other hand, the situation of its medical knowledge was quite different. For one thing, by comparison with the Arabic world, the residues of ancient learning were fewer, less accessible because of the loss of the Greek language, and without extensive cultivation in formal institutions of learning. In addition, Wallis draws our attention to two other curious differences: the apparently deliberate decanonization of the medical texts; and the striking omission of the theoretical parts from this ancient medical lore.

Wallis argues that the exclusion of theory was because pagan world views conflicted with Christian doctrine. However, in the course of their

---

[19]   Though not, of course, Gnosticism.

highly selective, and at times quite irreverent gatherings of ancient texts, these early European scholars also tell us much about their own epistemological attitudes. On the one hand, to cultivate (i.e., translate and put together) the practical parts was to invest this ancient knowledge with some sort of value. On the other hand, such texts were not sanctified. They served merely as quarries to be mined, the useful ore to be separated from the pagan dross of a divine nature that did not need God.

What is also striking about these texts is that they are not so much epistemologically passive as indifferent. Along with an absence of natural philosophy is an absence of epistemology altogether. Discontinuous bits of ancient medical knowledge are harvested as ingredients for distinctively medieval recipes of knowing (the *florilegia* or anthologies), so that, even more than in the Arabic world, the 'self-consciously anti-theoretical and anti-canonical textual practices' of early medieval Europe (p. 126) do not fit a neat pattern of medical knowing that is either gnostic or epistemic in character.

On the strength of this example our sharply contrasting notions of gnostic and epistemic need not only to be gradated towards each other, but also to be brought into triangular relation with a third pole – that of pragmatic eclecticism where there really isn't that much explicit concern to justify knowing one way or another. This is surely the most common approach to knowing in most societies, West or East, most of the time. Its absence from our discussion up to now is largely an artefact of our focus on scholarly knowing.

Now we come to the closing centuries of pre-modern Europe. Given that this is the era of Scholastic Galenism, and given the rhetoric of the 'scientific revolution' that came after, we are accustomed to perceiving it as *the* Western example of a text-based tradition of what I am here calling gnostic knowing. According to this stereotype, Aristotle, Hippocrates, Galen and the wise sages who followed, like Avicenna, are the revered authors, if not of the truth then at least of the next best thing. The historical record, however, does not entirely support this caricature.

In the first place, throughout Islamic society and the European Middle Ages medical knowledge was subordinate to the knowledge of nature and both were below religious certainties in the hierarchy of cognitive privileges.[20] As Amos Funkenstein points out in his commen-

---

[20]   Indeed, the very fact of this hierarchy is evidence of an epistemic and characteristically Western intellectual climate (Funkenstein's 'Commentary', this volume). For the status of medicine among the 'sciences' in Arabic scholarship, see Dimitri Gutas, *Avicenna and the Aristotelian Tradition* (Leiden: E.J. Brill, 1988), pp. 150–2.

tary (p. 352), medieval Scholastics looked upon medical knowledge as a *scientia media*, and, as such, not as worthy of the epistemological scrutiny of disputation.[21]

Indeed, Luis García-Ballester makes clear that one of the great movements of university medicine in the High Middle Ages was to give medicine (i.e., Galenism), hitherto looked upon as a practice and an art, the social status of natural philosophy, regarded as an intellectual activity. Even so, it was acknowledged that medicine could achieve only the accuracy of the senses while it was left to natural philosophy to discover the truth (p. 143). In other words, there was a good deal of epistemic sensitivity reflected in debates over the status of medical knowledge.

At the same time, García-Ballester's account illustrates another point: while the texts of Galen and Aristotle, for instance, were sufficiently privileged that no Scholastic would presume to set himself[22] up in authority against them, they were still not absolute authorities in a thorough-going gnostic way. Differences between the two authors, for example the celebrated debate over the relative importance of the brain, heart and liver, led to endless disputes between the Aristotelian natural philosophers and the Galenic physicians.[23] Consistent with an epistemic attitude, it was chiefly the virtues of the Aristotelian and Galenic *arguments*, and not so much the virtues of the *authors* themselves, that were relevant to the debate. In short, Galenism was more a medical philosophy than a gnostic tradition based on Galen.[24]

On the other hand, this same behaviour also reflects a good deal of gnosticism. After all, Aristotelian philosophers and Galenic doctors still took those ancient writings as canonical. In fact, Avicenna had suggested reconciliation through a 'double truth'. The physician, guided by sense perception, should subscribe to the proofs of Galen's anatomical evidence while the philosopher should follow the higher truth of Aristotle that is perceived by the intellect.[25] The details of Avicenna's solution are epistemic; the sense of need to reconcile the writing of the two ancient sages is gnostic.

[21] This is, of course, an oversimplification. See also p. 350, and, for example, Michael McVaugh, 'The Nature and Limits of Medical Certitude at Early Fourteenth-Century Montpellier', *Osiris*, sec. ser. 6 (1990), 62–84. Disputation was enthusiastically taken up by the philosopher-physicians of Renaissance Italy. See J.J. Bylebyl, 'Medicine, Philosophy, and Humanism in Renaissance Italy', in John W. Shirley and F. David Hoeniger (eds.), *Science and the Arts in the Renaissance* (Washington: Folger Books, 1985), pp. 27–49, esp. p. 31ff.

[22] I use 'himself' advisedly.

[23] For a brief overview of this argument see Bylebyl (note 21), pp. 29–31; also McVaugh (note 21), pp. 75–82.

[24] As the very title of Temkin's book (note 18) makes clear.

[25] Bylebyl (note 21), p. 30f. See also García-Ballester, this volume, pp. 142 and 144.

Turning to early modern England, Andrew Wear explores the decline of Galenism in the social context of seventeenth-century England. It is as if there was built right into that philosophy the seeds of its own demise. As Wear demonstrates, for instance, within the general framework of Galenism, *and provided for in its very epistemology*, there was a good deal of room for adjustment and even explicit disagreement arising from personal judgement and experience. In addition, much knowledge was, as it had been from the time of the Hippocratics, what Wear calls 'declaratory' and 'aphoristic' in that it carries no implied or stated warrant for believing it, nor any sense that such a warrant is needed. It is simply matter of fact. And finally, since the Galenic system emphasized the relevance of local conditions – geography, environment and weather – to variations in disease conditions, diagnosis, treatment, and the availability of medicinal herbs, these conditions could argue against the relevance of even Galenism itself, especially in a time of growing nationalism.

Moreover, the canonical Galen was not the only gnostic feature of Galenism under attack. After all, it was as much the institutional setting (Latin, the university and Scholastic practices) that constituted the accrediting source for Galenic medical knowledge as it was the ancient and not so ancient authorities. In good gnostic fashion, in other words, it was the *learnedness* of the medicine (in contrast to 'empiric' medicine), that was called upon to privilege the knowledge of the so-called 'Galenist'.[26] As Wear makes clear, though, it was just as much the social and especially economic assault on those institutions of learnedness as it was the epistemic challenge to Galenic theories and concepts themselves that was leading to Galenism's decline.

From even this sketchy account of the migration of Galenic medicine around the Mediterranean basin it is clear, then, that we do not ever have a really pure example of a gnostic approach to knowing, at least where medicine is concerned. What we do have, though, is a variety of approaches to the warranting of ancient knowledge and its authors, and, by the late Middle Ages, a very scholarly approach with strong gnostic overtones.

Apart from Galen's reverential treatment of Hippocrates, the Hippocratic and Galenic texts do not, by themselves, cultivate the idea that their contents are the revelations of transcendent authorities. This contrasts with both Chinese and Indian texts which either implicitly or often explicitly cultivate the reader's belief that they are the revealed words of some superior knower(s). For example, in his 'Text and Experience in Classical Chinese Medicine', Nathan Sivin uses two such

---

[26] See also note 38, below.

texts as the sources for his description of the gnostic way in which medicine was taught. In other words, quite apart from the social institutions and practices that were designed to foster gnostic attitudes to the texts in question, and quite independently of any changes in geographical and cultural context, the very texts themselves promoted this alternative way of knowing.

Let us now turn specifically to Chinese textual medicine. In a passage from his original paper as it was presented at the workshop, Sivin summarized a tradition that 'evolved round a cumulative tradition of written texts' that 'began with charismatic scriptures ... embodying the perfection of a lost golden age'. He went on to say that 'personal teaching by a master and the study of later writings were essential to comprehend the insights of the founding sages. The text was conveyed by master to disciple, locating both in a lineage patterned on blood descent.' In the conclusion to his chapter as it appears in this volume, moreover, Sivin says that 'the criterion of the true practitioner is thus inseparable from that of true knowledge ... both are settled by member-ship in a lineage of properly initiated masters who transmit authentic, written medical revelations' (p. 199f.). For Chinese medicine, 'philo-sophy or conscious epistemology ... remained occasional but marginal indulgences' (p. 198). And again, 'epistemology was not necessary to true knowledge. That was settled ... by initiation' (p. 200).

Here is a profound difference that begins with the earliest records. So it is with Āyurvedic medicine.[27] In an earlier work,[28] Francis Zimmermann makes clear that the classical Āyurvedic way of knowing is gnostic in the sense in which I am using that term. As with the classical Chinese, knowing is centred on the knower, with a concomitant concern for lineages, discipleship and orthodoxy.[29]

Unfortunately, it is not possible for me to fill in the detailed, post-classical history of Chinese and Āyurvedic textual traditions in a way that would offer a satisfactory comparison with their Western counter-parts. But it does seem reasonable to suggest that, after all variations and exceptions have been granted, there remains this thread of gnostic continuity in the two Eastern traditions,[30] which has its counterparts in,

---

[27] Just how much these differences are rhetorical and to what extent they meant real differences in the way healers went about their work will be considered later.

[28] 'From Classic Texts to Learned Practice: Methodological Remarks on the Study of Indian Medicine', *Social Science and Medicine*, 12 (1978), 97–103; p. 97.

[29] See also Zimmermann, this volume, p. 299; Cohen, p. 330; and P. Kutumbiah, *Ancient Indian Medicine* (Bombay: Orient Longmans, 1962), 'General Introduction', pp. i–liv.

[30] For present-day China, see Farquhar in this volume and also the discussion of her paper, below. For contemporary India, see Charles Leslie, 'Modern India's Ancient Medicine', *Trans-action* (June, 1967), 46–55.

say, Islamic or Christian *religion*, but which is less strongly manifest in Galenism or in Western *medicine*, generally.[31]

Learning and experience

So far, I have been talking about traditional medicine largely from the point of view of texts. What about experience? Any sophisticated system of knowing makes provision for the fact that learning and experience are closely interactive: what we experience is influenced by what we have learned, but we also need to believe that what we have learned coheres with what we experience. This being so, perhaps the most consequential feature of the different ways of knowing is their differing answers to the question, 'What are the respective roles of learning and experience in the constitution of what we know?'

In their idealized forms, gnostic and epistemic knowing have already implied answers, or at least initial positions from which any discussion of the question subsequently flows. For gnostics, experience, however novel, is ultimately understood within a framework of basic principles that have been learned from superior knowers, while for epistemics the lack of any such constraining framework at least leaves open the possibility that experience will be claimed to have some autonomous role in the constitution of knowledge.[32]

That the role of experience (mostly in the form 'What else besides experience?' or 'In what way experience?') was controversial in the West from classical Greek times on is evident from what Lloyd tells us. And Hankinson's paper is all about the subsequent development of a full-fledged philosophical debate over the matter. Indeed, not only was there the very idea that experience *can* have an autonomous role in the constitution of knowledge, some empiricists offered the radical suggestion that *only* experience can produce knowledge.[33] And, as Funkenstein emphasizes (p. 352f.), the possibility that experience could contradict theory persisted at least as a claim, sometimes more, sometimes less, throughout the history of Western thought.

[31] With respect to religious canons, see John B. Henderson, *Scripture, Canon, and Commentary: A Comparison of Confucian and Western Exegesis* (Princeton: Princeton University Press, 1991).

[32] According to Hankinson (p. 74f.), empiricists regarded certain theoretical disputes among dogmatists as 'undecidable' since there was no independent arbiter to appeal to. I am grateful to Nathan Sivin for suggesting the word 'autonomous'. It means, of course, autonomous from *their* point of view.

[33] To say nothing of the even more extreme argument of some sceptics that *not even* experience can produce knowledge.

This is in striking contrast to what Sivin tells us. In the idealized form of ancient Chinese medicine, at least, experience corroborates, elaborates and extends rather than criticizes and contradicts what has been learned. Nor is the role of experience a matter for dispute. However, this idealized view, derived from classical texts, invites comparison with what we learn from other sources.

Lesley Dean-Jones and Francesca Bray compare examples of how experience entered into actual practices among certain Greek and Chinese doctors, respectively. Specifically, they contrast the ways in which male healers experienced and knew the bodies of their female patients.

The comparison produces a seeming paradox. On the one hand, it was apparently quite acceptable for the male Hippocratic physician to do an internal, gynaecological examination on his female patient. Yet such an examination was not enough. In addition, he felt obliged to rely on her testimony for information which only she could know, as a woman, through experiencing her own body. Conversely, the Chinese doctor, with virtually no access to his female patient beyond questioning (often through an intermediary), and her pulse (sometimes through a cloth draped over her wrists), invested the patient's own testimony with no special significance based on the fact that she was a woman.

But the difference, here, is not one of differing attitudes towards the role that experience plays in the assessment of a patient. Rather, it is one of differing ideas about what constitutes relevant experience. Superficially, this distinction arises out of differing concepts of disease, of the role the healer plays in its treatment, and especially out of different conceptions as to how the sexes differ.

However, as we learn especially from Shigehisa Kuriyama's chapter on visual knowledge in classical Chinese medicine, at a deeper level there is an even more profound difference in the respective notions of what constitutes experience, a difference, moreover, that distinguishes Chinese from Western healers, more generally. This has to do with fundamental differences in the way we understand the body. According to Kuriyama, 'the differences in how Greek and Chinese physicians looked at the body, as an external object, derived in large measure from differences in how they conceived and experienced themselves from within, as persons' (p. 227). Greek anatomical study is centred on models of the body as 'articulation of intentions' and 'manifestation of the will', while a crucial model of Chinese self-definition is that of the 'growth and health of plants' (p. 230).

As a result of this, when they looked at the body of the patient, Chinese doctors neither saw in the same way as their Greek counterparts, nor granted the same salience to the same things when they saw.[34] As Kuriyama puts it, 'how we see something is influenced by what we imagine the thing to be' (p. 227). In other words, there is the epistemic question, 'Is experience autonomously constitutive of certain kinds of knowledge (and, if so, to what extent)?' and there is also the essentially aesthetic question '*How* do we experience?' Besides different ways of knowing, there are different ways of experiencing.

Now, in any learned tradition of medicine, learning and experience are interactive, but the whole approach makes it likely that the influence of learning will be especially strong. As Zimmermann explains in the final section of his paper on Āyurvedic medicine (pp. 310–19), the practices of diagnosis and therapy bring experience into intimate, dynamic interplay with culturally constructed theories of disease, categories of drugs, and the 'universals' of tropical botany. 'Empirical observations are couched in humoralistic terms. Plants and other crude drugs are mirrors of men' (p. 318), and 'modern Natural History was born from a combination of field studies and indigenous scholarship' (p. 312).

Zimmermann is here referring to Āyurvedic medicine, but he makes clear that his remarks apply to any traditional medicine. 'What is at stake in the scholarly traditions of humoral medicine is the discovery of collective patterns of sensibility.'[35] Nevertheless, Zimmermann also puts the case much more forcibly with respect to the very gnostic system of classical Āyurvedic medicine. 'The Āyurvedic physician is a professional trained by a teacher. Nothing is seen with the eyes which has not been said in the texts.'[36]

With gnostic knowing, then, experience is not necessarily less privileged than learning, it's just that learning is particularly influential. Moreover, experience, like knowing, is often hierarchical. It becomes a matter of *whose* experience counts most – that of the master more than the student's, that of the transcendent authority more than the master's. But even the authority of the most superior knower may rest, in part, on experience or a superior capacity to learn from experience. (See Sivin, pp. 184 and 189.) The bottom line, though, is that experience is rarely if ever understood in such a way as to contradict a knower further up the line of knowing authority.

---

[34] In an earlier work, Kuriyama describes how, in the act of taking the pulse, the very sensation of touching could be different for the physician trained in Galenic pulse lore as compared to the 'haptic experience' of the Chinese doctor ('Varieties of Haptic Experience: A Comparative Study of Greek and Chinese Pulse Diagnosis', unpublished Ph.D. thesis, Harvard University (1986)).

[35] p. 319. See also Judith Farquhar, *Knowing Practice: The Clinical Encounter of Chinese Medicine* (Boulder: Westview Press, 1994), esp. ch. 5, pp. 147–74.

[36] p. 300. Also see p. 305

This could even be said of the more weakly gnostic knowing of medieval Galenism where, for example, anatomists took seriously Galen's admonition to be guided by experience, and yet to see 'through his eyes', so to speak. In one well known instance of this, Galen described the human liver as having five lobes, like that of the dog. Later medieval Galenists, not knowing that Galen had dissected only animals, dutifully dissected humans in order to follow Galen's admonition to 'see for yourself'. Just as dutifully, they 'saw' the human, two-lobed liver as having five lobes.[37] Indeed, it is just this sort of behaviour on the part of Scholastic Galenists that led later historians to accuse them of having 'slavishly' followed Galen.[38]

Perhaps at this point it would be useful to summarize the overall argument of this essay to date. On the one hand, *any* scholarly medical tradition is going to be significantly gnostic, by definition, because by 'scholarly' and 'tradition' we usually just mean a learnedness that reveres the past. But that does not require that all three medical traditions were gnostic to the same degree, nor, conversely, devoid of epistemic features to the same degree. The classical traditions started off differently – the Greek in a largely epistemic mode and the Chinese and Āyurvedic in a gnostic mode. Relatively early, the Western tradition evolved along more (and sometimes less) gnostic lines until, in the time of Scholastic Galenism, it had become markedly gnostic in character. Conversely, it can no doubt be argued that the Chinese and Āyurvedic traditions had their epistemic side to them as well.

However, having said that, one gets the impression that Western medical traditionalism, throughout most of history, never embraced a gnostic way of knowing that was fully comparable with that of its Eastern counterparts (nor even with that of its own religions on occasion). Admittedly, there were times when the three traditions exhibit one or more specific characteristics in common – the use of texts, archaism, an emphasis on learnedness, attitudes towards experience, etc. But, when one checks out the broader constellation of ideas embraced by the concepts of gnosticism and epistemicism, there does seem to be a persisting difference. Western traditional medicine remains more epistemic *by comparison* with its Chinese and Āyurvedic counterparts while they, in turn, remain more gnostic *by comparison* with the tradition in the West.

[37] See Temkin (note 18), fig. 5, opposite p. 108. For Vesalius' comments on this curiosity, see Andreas Vesalius, *De humani corporis fabrica libri septem* (Basel, 1543), bk. V, pp. 506f.

[38] The intellectualizing of university Galenism that García-Ballester describes, and the attitudes it fostered with respect to the role of experience, also added to its gnostic flavour (pp. 138f.). Also see Wear (p. 165).

Of course, this whole idea is impressionistic and would no doubt need to be substantially revised in the light of more historical evidence. But, as I said earlier, my point is not so much to insist on the argument's validity as to suggest a framework for thinking about the different ways of knowing in the three traditions and how they might be compared.

Scholarly medicine in society

Until now, I have dwelt chiefly on the role of the text and the place of experience in the claims made for scholarly medical knowing. A number of our contributors have taken a broader view of the role of society in shaping traditional medical knowledge. For example, although avowedly speculative, Margaret Trawick's reflections on Chinese and Indian medicine offer us a way of imagining how cosmology and society might have given birth to each other (pp. 289f.). Using Victor Turner's concept of 'root metaphor', Trawick argues that in both classical Chinese and Hindu medicine we can see how ruling élites made the body meaningful, in health and disease, by 'explaining' it through the language and experiences of agrarian societies living under central political control.[39] Historians of Western medicine will immediately recognize the potential of her vision for their own story about Galenism, because similar metaphoric resources were apparently called upon by the ancient Greeks. For example, the veins were perceived as an irrigation system.[40] Part of the argument over the primacy of brain, heart or liver had to do with their relative 'nobility'.[41]

With respect to the handling of Greek medicine in Arabic culture, Lawrence Conrad's central argument is that 'socio-cultural forces ... play a crucial role in the process by which ideas ... established within a scientific tradition gain assent as truth and their relative value or importance in that tradition' (p. 86). He goes on to recount a long-running polemic between two Arabic physicians: a well-established Galenist in Egypt against an Aristotelian newcomer from Baghdad. The thin disguise of a 'scholarly' debate over whether 'the chicken is of a warmer nature than the young of the bird' (p. 92) cannot hide their highly competitive war of words. While the rules of engagement were putatively gnostic, the actual fighting was downright nasty. Each side mobilized a host of social and psychological weapons to win communal

[39]   See also Sivin, pp. 188 and 195.
[40]   I. M. Lonie, 'Erasistratus, the Erasistrateans, and Aristotle', *Bulletin of the History of Medicine*, 38 (1964), 426–43; p. 426.
[41]   See, for example, Aristotle, *Parts of Animals*, III, 4, 20. Ancient Greek accounts of digestion speak in terms of cooking and the kitchen. For a general comparison of the intellectual climate in ancient Greece compared to ancient China, see Lloyd (note 11).

'affirmation' for the claimant and 'confirmation' for his scholarly writings, rather than epistemic weapons to justify the knowledge claimed. So, while the writings of both combatants 'serve in their own small way to confirm the authority of Aristotelian science and Galenic medicine ... it is at other levels that their essential disagreement must be sought' (p. 100). Clearly there is lots of room for debate and competition within a largely gnostic system without it thereby becoming epistemic.[42]

Shifting now to the very recent past, anthropologists Farquhar and Cohen look at the contemporary scene in China and India, respectively.

One might have thought that, in the traditional Chinese medicine of post Cultural-Revolution China in the 1980s, talk of scientific Marxism and historical and dialectical materialism would have erased any vestiges of the gnostic way of knowing. But, as Farquhar's 'Re-writing Traditional Medicine in Post-Maoist China' richly suggests, the centring of knowing in the knower has reappeared in the language of that 're-writing'. The values of lineage, genealogy, 'filiality' and continuities are all there. (Also see Sivin, pp. 197f.)

Farquhar's account is valuable not only as a glimpse into a present-day version of gnostic knowing in action, but also because it highlights features of that style which are not as apparent in textual traditions that hail back to transcendent authorities. I am referring to the strong emphasis on contingency and localism.[43] As a concomitant to person-based knowing, this emphasis should hardly surprise us, especially when the persons involved are themselves so carefully situated in time and place, 'adept personages' (p. 275) moreover, who are prized for their connoisseurship and their virtuoso performances.[44] Similarly, there is a deliberate personalizing of knowledge which, in turn, engenders discipleship among those who come to share the master's individualized insights and 'positions' (pp. 271–3).

Nor are these features of contingency and individuality, ascribed to both the knower and the known, unimportant in the current rhetoric of Chinese gnostic knowing. As Farquhar herself notes, although the 'idea that an ancient form of medical practice should be more embodied than

[42] Regarding this same point in Āyurvedic medicine, see Kutumbiah (note 29), p. xxvf.
[43] Passim, but see especially pp. 272f.
[44] Farquhar herself refers to the 'therapeutic virtuoso' (ibid.), and, in a personal conversation, suggested that the Chinese practitioner is a 'connoisseur'. For some background on the use of 'connoisseurship' see James Hevia and Judith Farquhar, 'The Concept of Culture in Post-War American Historiography of China', *Positions*, 1:2 (1993), 486–525; p. 497. Although Kuriyama does not actually use the term, he very clearly alludes to connoisseurship in his 'Pulse Diagnosis in Greek and Chinese Traditions', in Yosio Kawakita (ed.), *History of Diagnostics* (Osaka: The Taniguchi Foundation, 1987), pp. 43–67; p. 57.

recorded ... is not new in anthropology ... there are still voices in China, not all of them elderly, who assert that this embodied medicine ... *is* Chinese medicine's essence' (p. 274).

The localism and personalism that Farquhar finds in current expressions of traditional Chinese medical knowing has an interesting resonance with recent trends in social science scholarship in this part of the world. For example, current talk of 'tacit' and 'embodied' knowledge reflects our own attempt to put knowledge back into the knower, to return the known to the only thing that can experience and know – the living body.

Perhaps we should add some further complexities to our categories of gnostic and epistemic, for it would seem that both gnosticism and epistemicism have their local and their universalistic varieties. Local gnosticism, of the kind Farquhar identifies in certain biographical texts of the 1980s, has the characteristics of connoisseurship and virtuoso performance. Knowledge is embodied in this particular body, as compared to that. Then there is the more classical gnosticism, of the kind elaborated upon by Sivin, or referred to by Zimmermann, which is embodied in the body or bodies of transcendent authorities.

Similarly, epistemicism seems to come in at least two varieties: the disembodied and universalized kind that we typically associate with science, in which knowledge has been separated from the knower; and the recently rediscovered, local kinds of embodiment and tacitness. But, even here, the localism has a certain universalistic quality about it insofar as it refers more generically to *bodies* than to particular persons with proper names.

Moreover, comparing our studies of the scholarly medical traditions with current social science studies of knowledge makes clear that our double-axis scheme for ways of knowing must make room for a third. Not only is there gnosticism vs. epistemicism; not only is there localism vs. universalism; there is also a polarity between scholarly commitments to ways of knowing and actual practices.

As the titles of both the volume and this essay suggest, we are concerned here with *scholarly* ways of knowing. These constitute organized, rhetorical and institutional expressions of cultural values with respect to knowing. They do not give us a full account of how people actually behave, relative to the business of knowing. Yet, as Young makes clear in his commentary, for anthropologists it is these practices that tend to be the focus of their attention.[45]

---

[45] See also Allan Young, 'The Creation of Medical Knowledge: Some Problems in Interpretation', *Social Science and Medicine* (1981), 15B, 379–86. Young points out that, whatever the rhetoric, people's medical knowledge is 'not epistemologically homogeneous'.

This brings me to Lawrence Cohen's contribution about 'the epistemological carnival'. Cohen wants us to think about the conflict between international studies of Āyurvedic medicine, where scholars' 'epistemology can remain a clean realm' (p. 343), and the lived daily experience of those who actually practise Āyurvedic medicine. When these come together in the same place and time, as they did at the third International Conference on Traditional Asian Medicine in Bombay, in 1990, the epistemological result, Cohen suggests, is a carnival.

To this he adds that 'the missing piece in all grand theoretical debates between structure and practice' is a contingency, and that contingency 'is the body. For the lived and mindful body is not the stable universal which both cultural and practical accounts tend to assume ... It resists its reduction to any one totalizing frame' (p. 321).

From our earlier reflections on scholarly ways of knowing, we are already familiar with the idea that knowledge and the body are problematically related, and, as we have just noted, problematic even *within* the broad categories of gnostic and epistemic knowing. For Cohen, it is this problem of the contingently knowing body that is part of the reason for the carnival, and the 'epistemological anxiety' that consequently arises.

But Cohen also draws attention more specifically to medical knowing. The contingency he speaks of 'problematizes the monoglot coherence and stability of any medical inscription of the body ... Apparent continuities in a medical tradition, in articulating knowledge of and relationships to bodies in shifting symbolic and political contexts, disguise points of deep disjuncture and conflict.'[46] Scholarly medical knowledge is contingent upon the contingent body, because that knowledge is scholarly, because it is medical, and because it is knowledge.

Although Cohen is not the only one to raise an eyebrow in this volume, his challenge to the whole enterprise of comparing ways of knowing in the different scholarly traditions of medicine is arguably the most radical. Never mind that we are presuming to compare 'cultures', or trying to study 'traditions' as if they are out there, ontologically. Cohen reminds us that we are also presuming to study scholarship using scholarly methods; that we are counting on producing knowledge about knowers and the known; and that we are bodies earnestly expecting to transcend our local and individual selves.

---

[46] p. 321. One such disjuncture was already recognized by Galen. As Stephanus, a sixth-century commentator on Galen, observed, 'there is no science of the individual', and, 'medicine suffers from a fundamental contradiction: its practice deals with the individual while its theory grasps universals only' (paraphrased by Owsei Temkin in his *The Double Face of Janus* (Baltimore: The Johns Hopkins University Press, 1977), p. 446).

With this thought we shall leave the reader to examine the various contributions and to draw her or his own conclusions in an atmosphere of unresolved (and apparently unresolvable) but fruitful tension between the local here and now from which there is no escape and the transcendent knowing through which we strive, however imperfectly, to understand and to accommodate the other.

Part 1

Scholarly medicine in the West

2 Epistemological arguments in early Greek medicine in comparativist perspective

G.E.R. Lloyd

'Epistemology' is a term that can be used in a looser, and in a more strict, acceptance. In the looser one, which a number of contributors to this volume appear to have in mind, it may be used of any statement or position that may be thought to imply a claim to know or that allows one to investigate how such a claim might have been sustained, for example, by reference to what is represented as the correct method to adopt. All uses of expressions for cognitive states or processes, all methodological observations, have, on this view, an epistemological component. In a stricter acceptance, however, epistemology relates solely to explicit statements that directly address such questions as the criteria of knowledge or the conditions that have to be met for a knowledge claim to be justified. While clearly no hard and fast distinctions are to be drawn between the two ends of the spectrum indicated by these acceptances, I shall be concerned here with the strict, or stricter one, that is to say with explicit discussions of the nature of knowledge and of the basis of claims to have secured it.

It is well known that extant Greek medical texts from the fifth century BC onwards offer many examples where the authors reflect self-consciously on the status of medicine. Can it be said to be an art, *technē*, or a branch of knowledge, *epistēmē*, and if so, why? What distinguishes the true practitioner from the lay person or the quack? What can justify a doctor's claim to know, for example, what the causes of diseases are or how to cure them, whether in general or in any particular case? Such questions are already frequently addressed in texts in the Hippocratic Corpus and they are at the centre of debate between rival medical sects or groups in the Hellenistic period.

The aim of this brief discussion is threefold. First I shall attempt to survey some of the key texts from the fifth and fourth centuries to examine, in particular, how explicit they are on epistemological questions in the stricter acceptance I have spoken of. Second, in a brief

For a list of bibliographical abbreviations, please see the end of this chapter.

interlude, I shall try to take stock of *some* of the comparisons and contrasts that might be drawn with another developed, literate, medical tradition, namely the ancient Chinese, though what I have to say on that topic has no ambitions to be comprehensive. Third, in the more substantial part of this paper, I shall examine how far we can get towards understanding *why* epistemological interests developed in the way they did in early Greek medicine. How far was this primarily just a response to the problems encountered in clinical practice? How far did those interests reflect the influence, on medicine, of contemporary developments in philosophy? How far were they developed independently in medicine specifically for polemical purposes, that is for the construction of arguments directed at undermining the ideas and practices of rivals – which could be rejected as unsound on the basis of their unsound epistemology? Those three suggestions are, of course, not mutually exclusive and it is often difficult to see what weight to attach to each one. However an attempt to evaluate them can and should be made, not least in view of the comparative questions raised in the second part of our discussion.

First, then, we should review some of the main evidence for explicit epistemological concerns in early Greek medical writings and we can do no better than to start with one of the most sustained discussions, in the Hippocratic treatise *On Ancient Medicine*. This sets out a detailed confrontation between the author's preferred conception of medicine and that of certain unnamed opponents. Who precisely these opponents may be is disputed,[1] but that need not concern us here since the author's statement of the position he wishes to attack is clear. They attempted, so we are told, to found medicine on a small number of 'hypotheses', that is postulates, such as hot, cold, wet or dry. It is not that the author thinks such factors have no role in the body, but he argues that they are among the least important 'powers' (chapter 16). What he objects to in his opponents' procedures is that they 'narrow down the causal principle of diseases and of death' (chapter 1). He contrasts the situation in the study of 'things in the sky and below the earth', where postulates are unavoidable. Yet what is the effect of their use? 'If anyone were to speak and declare the nature of these things, it would not be clear either to the speaker himself or to his audience whether what was said was true or not, since there is no criterion to which one should refer to obtain clear knowledge' (chapter 1).

---

[1]   For a first orientation see my article 'Who is attacked in *On Ancient Medicine*?', *Phronesis*, 8 (1963), 108–26, reprinted in *MP*, ch. 3, and see most recently R.J. Hankinson, 'Doing without Hypotheses: the Nature of "Ancient Medicine"', in J.A. López Férez (ed.), *Tratados hipocráticos* (Madrid, 1992), pp. 55–67.

What the author himself offers as an alternative is what he represents as the old, tried and tested, method, based on experience and research. Medicine, he claims (chapter 2), has long had its principle and the way it has discovered: it is the result of inquiry and investigation – the terms *skepsis, heurema, zetema* and cognates recur throughout the work. He even offers an account of the origins of medicine, which developed, he suggests, from dietetics (chapter 3, 37.26ff.). People observed the bad effects of eating strong or uncooked foods and counteracted these by trying out various ways of cooking and blending them. That is just like medicine itself, he says, and indeed a large part of his discussion of medical therapies in the bulk of the treatise (chapters 5–14) consists in an examination of the various problems associated with the adjustment of a patient's diet.

He acknowledges that medicine is not exact. There is no measure, neither number nor weight, by referring to which you will know what is exact, and no other measure than the feeling of the body (chapter 9, 41.20ff.). But that is no reason to conclude that the art does not exist, just because it has not attained exactness in every item. Rather one should admire the art for the discoveries it has made, which are true discoveries based on reasoning and experience, not just a matter of luck (chapter 12, 44.2ff.). There are good practitioners as well as bad ones, a sure sign that we are dealing with an art (chapter 1), though again he concedes that most actual practitioners are no good: they are like bad pilots whose lack of skill is not revealed in fine weather but becomes clear in a storm (chapter 9).

Correct practice depends on the investigation of the causes at work, and he states the criteria that a cause should fulfil. 'We must, therefore, consider the causes of each condition to be those things which are such that, when they are present, the condition necessarily occurs, but when they change to another combination, it ceases' (chapter 19, 50.7ff.). Causes then should be carefully distinguished from mere concomitants (chapter 17), though most practitioners, like lay people, tend to assign the cause to anything unusual that has happened to the patient near the onset of the disease (chapter 21, 52.17ff.).

While much of the writer's defence of medicine consists of an analysis of its positive features, he returns to the contrast between medicine and other inquiries in chapter 20. Here he explicitly distances medicine from 'philosophy', explained as the 'inquiry concerning nature'. Some doctors and 'sophists' assert that it is impossible to know medicine unless you know about the constituents of the human body. But the writer counters that they have got it round the wrong way. So far from medicine needing to turn to philosophy for knowledge about' the constituents of the body and about nature in general, medicine itself is the only sure source for such knowledge.

The treatise *On Ancient Medicine* thus presents a number of detailed arguments relating to the status of medicine and to the basis on which knowledge claims can be made in diagnosis or therapy. But many of these themes are echoed in other works, both those that can be dated to the fifth or early fourth centuries, and others, such as *Precepts*, for which a later date is likely. The topics of the distinction between the lay person and the practitioner, and of the further contrast, within the latter, between the true physician and the quack, recur in many works from the earlier period.

The treatise *On Regimen in Acute Diseases*, for instance, opens with a criticism of a rival work, the *Cnidian Sentences* (itself now lost), for merely giving an account of the symptoms that patients suffer from and the outcomes of their diseases. But anyone, the writer protests, could manage that, if they questioned the patients. What requires real medical knowledge and skill turns out, as in *On Ancient Medicine*, to depend on knowing the causes of diseases and on an appreciation of when precisely a change in regimen is needed. This writer points out that the same condition may arise from different causes (chapter 11). Not recognising this, physicians often give the wrong treatment, and when someone else, maybe a lay person, suggests something different and the patient is cured, the original physician becomes a laughing-stock (chapter 11) and medicine itself seems no better than divination (chapter 3). His opponents are mistaken both because they tend to consider conditions with even the slightest variation as different diseases and because they use too few types of remedy – purges and whey and milk (chapter 1). But he also criticizes lay people as well for being impressed by any doctor who introduces new or strange cures (chapter 2); that is an interesting objection since a variety of other texts in the Hippocratic Corpus indicate that innovation in medical practice was often cultivated as a way of making a reputation. Some practitioners evidently went all out to *amaze* their patients, even while others shared some of the misgivings expressed in *On Regimen in Acute Diseases* about the adverse effects of the pursuit of novelty.[2]

A further theme that recurs in a number of works is the contrast between the effects of medicine and those of mere chance. The treatise *On the Art*, in particular, develops some subtle arguments on the point. In chapters 4ff. the writer considers the objections (1) that patients can

---

[2]   The evidence for both the positive ambition to innovate and the negative reactions that this provoked is set out in ch. 2 of my book *The Revolutions of Wisdom* (Berkeley, 1987).

and do sometimes recover even without medical treatment, (2) that when they are treated, they do not always recover, and (3) that when they are treated and do get better, that is not necessarily because of their treatment. To this the writer counters that there are *causes* at work, in recovery and indeed also in death, in any event. Even when medical practitioners do *not* intervene, the reasons for the patients recovering, or dying, are not a matter of *chance*. 'Everything that happens will be found to have some cause, and if it has a cause, the spontaneous can be no more than an empty name' (chapter 6, 13.2ff.). Again the positive argument is that medicine, based on reason and experience, can and does achieve cures.

There is, of course, far more to early Greek medical epistemology than this brief sketch can convey, but it provides, I hope, enough evidence of some recurrent Greek preoccupations. With this as our basis, we may now turn to the second section of our discussion, the comparisons and contrasts with classical Chinese medicine. It is certainly not the case that explicit epistemological concerns are quite absent from classical Chinese thought. As Graham has pointed out in his discussion of the Mohists,[3] they spoke of three sources of knowledge, report, explanation and observation. In a well-known passage in *Mo Zi* (chapter 31) the existence of ghosts and spirits is argued on the basis that people say they have seen and heard them. The Mohist criteria are, in turn, attacked, for example by Wang Chong, in his *Lun Heng* (chapter 67), on the rather tendentious grounds that they ignore the element of reasoning. As usual in Chinese philosophical argument, basic ethical questions are implicated, both in the Mohist defence of the belief in spirits, and in Wang Chong's counter. But the epistemological elements, on both sides of this debate are unmistakable.

Again where Chinese medicine is concerned, there are many texts, both in the various recensions of the *Huang Di Nei Jing* and in our other sources, that illustrate an interest in problems to do with the correct methods, in diagnosis and in treatment. In the exchanges between the Yellow Emperor and his various respondents, Qi Bo, Shao Shi and the rest, the discussion often turns to the efficacy of different remedies for different complaints and how the remedies are correctly applied. Thus questioned at one point on why different techniques may be effective for the same illness, Qi Bo reflects on their origins in different regions. Stone therapy comes from the East, powerful drugs from the West, moxa from the North, needles from the South, while exercise and massage originate in the Centre, but all may be efficacious.[4]

---

[3]   See A. C. Graham, *Later Mohist Logic, Ethics and Science* (London, 1978), pp. 30ff.
[4]   *Huang Di Nei Jing su wen*: 12.

The interlocutors in the *Huang Di Nei Jing* sometimes appear to reflect divergent view-points on questions to do with medical practice. But direct rivalry between doctors is more explicitly referred to in another early source, the biography of Chunyu Yi in Sima Qian's *Shi Ji* (chapter 105).[5] This material is exceptional in that it represents a doctor's own apologia for his practice, where he justifies his diagnoses and treatments in a series of individual case-histories. He explains how he was trained, what he owed to his teachers and to the books he studied, but he also refers critically, from time to time, to rival doctors, sometimes unnamed but on occasion named, where it is not a question of easily dismissed members of marginal groups, but of learned practitioners some of whom held responsible official positions.[6]

One such text serves to underline the importance, in Chunyu Yi's view, of experience as well as of appeals to learned authority. In case 22 he treats a patient who is himself a doctor called Sui, who had actually set about treating himself with the five stone therapy. Chunyu Yi comments that that is inappropriate, whereupon Sui cites the famous doctor Bian Que as his authority. That in turn elicits from Chunyu Yi the response: 'how far your account is [from the truth]'. Though Bian Que spoke as he did, there is a whole range of diagnostic questions that have to be evaluated. There are certainly rules for examination, but when the practitioners who try to apply them are ignorant, they are no use at all. Knowledge of the learned texts by itself is evidently not enough to be a successful practitioner.[7]

Thus the points of similarity that may be suggested between classical Chinese and classical Greek medicine include (1) a certain self-consciousness about methods, and (2) a certain spirit of rivalry not just between the learned medical elite and non-learned medical traditions, but also *within* the former. However what is harder, or rather, I believe, impossible to find in the classical Chinese medical texts, is any sense of the need to defend the very existence of medicine itself by way of a justification of its grounds to be able to claim to be a branch of knowledge, skill or art. Chinese writers generally take it for granted that medicine is possible, even though they indubitably recognize its difficulties and complexities, and even though they often contrast modern practitioners unfavourably with the sages of past times.

This short interlude on some Chinese evidence may suggest various points of entry for an examination of the chief problem I wish to raise in

5   See N. Sivin, 'Text and Experience', this volume.
6   This is the case with doctor Sui, discussed below.
7   See Sivin (note 5), pp. 195–8.

relation to the Greek texts, namely why it should be that, comparatively speaking, foundational epistemological debates figure so prominently in them. I must stress at the outset that any answers that we might offer must be considered in the nature of conjectures. However, an attempt may be made to evaluate the various suggestions I outlined at the start of this paper.

First, how far does a stimulus to raise fundamental epistemological questions relating to the status of medicine itself come directly from the particular problems encountered in day-to-day clinical practice? Those problems may, to be sure, be the occasion for reflecting on such questions as how sure a doctor may be, on the diagnosis of this or that disease, on the treatment to adopt, or again, more generally, on problems to do with the classification of diseases as a whole. We saw that the author of *On Regimen in Acute Diseases* raises such issues. Yet it is to be remarked that he does so particularly in two related connections, first his concern to distinguish proper medical practitioners from mere lay people, and second his desire to contrast his own position with that of his opponents, chiefly those represented in the lost work *Cnidian Sentences*.[8] Similarly *On Ancient Medicine* has much to say about how one can determine which are the potent factors whose imbalance in the body causes diseases. But again the polemical context is provided by the rejection of the 'new-fangled' method of trying to base medicine on postulates and by the perceived danger that medicine will turn out not to be an art at all.

Similar points emerge in texts from other treatises. A sequence of chapters (5–9) in *On Diseases* I, for instance, discusses problems to do with what happens spontaneously or automatically. The author recognizes that this occurs, and when it does, the doctor's own knowledge or ignorance has nothing to do with it (chapter 7). Thus doctors may follow a course of treatment that is accompanied by chance effects. There is no proven starting-point or principle valid for the whole of medicine that can serve as the basis for everything the doctor says and does (chapter 9). As in *On Ancient Medicine* medicine is said not to be an exact branch of knowledge (chapter 5). But these reflections on the status of medicine are not just a series of observations that occur to the writer on the basis of his clinical experience, though of course they draw on that. At least chapter 8 brings the argument for the effects of

---

8   It is notable that *On Regimen in Acute Diseases* refers to the authors (in the plural) of the work *Cnidian Sentences*, and indeed to those who later revised that book: E. Littré (ed.), *Œuvres complètes d'Hippocrates*, vol. 2 (Paris, 1840), ch. 1, pp. 225.1 and 226.8. Plural authorship may be suspected for several of the Hippocratic treatises themselves, as I argued in 'The Hippocratic Question', *Classical Quarterly*, 25 (1975), 171–92, reprinted in *MP*, ch. 9.

chance to bear to defend the doctor against unfair accusations of failures for which he should not be held responsible. As in some other Hippocratic works, the view that medicine is not an exact branch of knowledge has both a negative and a positive side: it should not be blamed for *failure* in exactness, but it *is* a branch of knowledge nevertheless.

On Affections is another treatise that refers to what may happen by chance. In chapter 45 the writer concedes that some remedies are discovered by chance and that lay people might stumble on them just as much as doctors. But again an underlying concern with the defence of medicine as an art is discernible in the continuation, for the writer goes on to contrast what comes about by chance with what belongs to medical reasoning, with what he says can be learnt only from those who can distinguish what belongs to medical art.

Yet another work that exhibits a similar defensiveness but that produces a very different solution to the problem is *On the Places in Man*. Chapter 46 opens with the claim that the whole of medicine has already been discovered. The doctor who understands has least need of chance: indeed what passes as good fortune and bad really reflects the knowledge or ignorance of the practitioner. Successes just reflect the doctor's knowledge and ability, and the writer accepts that the converse is also true, that failures stem from the doctor's lack of understanding.

The question of the nature of the knowledge on which medicine is or should be based is one that receives a range of different answers in different Hippocratic works. Many writers acknowledge that what happens to their patients does not solely depend on what the doctor can claim to do on the basis of his knowledge. But one concern that all the texts we have just cited exhibit is to secure at least *some* area of operation, whether larger or smaller, over which the art of medicine can be said to be in control.

But how far, we may now ask, does it appear that the epistemological preoccupations we find in Greek medicine stem directly or indirectly from influences coming from contemporary Greek philosophy? Of course, from the late sixth century BC onwards, epistemological questions are often at the centre of Greek philosophical debate. In the early fifth century Parmenides' insistence that reason or argument alone is to be trusted had a radical impact, and not just on later Presocratic philosophers. Several of them sought to reinstate perception as a source of useful information, even while usually conceding that the deliveries of the senses cannot always be relied on. Again questions to do with the very possibility of knowledge, about the underlying realities or about the domain of the obscure or more generally, were raised by Xenophanes and echoed by, among others, Democritus.[9]

The extent to which those engaged in medical practice were aware of these philosophical debates should not be exaggerated. But as we have seen we have some direct evidence that they sometimes were. As we noted, chapter 20 of *On Ancient Medicine* criticizes those – both doctors and 'sophists' – who argued that medicine must be based on general knowledge about the nature of the human body and about nature itself. This leads into 'philosophy', the term which the author uses – though scarcely with approval – of the study of nature. His own position, as we saw, is that knowledge of nature should, if anything, be derived from medicine, not be brought into medicine from outside. Again in his attacks on the use of hypotheses or postulates he identifies such investigations as those into things in the sky or under the earth as the type of inquiry where postulates may be needed – not that he approves of them, even in that context. Rather, the very fact that such inquiries have to be based on postulates is evidence, in his eyes, of their irredeemably speculative character.

On Ancient Medicine refers to the inquiries that formed part of natural philosophy primarily in order to *contrast* them with his own conception of the art of medicine, based on the ancient tried and tested methods. However, it is not as if his own ideal owes *nothing* to philosophy, which remains an *indirect* influence precisely insofar as it is by way of a contrast with it that he seeks to define his own view of medicine. It may thus be that the philosophical debate provides a stimulus to the exploration of the status of medical knowledge here, even if that stimulus provoked a negative reaction to the styles of reasoning of the philosophers themselves. As for the medical rivals envisaged in *On Ancient Medicine*, the doctors whom the writer criticizes for trying to base their practice on postulates, in their case the philosophical influence is more probably direct, for if we ask where they got their idea that medicine should somehow be able to derive all that it needed to know from a few basic principles, it is clear that the deductive systems which, from the mid-fifth century onwards, were being developed – in both philosophy and mathematics – provided the main possible models.[10]

Two other Hippocratic treatises also exhibit a certain defensiveness concerning the relationship between philosophy and medicine, namely

[9] For a recent overview of Greek philosophical epistemology from the Presocratics onwards, with an up-to-date bibliography, see Stephen Everson (ed.), *Epistemology* (Cambridge, 1990).

[10] The possibility that the method of hypothesis attacked in *On Ancient Medicine* owes something to contemporary mathematics is explored in *MP*, ch. 3. See also C. Huffman, *Philolaus of Croton* (Cambridge, 1993).

On the Nature of Man and *On the Art*. Other works, however, adopt a more positive attitude: works such as, for example, *On Regimen* I, the author of which is happy to accept what *On Ancient Medicine* rejected, namely that the study of human regimen should be based on a general inquiry into the fundamental constituents of the human body[11] and who, in his own elaboration of how the two elements – fire and water - interact in the body, draws heavily on doctrines originally developed by such Presocratic philosophers as Heraclitus and Anaxagoras.[12]

The author of *On the Nature of Man*, for his part, offers his account of the elements in the body, but his opening chapter is devoted to criticism of those who discuss the nature of humans beyond what is relevant to medicine. He is particularly concerned to refute those who argued that all the constituents in the human body are modifications of a single elementary substance, a position that bears obvious similarities with the monistic physical theories ascribed to Anaximenes or set out in Diogenes of Apollonia. The very fact that those who advocate such monistic views disagree so much with one another, not least on the nature of the single primary element, undermines their whole case. Indeed he claims that the effect of their disputes is to tend to establish the position of Melissus, the Eleatic philosopher who asserted 'the one', but denied the evidence of the senses and argued that neither coming to be nor change occurs.[13]

As for the treatise *On the Art*, the writer explains his mission, in the opening chapter, as the defence of medicine against those who 'make an art' out of denigrating the arts. It is clear that their attack is not just directed at medicine, for the writer says that he will leave to others the defence of other arts. While we cannot identify precisely who these denigrators were, there is other evidence for debates concerning the status of a variety of different inquiries in the fifth and fourth centuries. Some of this is associated with those whom Plato labelled 'sophistic', men such as Protagoras, Hippias and Prodicus. But Plato himself provides plenty of insight into the kinds of claim and counterclaim made with respect to the viability of different types of inquiry. Plato's own primary concern is often to dissociate his own ideal of philosophy from 'rhetoric', 'sophistic' and 'eristic', criticized both on moral grounds and on the score of whether indeed they had a right to be called *arts*. In several of the texts in which he discusses this, the status of medicine itself is in question. Thus in the *Gorgias* (464b ff.) there is a contrast between certain genuine arts – which include medicine – and their

---

[11]   *On Regimen* I, ch. 2: *CMG* I 2.4, 122.22ff.
[12]   *On Regimen* I, chs. 4 and 5 especially: *CMG* I 2.4, 126.20ff., 128.12ff.
[13]   *On the Nature of Man* refers to Melissus in ch. 1: *CMG* I 1.3, 166.11. For Melissus' own views, see especially Fr. 1, Fr. 7 and Fr. 8.

spurious counterparts. In the *Phaedrus* (260e) the proper practice of medicine as an art is contrasted with its practice merely as a knack and by experience, and in the *Philebus* (55e ff.), where the arts are graded according to their degree of exactness, medicine comes in the lowest category, along with music, farming, navigation and generalship, below carpentry, which makes more use of instruments designed to achieve exactness.

It is not that the author of *On the Art* has Plato in mind. Yet the concerns that the Hippocratic work expresses relate to a general debate in which a variety of claimants to intellectual leadership and prestige participated, a debate that stretches far beyond the confines of those who considered themselves primarily as medical practitioners. Once again we may conclude that the epistemological twists to the arguments in this treatise do not *just* spring, and may not even primarily spring, from reflections on the problems of clinical practice, but relate in part to these wider issues of justifying the claims of medicine as a respectable art. Here too it is the characteristically Greek competitiveness between rival 'masters of truth' – a competitiveness exhibited in far more aggressive polemic than was customary in China – that may have acted as the primary catalyst to epistemological self-justification in the early medical writers.[14]

However, while some of the Hippocratic writers are evidently concerned with what they perceived to be threats coming from *outside* medicine, others are more preoccupied with polemic *with other practitioners*. It is time now to try to evaluate this third factor, and again our chosen texts yield direct evidence to the point. Take the writers of *On Ancient Medicine* and *On Regimen in Acute Diseases*. The former is critical of what he calls 'philosophy', but not just in itself: he is chiefly concerned that *doctors* should not be taken in by the 'new-fangled' method of hypotheses or postulates. The latter opens, as we have noted, with an attack on the trends set by those represented in the *Cnidian Sentences*.

We should be careful not to suppose that these Hippocratic debates were between clearly distinguished and well-organized medical sects such as we know existed from the Hellenistic period. The notion that there were two such sects in the fifth and early fourth centuries, the school of Cos and the school of Cnidos, is, as Smith and others have shown, largely an artefact of the commentators – ancient and modern.[15]

---

[14] See M. Detienne, *Les Maîtres de vérité dans la grèce archaïque* (Paris, 1967). See also my *Magic, Reason and Experience* (Cambridge, 1979), ch. 1.

[15] See W.D. Smith, 'Galen on Coans versus Cnidians', *Bulletin of the History of Medicine*, 47 (1973), 569–85. See also I. M. Lonie, 'Cos versus Cnidus and the Historians', *History of Science*, 16 (1978), 42–75 and 77–92.

At least 'school' is potentially a highly misleading term to use in either the educational or the dogmatic sense. The medical education on offer in any Greek city-state was a matter of what individual practitioners provided for those apprenticed to them. As for school in the sense of shared doctrines, it is clear from the medical history preserved in Anonymus Londinensis that doctors from Cos disagreed as much among themselves as they did with other doctors. There was no orthodoxy among those associated with Cos, or indeed with Cnidos, though, as we have seen, that did not stop the author of *On Regimen in Acute Diseases* attacking the authors and revisers of the *Cnidian Sentences*.

The fifth- and early fourth-century polemics were very much a free-for-all. In the Hellenistic period more determinate groupings did come to be formed, and indeed one of their main functions was to serve as alliances, for offensive and defensive argumentative purposes, in the continuing polemics. Some groups were known from the doctor they followed or took as their ideal. There were, for instance, Herophileans, Erasistrateans, Praxagoreans, even Hippocratics.[16] But others were labelled, by themselves or others, by their methodology. Galen is one who distinguishes between Dogmatists, Empiricists and Methodists, but again caution is in order. Those called Dogmatists were united in the belief that medicine should be based on an understanding of causes, including the hidden causes of diseases. But otherwise they shared no set of concrete medical doctrines. The Empiricists and Methodists may have had rather more in common, the latter, for example, holding that what the practitioner should focus on, indeed all that he needed to investigate, was the three common conditions, the lax, the restricted and the mixed. But even the Methodists disagreed often enough among themselves, as we see from both our main extant Methodist authors, Soranus and Caelius Aurelianus.[17]

The point of interest for our present concerns in these later, Hellenistic, debates is that sometimes, at least, they related not to medical practice, but simply to the justification of that practice. In his work *On Sects for Beginners* Galen remarks that the Methodists rejected most of traditional Greek medicine, both the classification of disease entities and the use of the usual remedies. However, the Dogmatists and Empiricists, he says, disagreed not on points of medical practice, so much as on the account to be given of that practice or the methods that

[16] See 'Galen on Hellenistics and Hippocrateans', ch. 17 of *MP*.
[17] For the Hellenistic medical sects, see chs. 12–15 in M. Frede, *Essays in Ancient Philosophy* (Minneapolis, 1987), and H. von Staden, *Herophilus: The Art of Medicine in Early Alexandria* (Cambridge, 1989). I discussed differences of opinion between the Methodists in *Science, Folklore and Ideology* (Cambridge, 1983), pp. 185ff.

doctors should adopt. On his view, at least, where the Dogmatists and Empiricists differed was primarily on the types of epistemological question we have been concerned with, for example on the question of whether the investigation of hidden causes and underlying reality is possible or relevant, and, if so, whether a doctor should try to be in a position to deduce treatments from such causes, or whether all that he can and should focus on is what had proved efficacious in what appeared to be similar cases in the past. What this suggests is that, to Galen at least, this polemic between rival doctors was a polemic about epistemology more than one about practice.[18]

Now in our brief references to classical Chinese sources we found that Chinese doctors do not just criticize one another obliquely, but sometimes do so directly. Certainly there are rivalries in Chinese medicine, as there are in Greece. But the nature of some Greek rivalry may differ in this respect, that it was sometimes not just a matter of this or that individual being accused of ignorance or lack of experience, but rather of an analysis of the role of experience itself in medicine, or again a matter of the status or grounds of *any* knowledge claim. The goal of some Greek forays into epistemology was not just to provide yourself with firm foundations to validate your own medical practices, but comprehensively to demolish the opposition, your rivals. They must be wrong, you argued, since their methods are.

An attempt may now be made, in conclusion, to take stock of the provisional findings our inquiry suggests, and, given the highly selective nature of our survey, we must emphasize, once again, the tentativeness of those findings. It is not difficult, first, to point to similarities between features of the medical theory and practice for which we have evidence in classical Greece and those we find in classical China. These extend to points to do with a concern with medical methods themselves. We noted a certain self-consciousness about methods in both cases, and again a certain spirit of rivalry within both complex sets of medical traditions.

However, the intensity of concern with epistemological problems in some early Greek medical texts is exceptional. Some might see this purely in terms of the well-marked traits of curiosity or inquisitiveness that, ever since Aristotle, have been associated with Greek intellectual life. Yet as we have seen, the medical writers in question are not just reacting to issues that naturally arose in their day-to-day clinical practice. There is evidently far more to those epistemological interests than is captured by some gesture towards a presumed Greek natural curiosity –

---

[18]   Galen, *On Sects for Beginners*, especially ch. 6. See M. Frede, *Galen: Three Treatises on the Nature of Science* (Indianapolis, 1985).

a presumption that, in any case, raises questions rather than resolves them.

Two further factors in particular seem important, first the relations between medicine and other inquiries, especially philosophy, and second the internal dynamics of relations between groups and individuals within learned medicine itself. Chinese medicine too eventually has strong links with Chinese natural philosophy. Once the ideas associated with *yin* and *yang* and the five phases had become more or less systematized, in the Han, they were used in every branch of inquiry, medicine included. Yet Chinese learned medicine did not find itself impelled to justify its very existence in the way some Greek doctors did, in relation to attacks from outside or in competition with other masters of truth. Some of those attacks owed something to philosophical developments but the models provided by philosophical debate can also be said to have been adapted by the doctors themselves to defend their own positions and to stake out claims for the art of medicine as they practised it.

But secondly, and perhaps more importantly, there is the use of epistemology by Greek medical writers in internal polemic with rival practitioners. We even find, in the Hellenistic period, polemic concerned just with epistemology or methodology in contrast to therapies or practices.

The degree of epistemological interest in Greece reflects the intensity of competitiveness between and within different groups of claimants to intellectual prestige. But we can be more specific about the contexts in which that competitiveness flourished, for it did so in an institutional framework that again manifests certain contrasts with that within which Chinese intellectuals operated. The crucial difference may lie in this, that in Greece neither in philosophy nor in medicine were pupils required or expected to show life-long and unquestioning devotion to those who had taught them. True, the Hippocratic Oath illustrates that some doctors, as teachers, certainly wished to tie their pupils to them.[19] But even in the Hellenistic period, with the rise of some more or less well-defined sects, the allegiance of pupils or indeed of the existing members of the group was far from guaranteed. The Empiricist sect itself was founded by Philinus who had been a Herophilean.[20] The

---

[19] The Hippocratic Oath specifies that the pupil should treat his teacher like his parents: *CMG* I l, 4.5ff. Which groups of doctors swore to the oath in one or other version is disputed: see L. Edelstein, in *Ancient Medicine*, O. and C.L. Temkin (eds.) (Baltimore, 1967), pp. 3–63.

[20] The evidence for the followers of Herophilus is set out by von Staden (note 17), pp. 71, 101ff., who discusses the disputes between Herophileans and Empiricists. See also Frede (note 17), ch. 13.

Methodists, as we noted, disagreed not just with members of other groups, but also with those whom they considered to be Methodists like themselves. *A fortiori*, in the earlier classical period, it was even more a question of every medical theorist for himself. Similarly also in philosophy, there are plenty of instances of pupils criticizing their masters – as Aristotle did Plato – and ample evidence also of young philosophers attending the lectures of several different teachers before deciding which group to join or whether to found schools for themselves.[21]

The contrast with China is marked in that what are rather misleadingly called the schools of philosophers and others – the *Jia* (families or lineages) – had, as their chief and overriding aim, the transmission and preservation of the teachings of the master, that is, especially of the texts that encapsulated them. True, individuals could and sometimes did break away and found new groups. But it is unheard of for Chinese pupils to criticize their teachers in their lifetime, let alone attack them face to face. In the classical, and even in the Hellenistic period, Greek philosophers and doctors did not enjoy the benefit of the solidarity of anything like such stable associations. Correspondingly they had to work harder, as individuals, both to make names for themselves and to defend their positions against potential opponents. If Greek epistemological debate, in medicine as elsewhere, had the effect of clarifying the status of various inquiries and of developing alternative views on such topics as the roles of experience and of reasoning, we should not forget that the underlying motivation of some such explorations was to secure a tenable position in the face of intense competition and to undermine any rivals who might seek to threaten it. While it would no doubt be exaggerated to claim that epistemological debate in Greek medicine is *just* window-dressing, *just* a matter of the rhetoric of self-presentation, we should recognize that it was *partly* that and attempt to carry further the analysis of why that should have been so.[22]

---

[21] Thus Theophrastus is reported to have 'heard' Plato, but then to have followed Aristotle, whom of course he succeeded: see Diogenes Laertius, *Lives of Eminent Philosophers*, trans. R.D. Hicks, 2 vols. (Cambridge, 1979), V, 36; Euclid of Megara, ibid., II, 106ff., is said to have associated with both Socrates and Plato, but then to have formed the group known as the Megarians (or Eristics or Dialecticians). The founder of the Stoa, Zeno of Citium, was taught first by Crates the Cynic, then by Stilpo the Megarian, as well as by two successive heads of the Academy, namely Xenocrates and Polemo: ibid., VII, 1; and similar examples could be multiplied.

[22] The topics mentioned in the last two paragraphs are the subject of collaborative research currently being undertaken by Nathan Sivin and myself.

ABBREVIATIONS

CMG   *Corpus medicorum graecorum*
MP   G.E.R. Lloyd, *Methods and Problems in Greek Science*
          (Cambridge, 1991)

3   *Autopsia, historia* and what women know: the authority of women in Hippocratic gynaecology[1]

Lesley Dean-Jones

It is axiomatic that virtually all the extant medical treatises of Graeco-Roman antiquity were written by men,[2] but the extent of women's role in the compilation of these writings is debated. Paola Manuli believes the Hippocratics treated the female body as a dumb canvas on which to project their theories, while Aline Rousselle claims the Hippocratic treatises were little more than the written mouthpiece for the female oral tradition.[3] Needless to say, most scholars believe the truth lies somewhere between the two. G.E.R. Lloyd has drawn attention to the

For a list of bibliographical abbreviations, please see the end of this chapter.

[1]   This paper was written as a direct result of the workshop and as such stands as an example of how exposure to other traditions can make us question the assumptions of our own more closely. My original presentation had been on what and how the Hippocratics had learned from women. The Sinologists at the workshop wanted to know why the Greeks felt they had to learn from women at all. My naïve answer, 'Because it's gynaecology', met with the response, 'So?' For the purposes of this volume, therefore, I have addressed the question '*Why* did the Hippocratics think they had to turn to women as a source of knowledge for their gynaecology?' Owing to the circumstances of the generation of the paper, my comparanda will be drawn from classical Chinese gynaecology. I am particularly indebted to Francesca Bray for help in this aspect. I should also like to thank Ann Ellis Hanson, Elizabeth Asmis and Martha Roth who gave me valuable suggestions when I delivered an earlier version of this paper at the University of Chicago's Workshop on Ancient Societies in May 1993. Any mistakes I may have made in fact or interpretation are entirely my own responsibility. In this paper, I do not mean to indicate that the Hippocratics as a group had a self-conscious theory of knowledge (though obviously some treatises such as *VM* and *Morb. Sacr.* address questions of the foundations of medical knowledge directly: see Lloyd, this volume, pp. 26–9). However, I believe we can identify criteria which served to validate a piece of information as a fact for the Hippocratics, thereby supporting their theories and treatment. As with most ancient Greek theorists, they were more concerned with understanding or justifying a body of beliefs than with eliminating the possibility of being wrong: see Julia Annas, 'Stoic Epistemology', in Stephen Everson (ed.), *Companions to Ancient Thought 1: Epistemology* (Cambridge: Cambridge University Press, 1990), p. 184.

[2]   The exceptions are treatises attributed to Cleopatra and Metrodora (see below, pp. 47–8).

[3]   Paola Manuli, 'Donne mascoline, femmine sterili, vergini perpetua: la ginecologia greca tra Ippocrate e Sorano', in Silvia Campese, Paola Manuli and Giulia Sissa, *Madre Materia* (Turin: Boringhieri, 1983), p. 155; Aline Rousselle, *Porneia: On Desire and the Body in Antiquity*, trans. Felicia Pheasant (Oxford: Blackwell, 1988), pp. 25–6.

interplay between developing scientific medicine and folk medicine, and Ann Ellis Hanson divides women into two types: the inexperienced, whose knowledge of her own body is indeed shaped by the physician, and the 'woman of experience', who functions as an authoritative source for male physicians.[4] The very existence of this debate, however, indicates the recognition that for the ancient Greeks and Romans the epistemological basis of their gynaecology differs somehow from that on which the rest of their medicine is founded. Neither ancient authors nor modern scholars are so concerned to analyse the contribution of the male clientele to Hippocratic theories and treatment.

In practising clinical medicine the ancient physician recognized two sources of information: *autopsia*, his own observations, and *historia*, what he was told by other people.[5] We might assume that it was the social impropriety of a doctor examining a woman's body in an intimate manner which caused a different emphasis in the epistemology of the gynaecology by restricting the opportunities ancient physicians had for autopsia in the case of women's diseases, but this is not acknowledged as a problem by the Hippocratics. Various issues of deportment are dealt with in the deontological works, including, for example, how to dress, how to sit at a bedside, and the necessity of moving one's hands gracefully, but there is no instruction given for how to approach a female patient – instruction we might expect if a physician anticipated concerns of modesty to be routine.

The only concessions to the delicacy of the relationship are made in *Medic.* and *Jusj.*, which imply physicians routinely examined female members of a household.[6] Female genitalia are referred to as anatomical parts with which an author can assume a physician will have familiarity, e.g., the labia at *Mul.* I 40 (8.96.10) and *Loc. Hom.* 47 (6.344.7), or the

---

4   G.E.R. Lloyd, *Science, Folklore and Ideology* (Cambridge: Cambridge University Press, 1983), pp. 76–9; Ann Ellis Hanson, 'The Medical Writer's Woman', in David M. Halperin, John J. Winkler and Froma I. Zeitlin (eds.), *Before Sexuality: The Construction of Erotic Experience in the Ancient Greek World* (Princeton: Princeton University Press, 1990), pp. 309–10.

5   Once again, the recognition is implicit. I use the formulation of *autopsia* and *historia* as an hermeneutic device to illustrate where the Hippocratics share assumptions with other early Greek theories of knowledge (see below, pp. 57f.). That sense perception and listening to others' experiences are the foundations of medical knowledge is stated explicitly in *Praec.* 1–2 (9.250.1–254.9). In contrast to the clinical treatises, the theoretical treatises sometimes proceed as if trying to deduce medicine from basic principles: see Lloyd, this volume (p. 33).

6   'Into whatsoever houses I enter, I will enter to help the sick, and I will abstain from all intentional wrong-doing and harm, especially from abusing the bodies of man or woman, bond or free', *Jusj.* (4.630.12–15); 'At every moment [the physician] meets women, maidens and possessions very precious indeed', *Medic.* 1 (9.206.7–9), trans. W. H. S. Jones, *Hippocrates*, 4 vols. (Cambridge, Mass.: Harvard University Press, 1923–31), Vol. 1, p. 301 and Vol. 2, p. 313.

relationship of urethra and vagina at *Aër.* 9 (2.40.7–42.5).[7] Moreover, in
the gynaecological works where actual examinations of patients are
described, while the gender of the participles shows that the woman
often examines herself and reports back to the physician, the physician
just as often performs the examination himself. So, at *Mul.* I 20 (8.60.1)
a doctor who feels a membrane across the vagina with his finger is
instructed to introduce a pessary as far into the woman as possible (hōs
esōtatō) and *Mul.* II 163 (8.342.13) describes what a doctor should do if
on examination he finds the cervix so indurated that it will not admit his
finger. Among other measures he is to open the cervix with a probe and
his finger, as he is also instructed to do at *Nat. Mul.* 37 (7.380.6).[8]

Therefore, despite the cultural ideal of the secluded woman and the
possible objections of some individual women, lack of opportunity to
examine women patients was not the major stumbling block for the
Hippocratics in understanding the female body and diseases. In terms of
autopsia the basis for Hippocratic knowledge of male and female bodies
was comparable.

In practising clinical medicine an ancient physician would have two
different types of sources of historia: the observations made by others
attending the same or similar diseases (relayed orally or in writing), and
the descriptions of the subjective experiences of the patients he was
treating. In Greek thought there were recognized problems with
accepting second-hand information (reliability of source, distance from
the event, etc.), so generally historia would be considered a less reliable
justification for a belief than autopsia.[9]

It is perhaps in the light of this that sometimes a physician will report
what he learned through historia as if he had learned it through autopsia.
For example, the case histories of the seven books of the *Epid.* are related

---

[7]   The text of this last passage is extremely problematic: see Lesley Dean-Jones, *Women's
      Bodies in Classical Greek Science* (Oxford: Oxford University Press, 1994), pp. 80–1.
      For evidence that Aristotle did *not* recognize separation of urethra and vagina see
      Lesley Dean-Jones, 'The Cultural Construct of the Female Body in Classical Greek
      Science', in Sarah B. Pomeroy (ed.), *Women's History and Ancient History* (Chapel Hill:
      University of North Carolina Press, 1991), p. 127.

[8]   Other cases where a male doctor definitely performs the examination are: *Mul.* I 60
      (8.120.7–9), II 155–156, 160, 167 and 168 (8.330.13–21, 338.5, 346.1 and 346.20),
      Nat. Mul. 8, 13, 35–37, 39, 42, 45–6, 67 (7.322.13, 330.14, 376.23–380.7, 382.16,
      386.8, 390.4–17, 402.8). Some of these cases are duplicates of one another. See
      further Dean-Jones (note 7, 1994), pp. 35–6.

[9]   See Thucydides I 22. The Greeks also considered the sense of hearing to be less
      reliable than that of sight: e.g., Heraclitus B 101a: 'The eyes are more exact witnesses
      than the ears'; see Edward Hussey, 'The Beginnings of Epistemology: from Homer to
      Philolaus', in Everson (ed.) (note 1), p. 14, n. 10. Compare Bray, this volume: 'not
      vision, but hearing and touch turned out to be the most important source of knowledge
      for the physician himself' (p. 238).

for the most part as if the author himself had seen the symptoms he describes, but at *Epid.* I, 13, case 4 (2.692.14–15) on the eleventh day of the illness of the wife of Philinus (which began fourteen days after delivery and in which day-by-day observations of stools, convulsions, delirium, sleep, etc. had begun on the sixth day), the author describes the woman's urine in great detail and appends the remark, 'Such was the urine as I at least saw' (toiauta ourei hoia kagō eidon), as if he wished to vouch for this part of the report more strongly than the rest, though otherwise there is no indication that he had *not* seen the other reported symptoms.[10] The confidence of an ancient physician to report the general progression of an illness as if he had seen all the stages himself, when in fact he had not, may derive from the fact that in some cases he had left an apprentice in charge of the patient. *Decent.* 17 (9.242.9–13) suggests, 'Let one of your pupils be left in charge, to carry out instructions without unpleasantness and to administer the treatment ... He is there also to prevent those things escaping notice that happen in the intervals between visits.'[11] The only cases where symptoms which could be the subjects of autopsia are reported as historia are at *Epid.* I 13, case 5 (2.694.6) and VII 117 (5.462.23). In the first case the wife of Epicrates 'when near her delivery was seized with severe rigor without, it was said, becoming warm'. Three days later the woman had a normal delivery (though the author notes the baby was a girl),[12] and further pathological symptoms did not appear until the second day after delivery. It is presumably only at this point that the doctor was called in so he does not want to vouch for a symptom from five days previously as autopsia. In the second case the child (or slave) of Deinias is reported as suffering from a fistula in his abdomen through which his intestines were protruding and a worm occasionally issued. The intestines would not remain inside because of a cough. All this is reported as autopsia, but the author also adds that the unfortunate patient *said* that when he had a fever bilious matter flowed through the fistula too. Presumably, because this was a chronic disease, neither the doctor himself nor his apprentice could be present at the manifestation of every symptom, and so for one important aspect (voiding of bile) the doctor had to take the patient's word, though he feels compelled to let his reader know he would not vouch for this on the same level as the other

---

[10] See Helen King, 'Using the Past: Nursing and the Medical Profession in Ancient Greece', in Pat Holden and Jenny Littlewood (eds.), *Anthropology and Nursing* (London: Routledge, 1991), pp. 16–17.

[11] Jones (note 6), Vol. 2, p. 299. Chapter 13 instructs the doctor to make frequent visits.

[12] If the sex of a baby is noted at delivery it is usually female because the Hippocratics thought this helped explain the problems attendant upon the delivery: see Ann Ellis Hanson, 'Diseases of Women in the Epidemics', *Die Hippokratischen Epidemien, Sudhoffs Archiv* 27 (1989), 48 and Dean-Jones (note 7, 1994), p. 211.

symptoms. In most cases, though, how often the details recorded in the *Epid.* were the result of autopsia and how often they were the result of *historia* is impossible to tell. The authors assimilate them all as knowledge.

Similarly, in expounding most general theories, the Hippocratics are content to express them as generally accepted knowledge. When they explicitly attribute theories or forms of healing to others it is usually for purposes of disagreement.[13] So, in addition to the avowedly agonistic treatises such as *VM*, *Nat. Hom.* or *Morb. Sacr.*, we have the comment in *Fract.* 2 (3.418.7). A certain physician who splinted a broken arm in the position of an archer, because, *he said*, the extension of the elbow brought the bones of the forearm parallel to one another, would have done better, the comment says, to follow the natural instinct of the patient who presented it in a position of pronation. And in *Morb.* II 4 (7.10.15) the author brings to task those who *say* that small vessels can overfill with blood and cause disease, because, he argues, nothing bad can arise from something good like an abundance of blood. Anything with which the author concurs is not said to have been said by anyone other than the author.

There are signs that the strongest challenge from alternative healers came from practitioners of traditional women's medicine; the *Epid.* contains only half the number of female as male case histories, which suggests women resorted to other forms of healing more often than men.[14] Yet while the gynaecological works contain many criticisms of the practices of doctors other than those the authors themselves employ (e.g., in *Mul.* I, 2 (8.20.14–16) the author criticizes those doctors who incise a tumour in a woman's groin when it could be caused by suppressed menses),[15] the Hippocratic authors only once criticize the practice of women healers explicitly (at *Mul.* I 67 (8.140.15–16) where women are criticized for using too acrid pessaries in their treatments and thus causing ulcerations of the womb). Furthermore, the Hippocratic authors usually cite women's testimony as the source for beliefs in which they concur. For example, in explaining how his client knew she was pregnant, even though she had conceived only six days previously, the author of *Nat. Puer.* 13 (7.490.5–7) says:

Now this girl had heard the sort of thing women *say* to each other – that when a woman is going to conceive, the seed remains inside her and does not fall out.[16]

---

[13]   See King (note 10), p. 16.
[14]   See Lloyd (note 4), pp. 69–70; Dean-Jones (note 7, 1994), pp. 33–5, 136.
[15]   See Lloyd (note 4), p. 80, for further examples of criticisms of rival physicians in the gynaecological works.
[16]   *The Hippocratic Treatises 'On Generation', 'On the Nature of the Child', 'Diseases IV'*, trans. Iain M. Lonie (Berlin: Walter de Gruyter, 1981), p. 7.

And at *Carn.* 19 (8.610.2–4) the author, in describing what a foetus aborted at seven days looks like, remarks, 'Someone may ask how I know this.' He then proceeds to justify his claim by saying that he had seen the results of abortions of several prostitutes who knew when they had conceived. This implies that this author at least felt that while his knowledge could be challenged that of his female informants could not.[17]

The passage from *Nat. Puer.* and *Steril.* 220 (8.424.18–19), which says a woman will know she has retained the seed from her husband if he says he has ejaculated and she remains dry, imply that a woman's knowledge of whether she had conceived or not derives from the environment of the vagina after intercourse. Soranus, *Gyn.* I 44, says that a woman's knowledge of conception derives from her feeling a shivering at the end of intercourse, and Galen, *Nat. Fac.* III 3 149–50, from her sensing the *os uteri* contracting and closing. No Hippocratic author discusses such experiences, but *Septim.* 4 (7.440.13–442.4) reads:

One must not doubt what women say about childbirth, for they say what they know and they will always say so. They could not be persuaded either by fact or by logical argument to know otherwise than what goes on in their own bodies (to en toisi sōmasin auteōn ginomenon). Some may wish to argue otherwise, but women decide the contest and they give the victory prize concerning this argument. Women say and always will say that they bear seven and eight and nine and ten and eleven months' children, and that of these the eight months' children do not survive but the others do.[18]

The phrase 'what goes on in their own bodies' suggests that women's knowledge is of some activity in their bodies rather than of a passive state which could equally well be checked by a male should he happen to examine a woman directly after intercourse.[19] It is possible, therefore, that the signs cited by Soranus and Galen as indicative of conception were accepted by the Hippocratics also. Later in *Septim.* the author takes issue with women's claim that they bear eleven-month children, but he

---

[17]   On the other hand, *Epid.* II, sec. 3, 17 (5.118.1–3) asks whether pregnancy should be counted from conception or from the menses. This could suggest that the author questions the reliability of female claims to recognizing the time of conception, and *Epid.* IV, case 21 (5.160.15) tells of the wife of a certain Antigenes who did not know if she was pregnant, suggesting that not all women were, or expected to be, cognizant of conception. *Epid.* IV 24 (5.164.6–10) relates the case of the daughter of Tekomaios who became pregnant 'without any sign' (*asēmos*). Symptoms began in the second month with phlegmatic vomiting. The signs that were missing, therefore, were ones that were expected to have manifested very early indeed, and probably should be taken to include the woman's recognition of conception.

[18]   'The Eighth-month Child: Obsit Omen', trans. Ann Ellis Hanson, *Bulletin of the History of Medicine*, 61 (1987), 594.

[19]   See below, note 26.

argues that this belief stems from a mistake in calculation, not an error of perception of subjective experience.[20]

There are also signs that the gynaecological treatises attempt to co-opt some aspects of traditional female healing; a disproportionate amount of Hippocratic pharmacopoeia is contained in the gynaecology, mainly in long lists of alternative remedies, and it is the only type of Hippocratic medicine to recommend the use of animal excrement as a drug.[21]

Midwives continued to play a large role in female health care, primarily in the attendance of normal births. In Pliny and Galen many midwives and wise-women are named, e.g., Salpe, Lais, Elephantis, Olympias, Sotira and Antiochis. And although they do give occasional advice on male or general diseases, their contribution is basically limited to women's health.[22] This shows that as antiquity progressed the importance of these women was not lessened; that is, physicians view them as an ongoing source of information, not as an earlier repository of traditional wisdom which could be discarded after its useful knowledge had been drained into the scientific tradition.

Within the scientific tradition, too, women were vouchsafed some authority in understanding the female body.[23] Two treatises entitled *Diseases of Women* are attributed to women authors: to Cleopatra, who wrote around the first century AD and who is referred to by Galen, Aetius of Amida in the sixth century and Paul of Aegina in the seventh,

[20]   *Nat. Puer.* 30 (7. 532.14–534.8), however, says those women who think they have been pregnant for longer than ten months are misled by having suffered from flatulence accompanied by amenorrhea for some time before actual conception.

[21]   See Heinrich von Staden, 'Women and Dirt', *Helios*, 19 (1992), 9–13 and Hanson (note 12), pp. 40–1.

[22]   See Lloyd (note 4), p. 63, n. 11 and p. 70, n. 46. Soranus seems to view midwives within the tradition of scientific training: see King (note 10), p. 21.

[23]   I am not concerned here with the status of practising female physicians in the ancient world, because their authority as a group is not recognized within the written tradition. For female physicians see Sarah B. Pomeroy, 'Plato and the Female Physician *Rep.* 454d2', *American Journal of Philology*, 99 (1978), 496–500, and Mary R. Lefkowitz and Maureen B. Fant (eds.), *Women's Life in Greece and Rome: a Source Book in Translation* (Baltimore: Johns Hopkins University Press, 1982), pp. 26 and 161–2. There is a story recorded by Hyginus in the first century AD of a certain Hagnodike (or Agnodike) who became a physician, although it was against Athenian law for women to practise medicine, because her fellow women were dying rather than allowing themselves to be treated by male doctors. The story is without doubt apocryphal: see Helen King, 'Agnodike and the Profession of Medicine', *Proceedings of the Cambridge Philological Society*, n.s. 32 (1986), 53–77. As we have seen, there is no indication that female modesty presented a serious obstacle to the prosecution of clinical gynaecology. In this anecdote, Hagnodike's superior authority as a physician was gained not from her gender, but from studying under the male Herophilus. Herophilus' treatise *Midwifery* was influential in the field of ancient gynaecology because he had had the opportunity to dissect human cadavers and observe the reproductive organs of both men and women: see Hanson (note 4), p. 321.

and to Metrodora who wrote in the sixth century AD. In addition, when compiling his medical encyclopaedia, Aetius refers to the authority of an otherwise unknown Aspasia for his chapters on gynaecology and obstetrics more often than to any other author, including Soranus. These women are not cited because they are correcting mistaken points of view of men. In fact the text of Metrodora (the only original text attributed to a woman doctor which survives) is constantly referring back to Hippocrates. These women are in the same scientific tradition as male authors on gynaecology. They seem to draw their authority from their gender rather than from anything they have to add to the tradition.

Paradoxically, the explanation for this continuing deference to female authority in the scholarly tradition of Graeco-Roman medicine lies in the problematic relationship which existed between Hippocratic doctors and their female patients. The subtleties of this relationship are described in the now famous passage of *Mul.* I 62 (8.126.4–19):

All these diseases, then, happen more frequently to women who have not borne a child, yet they also happen to those who have. These diseases are dangerous, as has been said, and for the most part they are both acute and serious, and *difficult to understand because of the fact that women are the ones who share these sicknesses* [my emphasis]. Sometimes women do not know what sicknesses they have, until they have experienced the diseases which come from menses and they become older. Then both necessity and time teach them the cause of their sicknesses. Sometimes diseases become incurable for women who do not learn why they are sick before the doctor has been correctly taught by the sick woman why she is sick. For women are ashamed to tell even if they know, and they suppose that it is a disgrace, because of their inexperience and lack of knowledge. At the same time the doctors also make mistakes by not learning the apparent cause through accurate questioning, but they proceed to heal as though they were dealing with men's diseases. I have already seen many women die from just this kind of suffering. But at the outset one must ask accurate questions about the cause. For the healing of the diseases of women differs greatly from the healing of men's diseases.[24]

This passage indicates that there is a culturally induced problem: women feel shame when discussing their gynaecological ailments with men. Elsewhere in the Corpus we see that the physician may be unable to ask all the questions he would like to because of the delicacy of the situation. In *Epid.* V, case 53 (5.238.4–5) the author states:

The wife of Simus aborted on the thirtieth day. This happened either upon her drinking something or spontaneously.

Epid. IV, case 26 tells of the niece of Temenes. The doctor attending her says he was not sure if she had had a baby or not. Obviously,

[24]   Trans. Ann Ellis Hanson, 'Hippocrates: *Diseases of Women* 1', *Signs*, 1 (1975), 581–2.

although this piece of information would have been extremely valuable when considering treatment, he did not feel he could simply ask, or if he did, he felt he had not received a satisfactory answer.

As a woman may be reluctant to confide in a man, so a man may be reluctant to trust the testimony of a woman. At *Epid.* IV, chapter 6 (5.146.9–12) the doctor was called to attend the wife of Acheloos after she had aborted. The physician notes that he could not tell how many months the foetus was, but that the woman told him she had aborted a second baby, a male, about the twentieth day [of her pregnancy?]. He remarks, 'If she was telling the truth, I do not know.'[25] In chapters 20 and 22 (5.160.6–7 and 162.4–8) he similarly casts doubt on the information given him by a certain Tenedia (one of the very few named women in the Corpus) and by the sister-in-law of Apamantos, who tell him they had aborted a male of thirty days and a female of sixty days in gestation respectively, by reporting their statements with the words 'so she said'.[26]

The occasions on which the Hippocratics suggest their male patients may be less than trustworthy are confined to whether or not they are following the doctor's instructions. *Decent.* 14 (9.240.12–16) says that patients sometimes lie about whether they have taken unpleasant remedies and die as a result, for which the doctors are unfairly blamed.[27]

So there were social constructs which made communication between a doctor and his female patient, and therefore female historia, more problematic than autopsia of the female body. But the passage in *Mul.* I 62 indicates that there is a more fundamental problem in understanding women's diseases. The Greek of the italicized phrase reads 'chalepa xunienai dia touth' hoti hai gynaikes metechousi tōn nousōn'. Literally this translates, 'difficult to understand on account of the fact that women share [the] diseases'. In a paraphrase E.D. Phillips says the diseases are 'difficult to understand because they are peculiar to women'.[28] Littré translates, 'parce que les femmes partagent les

---

[25]   The fact that the author questions the truth, *alēthea*, and not simply the correctness of the woman's observation, shows that he thinks the woman could be lying to him, for whatever reason, not miscalculating.

[26]   Compare pseudo-Aristotle *HA* 10.7, 638a5ff., trans. and ed. Jonathan Barnes, *The Complete Works of Aristotle*, 2 vols. (Princeton: Princeton University Press, 1984), Vol. 1, p. 991: 'We can determine whether those women tell the truth who say that when they have erotic dreams they wake up dry.' Presumably Aristotle thought men could confirm this through *autopsia*, though of course they would still have to take the woman's word that she had actually had an erotic dream.

[27]   In contrast, a woman of Cyzique simply refused to obey the doctor's instructions: *Epid.* III, ch. 17, case 14 (3.140.18). *De Arte* 7 (6.10.15–12.13) explains the death of patients under the treatment of a properly trained doctor as due not to any shortcomings in the art of medicine but in the *inability* of patients to properly follow instructions.

[28]   E.D. Phillips, *Aspects of Greek Medicine* (New York: St Martin's Press, 1973), p. 109.

maladies [communes], difficiles à comprendre,' and Manuli renders the phrase 'difficile diagnosi, perché le donne partecipano delle malattie comuni'. Where Littré indicates by square brackets that the term 'communes' is an addition, Manuli does not. Manuli understands this term to mean that women have a share in both male and female diseases.[29] She herself thinks there is no such thing as 'male diseases' and thinks that by this term the author means to indicate communal diseases. However, after the Greek verb 'metechō', 'share', we would expect a noun in the dative case indicating with whom the diseases are shared. Since none occurs it is easier to supply the indirect object by assuming the verb is to be taken reflexively, i.e., women share them with each other, not with men as well. The point is that the diseases are restricted to women and this in and of itself causes problems. It is not just, or even primarily, that women will not tell men about them. As we have seen, the Hippocratics feel they were privy to 'what women say' (see above, pp. 45f.).

Now, gynaecological ailments are not the only diseases the Hippocratics found difficult to understand. Comments made in the *Epid.* and the surgical treatises in particular show that the Hippocratic physician often found himself at a loss.[30] But he does not justify his lack of understanding by saying that he has not shared in the diseases himself. No doctor, male or female, could be expected to have suffered every type of disease they treated.[31] While this might indeed render a physician more sympathetic to his patients, it would not do much to boost his practice. The treatise *Medic.* recommends keeping oneself as healthy as possible to attract new patients. (*Medic.* 1 (9.204.1–4): 'The dignity of a physician requires that he should look healthy, and as plump as nature intended him to be; for the common crowd consider those who are not of this excellent bodily condition to be unable to take care of others.')[32] In spite of this, when discussing common illnesses Hippocratic authors are not constantly referring to the authority of those who have suffered them to buttress their claims to knowledge. In these cases they feel justified simply in reporting as fact what they have learned from historia without drawing attention to the impossibility of vouching for all their statements from actually having experienced them.[33]

---

[29] Manuli (note 3), p. 159.
[30] Lloyd (note 4), p. 81, n. 80.
[31] Though in classical Greece midwives were expected to have given birth themselves: see below, pp. 57–8.
[32] Jones (note 6), Vol. 2, p. 311.
[33] See Lee T. Pearcy, 'Diagnosis as Narrative in Ancient Literature', *American Journal of Philology*, 113 (1992), 603.

Yet why should the suffering of the average layman in disease be any more accessible to a Hippocratic physician than that of the average laywoman? Surely it is not the case that most men were able to communicate only because they were always experienced in the diseases which drove them to seek medical help. At least one author, in fact, cites attempts at self-diagnosis as a problem.[34] Why should female suffering be so difficult to understand unless it was communicated to the doctor by a woman of experience?

Compare the situation in ancient Chinese medicine. Unlike Greek medicine, Chinese medicine was split into specializations, of which gynaecology was one, though it was still practised entirely by men.[35] It was not a speciality because of the difficulty of understanding the female body, but because such bodies had a different balance of *yin* and *yang*. There was no more a different epistemology behind gynaecology than there was behind the speciality of, say, febrile diseases. A specialist studied a certain type of disease, not a certain type of body. The Chinese gynaecologist had far less access to the female body than did the non-specialist Hippocratic. In China live female patients indicated the part of their anatomy in which they felt pain on a model of the female body.[36] The only time a doctor could lay his hands on a female patient was to take her pulse, and even then the woman's wrist was decorously covered with a handkerchief.[37] In fact, examination of women's reproductive organs was not conducted routinely until well into the twentieth century.[38] However, this does not seem to have led to a feeling that there was any problem in understanding the female body or women's diseases

[34] *De Arte* 11 (6.20.7–9). Similarly at *Epid.* III sec. 2, case 6, in the case of the daughter of Euryanax the author reports, 'They *said* the trouble was due to eating grapes', without committing himself to concurring in the reported diagnosis.

[35] Though there was, in fact, no separate branch of medicine dealing with women's disorders before the tenth century (Bray, this volume, p. 236, n. 2). Charlotte Furth, 'Blood, Body and Gender: Medical Images of the Female Condition in China 1600–1850', *Chinese Science*, 7 (1986), 43–66, sees the proliferation of gynaecological treatises from 1500 to 1900 as an aspect of the consolidation of a paternalistic patriarchy among the Chinese élite.

[36] Lloyd (note 4), p. 73, n. 56. Unlike Greek medicine, Chinese medicine did countenance the post-mortem dissection of both male and female bodies for forensic purposes.

[37] Bray, p. 239. This precaution proved useless in one case where the physician was so skilled he could tell everything about the woman from her pulse, fell in love with her, and eloped with her. (I have this tale by personal communication from Francesca Bray.) It is interesting that in demonstrating the prognostic value of the pulse in *Prog.*, Galen recounts a similar anecdote regarding his own practice. He diagnosed a woman as suffering from love sickness by the fact that her pulse speeded up when the name of a certain dancer was mentioned: see Vivian Nutton (ed.), *Galen: On Prognosis, Corpus Medicorum Graecorum*, 8.1 (Berlin: Akademie-Verlag, 1979), pp. 101–3.

[38] Bray, p. 238, n. 5. It should be noted that there was no routine examination of men either.

in general. Moreover, before administering any remedies for amenorrhoea Chinese gynaecologists assume the authority of confirming
whether or not a woman was pregnant through objective tests.[39] Up to
the fourth month the doctor would judge from reactions to certain drugs
– after that he could, of course, tell by pulse.

In classical Chinese medicine, as in ancient Greek, a detailing of
the symptoms of a case was needed to help in diagnosis, but those
derived from any particular female patient are not glossed as being
more opaque or less trustworthy, to the extent that a Chinese
physician had access to them, than those derived from a male.
However, in spite of the lack of opportunity to examine the female
body and the apparently greater credence given to female testimony,
in the scholarly tradition of Chinese medicine we do not have
constant references about what must be learned from women, nor
citations of midwives and female medical authors. In fact, as Bray
shows (this volume, p. 243), Chinese gynaecologists dismiss women's
explanations of amenorrhoea (menstrual blockage) as the least likely
explanation. This does not mean that Chinese gynaecologists did not
learn from and collaborate smoothly with midwives. But they did not
feel the need to cite female sources to validate their claims to
knowledge.

So, as I mentioned before, there is a paradox between on the one
hand the Hippocratics' access to autopsia of women's bodies and their
negative opinion of historia from women patients and, on the other
hand, their comparatively frequent deference to the authority of women.
I would like to suggest a further source of knowledge about the body in
addition to autopsia and historia which is implicitly recognized by the
Hippocratic authors and which could not be assimilated by a male
author however well he communicated with his female patients – that is
the innate consciousness of one's own body.

VM 9 (1.588.14–590.1) says, 'You will not find a criterion, neither
number nor any fixed standard, by reference to which you will know the
exact amount [of food, drink or medicines to administer], except the
sensation of the body (tou sōmatos tēn aisthēsin).' The term 'aisthēsis'
could signify an observer's perception of another's body, but in context
here it seems more likely to signify the sensation an individual has of
their own body. The author is discussing feelings of repletion and

39 Bray, pp. 246f. This does not mean Chinese women were totally without influence in
    questions of their own health care, simply that their influence does not appear explicitly
    in the scholarly tradition: see Francesca Bray, 'Meanings of Motherhood: Reproduc-
    tive Technology and its Uses in Late Imperial China', presented at the Workshop on
    Gender and Sexuality in East and Southeast Asia, UCLA, 10–12 December 1990, and
    Furth (note 35).

depletion, feelings which do not necessarily manifest themselves in bodily appearance, at least not for some time.

Confirmation that the Hippocratics did recognize an innate under-standing of one's own body is found at *Epid.* VI, sec. 8, chapter 10 (5.348.1–5). This occurs in a series of chapters which list for the physician tools he can use for his prognosis and diagnosis, e.g., the regimen a patient had been following, excretions, weather, dreams, etc. Chapter 10 refers to 'the things from knowledge, meditation, itself through itself apart from organs and things' ('tak tēs gnōmēs, xunnoia, autē kath' heōutēn, chōris tōn organōn kai tōn prēgmatōn'). The example the author uses to illustrate this is a woman, the housekeeper of Hippothoos, who knew what was going on in her illness by her own innate knowledge ('tēs gnōmēs autēs kath' heōutēn epistēmos eousa tōnen tēi nousōi epigenomenōn').[40] Stoics used a specific term for this innate awareness of one's own body (which they claimed was the first thing known): *suneidesis.*[41]

This suneidesis is behind the faith the Hippocratics place in women's self-examination. On occasion it is a woman's self-examination which leads her to seek professional help, as is the case with Phrontis (another of those rare women to be identified by her own name) whose case is reported at *Mul.* I 40 (8.96.16–98.5). She did not have her lochial flow after giving birth. Feeling pain in her vagina she examined herself, without being told to do so by a doctor, and found her vagina obstructed. She reported this, presumably to the doctor, was treated and cured. As is normally the case in the *Epid.*, we are not told what treatment she received.

More often the woman touches herself on the instructions of a doctor and reports to him if the womb is hard, soft, moist, deviating from its normal position, etc. In *Mul.* I 59 (8.118.3), the author details symptoms whereby a doctor can distinguish a case of dropsy from true pregnancy through autopsia. He says there is also a sign at the orifice of the womb; it will seem withered and moist to the woman when she touches it. Note that in this case at least the woman was not sufficiently experienced to be able to tell the doctor herself whether or not she was pregnant.

Steril. 213 (8.408.16–17) lists several states which can be recognized by a woman touching herself. The condition in which the womb is so

40   The treatise *Insomn.* suggests that when the sensory organs cease to relay information about the external world during sleep, the body can send messages about its state of health to the soul in symbolic form.
41   See A.A. Long, 'Representation and the Self in Stoicism', in Stephen Everson (ed.), *Companions to Ancient Thought 2: Psychology* (Cambridge: Cambridge University Press, 1991), p. 106. Again, I use this term to facilitate discussion; I do not want to argue that the Stoic concept of *suneidesis* originated in any way with the Hippocratics.

slippery that it cannot retain the semen can be identified both by the woman touching herself and by careful questioning to see if she has ever had any ulcerations of the womb (8.410.3–4). Similarly one can tell by touch if there is a portion of the menses left inside the womb (because it feels hard), or if a womb is more wide open than it should be (8.410.20–1 and 23). In these last two cases the text leaves open the question of who is doing the touching.

Sometimes a woman may report on the condition of her cervix and perform the requisite therapy herself[42] as at *Mul.* II 141 (8.314.16), where the woman is to straighten the orifice and draw it back to its normal place, and *Mul.* II 146 (8.322.3), where the cervix of the womb cannot be felt by touch. After placing a pessary in her vagina, the woman removes it the next day and says whether or not the cervix has straightened itself.

In the majority of cases, however, the woman reports on the state of her cervix but it is the doctor who proceeds to treat her and manipulate the cervix. *Steril.* 230 (8.438.10–11) describes a woman diagnosing the hardening of the cervix or its shutting by touching herself, but it is the doctor who applies the pessaries to the womb (8.440.23). *Mul.* II 133 describes in detail a very long course of treatment. At the beginning of the woman's illness the orifice of the womb is so contracted and dry that it is impossible to find (8.282.8–9). At one point the author says that during a fumigation, if the woman is able to examine herself, the doctor should order her to touch the mouth of the womb (8.286.16–17). Later in the course of treatment she is again to try to touch her cervix during a fumigation (8.288.8). After the fumigation, however, it is the physician who is to insert the pessary and a 'tent', with the aid of probes, into the cervix (8.288.12–290.16) and from that point on it is the physician who manipulates the cervix. *Mul.* II 157 (8.332.16) gives directions for a doctor to insert probes into the cervix if the woman, after a course of treatment, reports that the orifice of her womb is soft. *Mul.* II 119 (8.260.10–11) says that after a course of treatment (which involves the doctor himself administering seven clysters to the womb through the cervix (258.21–260.10)), if, on being asked, the woman responds that the mouth of her womb is hard and painful (here there is no reference to anybody touching), her womb should be irrigated again.

Steril. chapter 222 reads:

When you have filled the clyster, tie it off and give it to the woman to whom you intend to administer it. Let her, drawing out the stopper, place it in her uterus – she will know where it must go.

---

[42]   See Lloyd (note 4), p. 74, n. 62, for men involved in their own treatment.

After the woman has inserted the clyster, the physician performs the rest of the treatment. Here, as in the other cases, we should ask why there is a division of labour *within* a single case. There are no general indications in these cases that the doctor is always dealing with a woman of experience. Even in the last case where the woman is probably assumed to be one who has borne children, it is not clear that the knowledge of where to insert a clyster derives directly from the experience of parturition. It would seem that in these cases, although the physician is more knowledgeable in how to proceed with therapy, the woman has a better understanding of her own body. The physician's experiences with multiple female bodies did not necessarily help him to understand any particular female body. This difficulty is perhaps what is recognized at *Steril.* 230 (8.442.27–444.9):

Try to be an enquirer into nature, attending to the patient's physical appearance and strength, for there is no fixed standard of these things, but try to gather evidence from these things, using purgations and evacuations of the whole body and the head, and fumigations and pessaries of the uterus. These are your elements, and treatment of these [conditions] lies in the part of each of them.[43]

If some Hippocratic doctors did feel at a distinct disadvantage in coming to conclusions about any given woman's body it may be the *doctor's* preference to use a female intermediary at *Mul.* I 21 and *Nat. Mul.* 6 to gain better information than he could himself, rather than a doctor's concession to female modesty when he would really prefer to be doing the examination.[44] It should be noted that in later writers it was a midwife who performed the internal examination of female patients, not the doctor or the patient herself.[45]

So, despite reservations about the reliability of female testimony, the Hippocratics deferred to women's innate knowledge of their own bodies from which they were excluded by being men.[46] Nor was this knowledge restricted to the female reproductive organs. Among the directions on what to look for in observing a patient at *Epid.* VI 8, 7 (5.344.17–346.7)

[43] See Dean-Jones (note 7, 1994), pp. 121–2.
[44] Compare Lloyd (note 4), p. 73: '[The Hippocratic physician] sometimes entrusts to the patient herself or to a female attendant the verification of certain points that are crucial to his understanding of the case, and he relies on their reports on occasions where it would have been possible – and one would have thought desirable – to establish the facts directly for himself.'
[45] Galen, ed. Kuhn, Leipzig, 1824 (repr. Hildesheim, 1965), VIII 425.1f., 433.15ff. and Oribasius XXII 3 (Bussemaker and Daremberg III, 1858, 53ff. at 54.15f.). I learned of this reference from Lloyd (note 4), p. 72, n. 54.
[46] Under this rubric, *pace* Rousselle, we should *not* subsume the account of female orgasm in *Genit.* 4 (7.474.14–476.16). This derives entirely from analogizing the male experience: see Lesley Dean-Jones, 'The Politics of Pleasure: Female Sexual Appetite in the Hippocratic Corpus', *Helios*, 19 (1992), 82–4.

are 'the words which they say', but there are very few examples of the recording of any actual words from patients. I have found four remarks recorded as the actual *logoi* of women patients describing physical symptoms not open to the autopsia of the attending physician:

> *Mul.* II 123 (8.266.14)(compare *Nat. Mul.* 48 (7.392.10)): women say they feel pain in the veins in the nose and under the eyes when the womb turns towards the head.
>
> *Epid.* V, case 63 (5.242.10) (compare *Epid.* VII, case 28 (5.400.4–5)): it seemed to the wife of Polemarchos that something was collecting around her heart.
>
> *Epid.* VI, sec. 4, case 4 (5.306.14): the wife of Agasios seemed to hear cracking in her chest.
>
> *Epid.* VII 11 (5.382.15): the wife of Hermoptolemos claims her heart 'went lame' ('guiousthai') on her.

There are no comparable examples of logoi of male patients describing physical symptoms recorded in the Corpus. There is one after-the-fact report of the nature of pain in *Coac.* I 136 (5.610.19–612.1) when the author states that those who had suffered from lethargic fever, on recovering their senses, reported that they had suffered pains in the neck and a ringing in their ears. Even here the physical symptom is recorded along with a perceptual symptom as a memory of the patient. So in *Epid.* VII, case 45 (5.414.2–5) Mnesianax reports that he feels a heating around his hypochondria, but this is reported in conjunction with his saying that he feels fear and constantly sees sparks before his eyes – again, psychological and perceptual symptoms.

Elsewhere when men's actual words are quoted, as if the author wished to distance himself from the responsibility for vouching for the truth of the report, the symptoms described are psychological. *Epid.* VII 86 and 87 (5.444.13–21) (compare *Epid.* V 81 and 82 (5.250.10–17)) recount the cases of Nicanor and Democles who had come to the doctor together. Nicanor told the doctor he was afraid of the flute if he heard it by night when he was drunk, though he could listen to it during the day with no trouble, and he had suffered from this phobia for a long time. Democles told the doctor that he had for some time been afraid of banks and bridges and could not cross a ditch of any depth, though he could walk along the ditch.

Int. 48 (7.284.19–286.9) (compare *Dieb. Judic.* 3 (9.300.15–26)), reports as fact that a patient suffering from a certain type of disease arising from bile becomes deranged and believes he sees all sorts of beasts and reptiles, and lice crawling on his bed, and imagines himself to be fighting among hoplites. It is only after the description of this that the author says that he knows this is the case because after the patient comes to his senses he tells the doctor that he has been having dreams which correspond to the way he moved his body and the things he was saying in his delirium. At *Epid.* VII 89 (5.446.14) Parmeniscus suffered from suicidal depression and could not talk. Later he said he recognized people who had entered the room while he had been ill.

I recognize that such a small sample is not statistically significant, but the dichotomy of reported actual *logoi* into physical symptoms from women and primarily psychological symptoms from men suggests that the Hippocratics did not feel the same separation from the physical symptoms reported to them by men. Although these derived from *historia*, not *autopsia*, they could be reported as knowledge by doctors because they had the same innate understanding of body, or *suneidesis*, as their male patients, though they did not want to commit themselves to the same *suneidesis* for psychological symptoms; the idea of being terrified by a flute was too far from personal experience.

In the case of women, not all physical symptoms can be assimilated by male *suneidesis* because women have a different type of body of which to be aware. Women of experience or trained women are valuable intermediaries in Graeco-Roman medicine, but their experience does not lie in having gained a better understanding of their own bodies so much as in better understanding of how to relay this knowledge to the male physician. It is not the case that midwives or female doctors would have suffered all the ills that their female patients had. Soranus, *Gyn.* I 4, states:

And it is not absolutely essential for her [a midwife] to have borne children, as some people contend, in order to sympathize with those giving birth through a *suneidesis* of the pains, which [they say] is more characteristic of those who have given birth.[47]

This could be taken to imply that midwives could have a *suneidesis* of labour pains even if they had not given birth themselves. Women, even barren women, were better equipped by the nature of their own body to understand the manifestations of pain and disease in the female body than were men.

This is compatible with early Greek epistemological theories which assume humans can have knowledge about human affairs either through their own experience or through understanding from another's report what such an experience would be like. In Hussey's formulation *historia* could serve as a basis for knowledge as well as *autopsia* when

---

[47] Translation after Owsei Temkin, *Soranus' Gynecology* (Baltimore: Johns Hopkins University Press, 1956), p. 6, from the Greek text in Paul Burguière, Danielle Gourevitch and Yves Malinas (eds.), *Soranos d'Ephèse: Maladies des Femmes I* (Paris: Les Belles Lettres, 1988), p. 7.

'Whatever falls within the range of direct personal experience is in principle knowable by anyone who might experience it ... The necessary conditions for knowledge include not merely justified true belief, but verifiability by means of the appeal to personal or collective experience.' The Hippocratics could not fully understand female diseases because they did not share in the collective experience of the female body. For the ancient Greeks there was a cognitive break in the understanding of body which made the testimony of women indispensable to the scholarly medical tradition.

[48]   Hussey (note 9), p. 16. Compare *VM* and *Nat. Hom.*

ABBREVIATIONS

Aër.	*Airs, Waters, Places*
Carn.	*On Fleshes*
Coac.	*Coan Prognoses*
de Arte	*On the Art*
Decent.	*Decorum*
Dieb. Judic.	*Critical Days*
Epid.	*Epidemics*
Fract.	*Fractures*
Genit.	*On Generating Seed*
Gyn.	*Gynaecology*
HA	*History of Animals*
Insomn.	*On Dreams*
Int.	*Internal Affections*
Jusj.	*Oath*
Loc. Hom.	*Places in Man*
Medic.	*The Physician*
Morb.	*On Diseases*
Morb. Sacr.	*On the Sacred Disease*
Mul.	*On Diseases of Women*
Nat. Fac.	*On the Natural Faculties*
Nat. Hom.	*On the Nature of Man*
Nat. Mul.	*On the Nature of Women*
Nat. Puer.	*On the Nature of the Child*
Praec.	*Precepts*
Prog.	*On Prognosis*
Septim.	*On the Seven-month Child*
Steril.	*On Sterile Women*
VM	*On Ancient Medicine*

Citations are usually made to the chapter in a work, though occasionally it is also necessary to cite a book number and sometimes a section reference. Figures in parentheses after citations of Hippocratic works refer to volume, page and line number in the edition of Emile Littré, *Œuvres complètes d'Hippocrate*, 10 vols. (Paris, 1839–61) (reprint Amsterdam: A.M. Hakkert, 1961). Unattributed translations are my own.

4   The growth of medical empiricism

Robert James Hankinson

Over the past few years, historians of Greek philosophy have become increasingly aware of the importance of the Greek medical tradition for the understanding of ancient philosophy. Of course, the voluminous medical literature of late antiquity, from Galen on, has long been recognized as invaluable as a second-hand source of information regarding the doctrines of philosophers, most notably those from the early Stoa, which have otherwise perished in the wreckage of history. But more recently scholars have turned to the medical writings as sources for philosophy in their own right. They have come to see the great epistemological debates that formed the core of Hellenistic philosophy as being prosecuted just as vigorously in the medical schools as in the groves of Academe. That debate is the principal focus of this paper: but it is worth first briefly sketching the long history of Greek philosophical medicine.

Among the earliest Presocratics, Alcmaeon of Croton (*fl. c.* 575 BC) was a man of both medical and philosophical interests, giving an account of the physiology of perception, and of concept-formation. A century later, Empedocles combined a reputation for abstract physical speculation with a certain *réclame* as a medical man, and he too was interested in cognition and perception. Equally, several early Hippocratic texts deal with philosophical questions concerning the nature of knowledge and explanation. Later doctors of importance to the development of philosophical methodology include Herophilus and Erasistratus (*fl. c.* 260 BC), Asclepiades of Bithynia (*fl. c.* 120 BC), and Galen.

But perhaps the strongest and most durable connections are those which developed between Empiricist medical epistemology and

For a list of bibliographical abbreviations, please see the end of this chapter.

Scepticism.[1] Sextus Empiricus, our chief surviving source of Greek Scepticism, was himself a doctor and his very name attests to the depth of the interconnection I have described. It is no accident that Sextus paints the Sceptical programme as being essentially therapeutic in nature.

Empiricism and explanation

I shall begin the detailed history, however, with a fragment of the Sicilian doctor Diocles of Carystus:

(i) those who think that one should state a cause in every case do not appear to understand first that it is not always necessary to do so from a practical point of view, and second that many things which exist are somehow by their nature akin to principles, so that they cannot be given a causal account. (ii) Furthermore, they sometimes err in assuming what is unknown, disputed, and implausible, thinking that they have adequately given the cause. (iii) You should disregard people who aetiologize in this manner, and who think that one should state a cause for everything. (iv) You should rather rely upon things which have been excogitated over a long period on the basis of experience (*empeiria*), (v) and you should seek a cause for contingent things when that is likely to make what you say about them more understandable and more believable.[2]

Diocles (*fl. c.* 325 BC) was a rough contemporary of Aristotle's. And our text clearly betrays Aristotle's influence. In the opening chapters of his *Posterior Analytics*, Aristotle stresses that first principles, the *archai* or axioms of a science, cannot be proved or demonstrated, and hence cannot be given an explanation (*Post. An.*, 1, 2, 71b26ff.; 3, 72b19ff.). These truths are simply fundamental, and (in some sense at least) self-evident. For explanation has got to terminate somewhere in prior and

---

[1] I should stress that I use the term 'epistemology' in its original, and standard philosophical, meaning of 'theory of knowledge', and not as it is apparently employed in the social sciences to mean 'belief-system': confusion between these two quite distinct significations was a recurrent source of inter-disciplinary deafness at the workshop, and is I imagine to be held accountable for the first question I was asked after presenting this study, namely 'what has your paper got to do with the themes of the conference?' This flabbergasted me at the time, since my understanding was that the workshop was about medicine and epistemology, and that was, as far as I could see at least, the subject of my contribution. I should also note that this is a much-reduced version of my original paper: owing to exigencies of space I have had to sacrifice much of the scholarly backing for my case originally found in these footnotes.

By 'Scepticism', with initial capital, I mean the developed sceptical philosophies of the Middle and New Academies and of the Pyrrhonists, while I shall continue to use the lower-case 's' to designate anyone predisposed against credulity and gullibility, particularly in matters of scientific explanation. Similarly, I shall use the capitalized 'Empiricism' to designate members of the medical *hairesis* or school of that name while initial lower-case 'empiricism' is the methodological handmaiden of science.

[2] Diocles, in Galen, *On the Powers of Foodstuffs*, VI, 455–6.

unexplainable premisses in order to avoid both infinite regress and circularity (*Post. An.*, 1, 3).

Aristotle has isolated one of the basic problems of scientific epistemology. If science is a matter of explanation, and if one explains propositions by pointing to the more basic truths on which they rest, what are we to say about those more basic propositions themselves? Either they are themselves explained on the basis of yet more fundamental propositions or they are not. If they are, then the same question re-surfaces one level further down; if they are not, then they seem to be mere assumptions, whose groundlessness is transmitted to every proposition which derives from them. And in the former case, the procedure is either without end (in which case it can have no explanatory power), or it terminates in some assumption (in which case the latter considerations apply at that level), or it leads ultimately back to the proposition first considered (in which case the procedure is circular, whose structure can serve to ground none of its components).

Aristotle's solution to this difficulty is, in essence, to deny that the basic axioms need have the status purely of assumptions – he holds that they can be known to be true without their having to be derived from any other propositions: such is the kernel of any foundationalist epistemology.

Diocles knew that Aristotelian discussion, although precisely how is unclear. But he is not concerned with the resolution of theoretical difficulties in the concept of explanation. Rather he holds it to be of no *practical* use to try to aetiologize absolutely everything. (In this regard he is heir to an empirical tradition stretching back to the celebrated Hippocratic treatise *On Ancient Medicine*). Metaphysics aside, for ordinary, everyday, medical purposes explanation must stop somewhere. He is out to sketch a practical epistemology for medicine – some things must be *accepted* as being fundamental in order to articulate the science, even though they may not in fact be so. They fulfil the same *function* as the axioms of geometry, for instance, in providing a starting-point for inference – but that may be no more than a matter of mere convenience.

Diocles' second sentence makes a point more familiar (to students of philosophy at least) as the Fourth Mode of Agrippa (see Sextus, *PH*, 173), the Mode of Hypothesis, although it is implicit in Aristotle's discussions of *petitio principii*. Even so Diocles may have been the first person to make it explicit. Sentence (iv) invokes the type of empiricism which first surfaces in *On Ancient Medicine*: the scientist should be wary of grand rational construction with no empirical content, and should deal rather in experientially derived propositions. Diocles does not say just what the conditions on the adequacy of such empirical claims might be. His position is at best a sketch of a methodology. Finally, (v) gestures towards the even stronger contention that aetiology is often only of rhetorical use. If someone asks you for an explanation, you may invent one to please them – but whether or not it is true is a matter of total practical indifference.

In sum, then, Diocles' 'great fragment on method' suggests, although it does not elaborate upon, the rudiments of thorough-going empiricism, one that certainly goes further than Aristotle's. For while Aristotle thought that explanations were always in principle possible (except obviously for the basic *explanantia*, which may even so be securely known), and indeed practically available to the scientist willing and able to invest the requisite time and trouble in their discovery, Diocles is not ready to allow even that such explanantia must exist, much less that they are recoverable to the human intellect. Explanation is a luxury, an added condiment which may titillate the intellectual palate, but which contributes nothing to scientific nourishment.

Diocles is no true Sceptic. He is not even technically an Empiricist in the sense of affiliation with the Empiricist *hairesis*, or 'school', for the excellent reason that in his time there was no such school. But he clearly adumbrates the characteristic Empirical attitude towards causal theorizing of caution and circumspection.

The Alexandrians

Both of the great third-century BC Alexandrians, Herophilus and Erasistratus, contributed sceptical arguments to the discussion of causation.

Erasistratus was concerned in his causal theorizing solely with combatting a particular view of the pathology of fevers – he had no desire at all to undercut the entire business of causal ascription, although he refused to allow antecedent causes the title 'causes', on the grounds that they were not invariably followed by their effects, and in this he seems to have been responsible for a pattern of argument taken over and deployed by later Sceptics.[3]

Herophilus, by contrast, appears to have had a general programme in epistemology, one characterized by circumspection. Particularly striking is his tentative attitude towards the business of causal theorizing, summarized in two fragments. 'Whether or not there is a cause is by

---

[3]   Antecedent causes were defined in the medical and scientific tradition not merely as causes which preceded their effects, but which were also at most necessary (and not sufficient) conditions of those effects, and which were not necessarily still operative at the time the effects occurred: *PH*, 3, 16.

nature undiscoverable; but in my opinion I believe I am chilled, warmed and filled with food and drink' (Herophilus, in Galen, *CP*, xvi, 198). 'Some, such as Herophilus, accept causes "on the basis of a hypothesis"' (Galen, ibid., xii, 162). The most plausible reading of these controversial fragments has Herophilus adopt causal explanations not because they are certain, or even probable, but simply because they offer the most perspicuous and rationally satisfying reconstruction of the physical world; as such they function as heuristic devices. Herophilus' attitude to causal explanation is thus similar to Diocles' towards first principles. Let us consider one further, equally controversial, fragment. 'Let the *phainomena* be said [to be] first (*prōta*), even if they are not first.'[4]

Herophilus offers here a methodological injunction (possibly influenced by Aristotle's well-known distinction between the things which are primary or more intelligible to us and those which are primary or more intelligible in themselves)[5] to the effect that even if the fundamental constituents of reality are *adēla*, hidden, non-phenomenal things, none the less all we have to go on epistemologically are the appearances. There may, for all we know, be actual deep facts of the matter, facts that are *adēlon* at least to perception; but they must at best be inferred entities – and any such inferences will only be as secure as the phenomenal evidence upon which they are based.

Herophilus thus advocates as a *modus operandi* a certain procedure which he is quite happy to admit may not capture the way things really are. The limitations of our epistemological resources dictate such modesty – and the demands of a practical medicine may require no more. Thus we may discern in Diocles and Herophilus the outline of a methodologically sophisticated empiricism, one whose roots can be traced at least to Hippocratic treatises such as *On Ancient Medicine*, but which has become, as a result of the absorption of Aristotelian philosophy of science, far more than a simple, practical recommendation. Here are the real beginnings of a genuine empiricism in science.

The Empiricists

Herophilus was not, for all that, an Empiricist in the technical sense. One of his pupils, Serapion (*fl. c.* 225 BC), is generally credited with being the founder of the school known as the Empiricists.

As I have emphasized, empiricism in medical practice can be

---

[4]   Herophilus, in Anonymus Londinensis, *Iatrica Menonia*, 21.22.
[5]   For this distinction see *Post. An.*, 1, 2, 71b33ff.; *Top.*, 64; *Nic. Eth.*, 1, 4, 1095b2–4.

discerned at least as early as *On Ancient Medicine*, even in Alcmaeon of Croton. But it is with the development of the Empiricist school proper that these tendencies become entrenched in a coherent scientific epistemology, an epistemology which may reasonably be called sceptical. It is no accident that several of the individuals recorded by Diogenes in his list of Sceptical philosophers (*DL*, 9, 115–16) are known to have been Empiricist doctors (Menodotus of Nicomedia, Theodas of Laodicea, Sextus himself, Saturninus), while in several other cases identification is probable.

Empiricism was no codified orthodoxy, however. There is evidence of lively debate within the school concerning the legitimacy, scope, and applicability of certain methodological principles. These debates centred in particular on the admissibility or otherwise of a particular type of analogical reasoning, which Empiricists called 'transition to the similar' ('hē tou homoiou metabasis'). Transition was a means by which all but the most hard-line Empiricist doctors sought to extend the range of their empirically acquired knowledge, and we shall briefly examine its structure a little later on.

The most striking feature of the Empiricists' position, however, was their consistent refusal to let their theorizing take them beyond the realm of immediate experience and into the arcana of things by nature obscure, the 'hidden things' or adēla of later Greek epistemology. That is, to invoke the terminology of the parallel debates among the philosophical schools, they refuse to countenance indicative sign-inference. However, congruently with what Sextus at least presents as the official position of the Pyrrhonist Sceptics, they are perfectly happy to allow the type of sign Sextus at least calls 'commemorative', or recollective (*hupomnēstikon*).

The nature of the sign

Of matters, then, according to the Dogmatists,[6] some are (a) pre-evident (*prodēlon*), some (b) non-evident (adēlon); and of the non-evident, some are (i) totally (*kathapax*) non-evident, some (ii) temporarily (*pros kairon*) non-evident, and some (iii) naturally (*phusei*) non-evident. Pre-evident are those which come to our knowledge from themselves, e.g., that it is day; totally non-evident are those which are not of a nature to fall under our knowledge, such as that the number of the stars is even; temporarily non-evident are those which, although

---

[6] To be a Dogmatist, in this sceptical sense, is simply to espouse and embrace any theoretical commitment. The term is connected with, although not identical to, its cousin in the medical debates: there 'Dogmatist' (or the equivalent 'Rationalist') is a general term covering all of the non-sceptical schools of medical theorizing – those, that is, who believe in the possibility of causal aetiologizing.

they possess an evident nature, are now not evident to us because of certain external circumstances, as the city of Athens is to me now; while the naturally non-evident are those which do not possess a nature such as to fall under our evidentness, such as the theoretical pores. (Sextus, *PH*, 2, 97–8)

That is one of the three passages in which Sextus discusses the four epistemological categories into which, according to the 'Dogmatists' (in this case principally the Stoics), things may fall: things 'pre-evident' – (a), i.e., immediately evident without recourse to inference – on the one hand, and three sub-divisions of things non-evident – (b), adēlon – on the other. Signs fall into two classes:

the pre-evidents do not, they say, need a sign, since they are apprehended of themselves. Nor too do the totally non-evident, since they are at bottom inapprehensible. But things which are either temporarily or naturally non-evident are apprehended by means of signs, not of course the same ones, but the temporarily non-evident by way of commemorative signs and the naturally non-evident by way of indicative signs. (ibid., 99)

The members of class (a) are apprehensible without the mediation of signs; class (bi) is beyond all knowing; but the elements of (bii) may be apprehended by way of commemorative signs, and (biii) via indicative signs. Or so the Dogmatists affirm. Commemorative sign-inferences take us from one evident object to another object which is temporarily obscure, but which can be made evident. To use the standard ancient example, I see some smoke; I cannot yet see any fire, but knowing that there's no smoke without fire, I infer that there's fire down there somewhere. And of course I can check in any particular case whether that inference is accurate.

An indicative sign, on the other hand, 'is an antecedent proposition in a sound conditional, which is revelatory of the consequent' (*PH*, 2, 101). An indicative sign, in this originally Stoic definition, brings to light a hidden fact, one which could not have been discovered by observation alone. Hence the fact of sweating is an indicative sign of the existence of invisible pores in the skin: the pores themselves are not open to perceptual inspection, but we can know that they must exist in order for sweating to occur.[7] Sextus goes on,

there being, as we have said, two different types of signs, we do not argue against all types, but only against the indicative sign, as it seems to have been elaborated by the Dogmatists. For the commemorative sign is relied upon in ordinary life (*bios*), since when someone sees smoke fire is signified, and when he observes a scar he says that a wound has occurred. (*PH*, 2, 102)

[7] Unsurprisingly, the Sceptics fastened on to this claim to be able to infer with deductive security from phenomenal to non-phenomenal matters: e.g. *PH*, 1, 180–5.

The Pyrrhonian Sceptic, as Sextus repeatedly emphasizes, has no quarrel with the ordinary beliefs of ordinary life: he takes issue only with the pretensions of the Dogmatists.

A commemorative sign, then, is always capable of being confirmed or disconfirmed. The consequent in the sign-conditional is *temporarily* non-evident – if it weren't there would be no point in formulating it in the first place. But it is not something *in principle* beyond direct empirical verification. Nor is any genuine inference involved at all. The model is not that of noting that n instances of K have been F, and inferring inductively that the next K one comes across will be F; rather that past (observed) instances of K's have been F is a simple fact, but one which psychologically predisposes us to expect the next K to be F. The procedure involves no justification – it is simply noted as a fact of human psychological life. In the invocation both of constant conjunction and of psychological compulsion, the Sceptics anticipate Hume's celebrated account of causation.[8]

Sextus is reporting a debate among philosophers. But the lineaments of that debate are closely paralleled in those of the medical schools, and it is in fact plausible to imagine that they got their start there. Let us turn again to Empiricist methodology.

The Empiricist account of medical science

Our principal source for Empiricist doctrine is Galen, in particular the three short texts usefully translated by Frede and Walter in 1985.[9] They are his brief account of the differences between the major, rival, medical schools for beginning students, *On Sects*; his *Outline of Empiricism*; and a very early work, *On Medical Experience*. Crudely, the Empiricist account of scientific discovery goes as follows. We observe that affections (*pathē*) arise in people, sometimes with no obvious cause (as in some cases of epistaxis), sometimes with some evident occasion (as when falls or wounds cause bleeding). Moreover, we can also observe that in some cases further interventions produce (or are at the very least followed by) beneficial (or harmful) results. On occasion we are naturally driven, by a species of psychological compulsion, to test out some remedy. Sometimes it occurs by chance, and sometimes we simply try anything at random, improvisationally, in the hope that it may happen to be efficacious. When we have observed something beneficial to occur

8 David Hume, *Enquiry Concerning Human Understanding*, VII, II.
9 Galen, *Three Treatises on the Nature of Science*, trans. R. Walter and M. Frede (Indianapolis: Hackett, 1985).

following one or other of these types of reaction, we may test it out again when similar circumstances arise:

an imitative experience is one where something which has proved to be beneficial ... is tried out again for the same complaint. It is this kind of experience which has contributed most to the art: for when they have imitated, not two or three but very many times, what has turned out to be beneficial on earlier occasions, and when they then find out that, for the most part, it has the same effect in the case of the same diseases, then they call such a recollection a theorem. (Galen, *On Sects*, 2)

The Empiricist builds a collection of instances in which certain things are seen to follow upon certain others, which he calls an 'experience', or *empeiria* – and if the collection comes to contain enough members, it is sufficient to ground a general rule, or theorem. Indeed, the relations that hold between the items in such theorems need not be universal and positive; the Empiricists developed a five-fold typology of connection and disjunction according to whether things were seen to go together always, for the most part, half the time, rarely, or never (*Outline*, 2, 6). These categories stand in determinate logical relations (e.g., for the most part *p* if and only if rarely not-*p*); and all of these types of relations are valuable in commending some therapies as appropriate, and rejecting others as useless.

Thus personal experience, or *autopsia*, forms the basis of the Empiricist doctor's *empeiria*, but it was not the only available route to empirical knowledge. One could in addition take notice of the reports of others, *historia*, in arriving at a determination of therapy. The Empiricists were not, however, uncritical in their treatment of second-hand knowledge: they fashioned a detailed and sophisticated methodology for assessing the relative values of different items of historia, dependent on, among other things, the demonstrated reliability of the source on previous occasions, and its agreement with other, already tested sources.

Thus the Empiricists quite self-consciously apply Empiricist epistemological standards to the assessment of the reliability of their own *confrères* (*Outline*, 8), and they are very careful not to be trapped into any Dogmatic claims regarding the intrinsic likelihood or otherwise of any particular report. They do not hold, for instance, that widespread agreement among authorities is some kind of natural (indicative) sign that what those authorities say is deeply, metaphysically true. Rather, they treat it as commemorative: in the past, where such agreement has been found, the results of acting in accordance with it have tended to be beneficial – hence we are driven to expect that they may be so in this case (*Outline*, 8).

The important feature in all of this is that no claim of any kind is made about any alleged underlying features or dispositions of the patients in virtue of which these empirically derived cures are efficacious. The Empiricist simply bypasses such causal theorizing as being intrinsically undeterminable and in any case of no importance in therapy. Hence all the epistemological work is done for the Empiricists at the level of the phainomena, the appearances, and the concatenations upon which their therapeutics are based are all perfectly evident sequences of repeated, observable events. They describe 'experience' ('empeiria'), i.e., the understanding that such connections have indeed held, as 'the memory of what one has seen to happen often and in the same way' (*Outline*). All an Empiricist doctor needs is to be able to remember the way things have turned out in the past.

The Dogmatist attack upon Empiricism

However, at this point the Empiricists lay themselves open to attack from the Dogmatists. First of all, their method of building up an experience explicitly relies upon their being able to discern the similarities that unite different cases. But, as Galen has his Dogmatist point out in *Med. Exp.* (which is written as a dialogue, in which a Dogmatist attacks, and an Empiricist duly defends, Empirical medicine), every case is different from every other in some manner (indeed each is in some ways unique and *sui generis*), while cases which are specifically different and unrelated will nonetheless resemble one another in some, albeit taxonomically irrelevant, features. 'Is it your opinion, then', Galen's Dogmatist asks (after pointing out that reason tells us, in the case of triangularity, that there are only three basic types of triangle, and that this cannot simply be a matter of experience),

> that only in the subject with which physicians are concerned the memory has simply to deal with simple and isolated things, and that there are no combinations and varieties in it? If you do affirm this, we would say: what is more manifold, more complicated, and more varied than disease? In any case, how does one discover that a disease is the same as another disease in all its characteristics? Is it by the number of symptoms or by their strength and power? For if a thing be itself, then, in my opinion, it must be itself in all these characteristics, for if even one of them is lacking it is perverted and ceases to be itself, since it no longer possesses the quality lacking. (Galen, *Med. Exp.*, 3–4, 89)

Galen's Dogmatist reproduces in large part the anti-Empiricist views of Asclepiades of Bithynia; the Empiricist counterblast is probably derived from the second-century AD physician Menodotus. How, in the absence of theory, are we supposed to determine what are the salient features in virtue of which the basic items related by Empiricist theories may be declared to be relevantly similar (*Med. Exp.*, 3–6)? Every instance is in some way different from every other – any taxonomy relies on some theory of *relevant* similarity. Even if this can be bypassed, how can the Empiricist make reliable use of historia? 'How can a person determine whether what he sees at this moment is identical with that which someone else has seen before or is something quite different, unless he himself has seen both?' (ibid., 4). Again, how can the Empiricist know, in default of any theory of causal relevance, which antecedent factors are pertinent to the individuation of the disease and which are not? He cannot simply enumerate them all – but he has no criterion for selection among them either (ibid., 6).

Furthermore, even supposing that the Empiricist can provide an account of relevant similarity which will justify him in saying that he has indeed observed the same thing many times, and even allowing that his experience can be supplemented by that of others, how many times is many? Galen's Dogmatist deploys a soritical argument designed to undermine the coherence of the Empiricist's fundamental concept of an experience. One observation is not enough to constitute an empeiria – but if one is not, two cannot be, and if two are not, three cannot be, and so on 'until I reach a very high number' (*Med. Exp.*, 7). If one observation on its own cannot constitute an experience, then the addition of one to an already existing set cannot do so either.

The Empiricist has a number of replies to these objections, but the most important and radical follow similar lines in each case. In the case of similarity, the Empiricist urges, he has no *need* of any criterion. He is not making any Dogmatic claims concerning the basis of such similarities, or about the real nature of fundamental likeness. Rather, he simply acts on the basis of what *seem to him* to be similarities – an ailment observed today will strike him as being like one he saw last week – and he may well be able to say why and in what respect it does so. But that is all there is to it. He has no theory of relevant similarity; but, since he does not seek to *justify* his practice (except in purely pragmatic terms – i.e., it works), he does not need one. Similarly in the case of the sorites (*Med. Exp.*, 16–18), an Empiricist will not say how many times makes many; there is, in any case, no single answer to that question. It will vary from individual to individual, from case to case, since it is, at bottom, a matter not of logic but of individual psychology. The procedure of building up experience is not an inferential one – it just turns out that, after observing a certain number of particular experiences, the Empiricist comes to see that they exhibit a general pattern. Of course, such a pattern might prove to be misleading and chimerical (if it does it will be abandoned or modified in the light of experience): but past experience suggests that, at least in general, it will not do so. But, ironically, past experience does not *license* belief for the Empiricist – it simply conditions it.

Transition to the similar

Next I want briefly to consider the Empiricists' account of the procedure of 'transition to the similar'. This was not conceived by its practitioners as being in itself a means of generating knowledge, but rather as a useful and empirically tested way of throwing up new testable hypotheses. 'Transition' involves seeing that a particular case is, if not genuinely a recurrence of some previously observed type, then at least similar to it in ways which might be relevant. Suppose you have a dislocated knee – I have never seen one before, nor do I have any historia to go on. However, I have successfully re-set luxations of the elbow. I will reason as follows: 'knees are rather like elbows – hence the elbow-treatment might work for knees'. I then proceed to try it out – and if it works, I have a new medical experience (or am at least on the way to having one).

Moreover, transition can be employed on other items in the theorems – I might decide that some drug is pretty similar to one I have successfully used in the past in such cases, but cannot at present obtain (Galen, *On Sects*, 2). Indeed,

in the case of transference of one remedy from one ailment to another similar to it one has a greater or smaller basis for expectation of success in proportion to the increase or decrease in similarity of the ailment, whether or not historia is involved. And the same goes for the transference from one part of the body to another. (Galen, *Outline*, 9)

Transition is the better founded the greater the number of similarities between the tested and the contemplated cases: but to say that is not to make any metaphysical assumptions about the regularity of the universe of the type that fatally compromised the notion of induction for Hume.[10] It is simply a report of how things have turned out, and as such (in regard to its future projection) is merely provisional. The Empiricist should not be greatly surprised in any particular case if the results are disappointing, precisely because, unlike the Dogmatist, he will not think that he has uncovered the secret and hidden key as to why things behave the way they do. Indeed, as Michael Frede notes, the subjective epistemic terminology employed is suggestive – Empiricists will have

[10] Hume (note 8), VI, II.

hopes, expectations, intentional states of that kind with respect to future outcomes, but no great confidence, and no rash complacency.[11]

The Empiricists go out of their way to distinguish their practice from the superficially similar method of the Dogmatists.

> Logical [i.e., Dogmatic] transition based on the nature of things lays hold of knowledge by means of indication (*endeixis*).[12] But the Empirical variety relies on what is discovered by experience, not because it is persuasive or plausible that the similar should be productive of something similar, or require similar things, or undergo similar things; it is not on the basis of this, or anything else of this sort, that they think it justifiable to make the transition, but on the basis of the fact that they have discovered by experience that things behave this way. (Galen, *Outline*, 9)

That is, the empirical success of the past applications of transition itself provides the justification, via a meta-application of transition, for the application of the procedure to new cases; but not because it is, in any sense, rationally compelling.

Thus the Empiricist, armed with this not inconsiderable arsenal of weapons, can set about the business of building up a body of medical lore. However, it is apparent that not all Empiricists were in agreement about the status or the acceptability of the transitional procedure. Furthermore, there was a dispute as to whether the Empirical method made use of any genuine type of inference or not – and it is to these issues that I now turn.

Signs, inference, and the scope of Empiricism

It is clear that, depending on how many different types of item one is prepared to allow as being fit subjects for it, transitional inference can be a weapon of considerable epistemological power. But it is also easy to see that the more extensively it is used, the more it might seem to compromise the purity of the Empiricist method. Both the acceptability and the proper representation of the role of transition were matters of dispute among the Empiricist doctors themselves.

> The question has been raised whether Serapion also believes that transition to the similar is a third constitutive part of medicine as a whole. Menodotus thought that it was not, but that the Empiricist merely makes use of transition to the similar – and it is not the same thing to make use of something as to treat it as a part. Cassius the Pyrrhonean, furthermore, tried to show that the Empiricist

---

[11]   Michael Frede, 'An Empiricist View of Knowledge: Memorism', in Stephen Everson (ed.), *Epistemology* (Cambridge: Cambridge University Press, 1990), pp. 225–50, p. 246.

[12]   I.e., indicative sign-inference.

does not even make use of transition of this sort; indeed he has written an entire book on the subject. Theodas did better when he held that transition to the similar constituted reasonable experience. Yet others, though, have claimed that transition to the similar is more like an instrument. (Galen, *Outline*, 4)

It is clear that there was a lively and multi-faceted dispute about the nature, status, and role of transition. Presumably the point of the difference as to whether transition was actually a proper part of Empirical medicine, or whether Empiricists simply employed it, turns precisely on the degree if any of warranted confidence one may have in the outcome of any particular application of the method, and in its general effectiveness. The more genuinely sceptical an Empirical doctor is the less he will be prone to allow that transition has an official part in the practice of Empiricist medicine – although, in a purely descriptive sense and without commitment to it, he may recognize himself using it.

Cassius was described by the first-century AD medical encyclopaedist Celsus as 'the greatest doctor of our times' (Celsus, *On Medicine*, Pr. 69); and he is presumably the 'Cassius the sceptic', mentioned by Diogenes (*DL*, 7, 32). His even tougher epistemological line, the rejection of transition in any form, no doubt represents an attempt to purify Empirical practice from what he took to be unwarranted and unjustifiable Dogmatic accretions. And presumably this took the form of rejecting anything that seemed to involve reasoning and inference. For these tough-minded Empiricists, Empirical practice simply was that – practice. Any admission of inferential procedures at all would tend to blur the sharpness of the divide between themselves and the Dogmatists, and to undermine the coherence of their fundamental attack on theoretical reasoning.

Thus some Empiricists tried heroically (if rather hopelessly) to attribute the discovery of complex drugs to pure chance, unmediated by theory of any kind (Galen, *MM*, X, 163). Similarly, while Galen admits that Empiricists may become good doctors (*On Sects*, 4), he refuses to allow that complex remedies, or technical instruments such as the cupping-glass, could have been discovered by mere luck or improvisation (*Loc. Aff.*, VIII).

The pressing questions then become: (1) what was the nature of this hardline Empiricism? And (2) what could revisionist Empiricists do in order to make clear the difference between themselves and the Dogmatists? First of all, it is important to get clear what reason involves for the ancients. It appears that at least since Aristotle (and really since Plato), ancient theorists tended to conceive of reason as a power or faculty in the soul which allowed one to go beyond the immediate data of experience in order to formulate general, universal principles. Such, for all its obscurity of detail, seems true of Aristotle's account of the role of *nous*, or intuition, in *Post. An.* (2, 19). Now, at this juncture it is obvious where sceptical objections can get a grip – the inevitable gap between experience and rationally derived 'knowledge' can never be conclusively and uncontroversially bridged.

Here the Empiricists avail themselves of the standard Sceptical appeal to the existence of an irresolvable dispute among the Dogmatists (Galen, *On Sects*, 5), since it is a sign of 'the non-apprehensibility of things'. Furthermore, the Empiricists attack the notion of proof of the Dogmatists, who

> do not grant that there is such a thing as indication (endeixis) or that one thing can be known on the basis of something else, for one has to know everything on the basis of itself. Nor do they allow that there is such a thing as a sign of something which by its very nature is non-evident. Furthermore they argue that no art (*technē*) has any need of logic ... Then they talk about the fallacious modes of proof which the Dogmatists are accustomed to use and in particular about the class of analogisms ... Epilogism, on the other hand, which they describe as reasoning solely in terms of what is apparent, is of use in the discovery of things which are temporarily non-evident. For this is how they themselves call things which are by genus perceptible but which have not yet become apparent. (Galen, *On Sects*, 5)

Analogism (*analogismos*) is the Empiricists' term for indicative sign-inference, while epilogism is equivalent to the commemorative sign. Indication (endeixis) is the procedure whereby the Rationalist doctors sought to derive therapeutic information on the basis of a theory of pathology. What the Empiricists reject, on this account, is that collections of evident phenomena can ever justify an inference to some hidden condition: and they do so for familiar reasons. If such inferences were logically watertight, then there should be no disagreement about them. But disputes among the doctors were invoked by Sceptics as a classical example of the fragility of sign inference:

> in the case of fever patients, flushing and prominence of the vessels and a moist skin and increased temperature and quickening of the pulse and all the other signs of the same thing ... nor do they appear alike to all; but to Herophilus, for example, they seem to be definite signs of good blood, to Erasistratus of the transference of the blood from the veins to the arteries, and to Asclepiades of the lodgement of theoretical particles in the theoretical interstices. (Sextus, *M*, 8, 219–20)

That example is used to justify the claim that there is no such thing as a universally accepted indicative sign. It derives originally from the Empiricists' attacks on the Dogmatists' theoretical structures.

Disputes of this sort cannot be settled, since there is no independent
arbiter to be appealed to. Indeed, the Empiricists affirm that

inapprehensibility (*akatalēpsia*) is the cause of the undecidable dispute (*diaphōnia
anepikritos*), while the dispute is in turn a sign of the inapprehensibility. And they
note that it is the dispute concerning non-evident matters which cannot be
decided, not the dispute concerning evident matters. For in the latter case
everything, once it is apparent what it is like, confirms those who are right and
refutes those who are wrong. (Galen, *On Sects*, 5)

These passages no doubt reflect the state of the debate in Galen's time
or a little earlier: i.e., Empiricism as it was practised by the likes of
Menodotus and Theodas. There is no indication here of the genuine
hard line. These Empiricists will embrace a type of reasoning – but it is
of such a kind as to be testable at the tribunal of experience, unlike any
form of indicative sign-inference, the soundness of which will remain,
on their view, for ever obscure.

But surely, it may be objected, the soundness of indicative sign-
inference might be tested by anatomical investigation? No, say the
Empiricists – what we are interested in is how creatures function
internally under normal circumstances; but nobody would hold that an
animal undergoing vivisection is in a normal condition. And we can
never adjust for this non-naturalness of state, since we cannot know (as
we cannot see) what the normally functioning creature looks like on the
inside. Anatomy is thus useless – and vivisection mere pointless cruelty.

Thus we have at least a provisional answer to question (2): reasoning
is all right if it is susceptible of empirical confirmation. The Empiricists
will insist that commemorative sign-inferences are admissible simply
because, unlike those of indicative signs, they are potentially verifiable.

The earliest Empiricists, when called upon to offer a justification for
their position, did so in severely commonsensical terms. Their 'knowledge' consisted simply in their possessing a body of seemingly reliable
general beliefs which were caused by a sequence of perceptions stored in
the memory, and which were then 'accessed' when stimulated by an
appropriately similar condition. Of course, describing it in that way
apparently presupposes a theory of behavioural psychology – but it is
easy to see how that description could be reformulated by the
Empiricists in non-Dogmatic terms, as simply reporting some facts of
their psychological life.

A further feature of that psychological life is that the doctor who
proceeds on memorist lines will often be seen to make the right decision,
in the sense that what he does will be followed by the recovery of the
patient. Can he take the credit for that? Could not the patient simply

have recovered spontaneously? Do we not need a theory of medical aetiology to justify the belief that it was the doctor's intervention that was efficacious and not some completely adventitious factor? Perhaps – but that will cause Empiricists no loss of sleep. They will simply continue to behave on the basis of their (limited) beliefs. If those beliefs start to guide them in the wrong direction, then they will alter them: more readily, indeed, than any Dogmatist, since they have no deeply-rooted commitment to their truth.

As regards any explanation of the persistent, apparent success of some beliefs, there may or may not be a causal story to be told – but at any event the Empiricist does not care if there is. Empiricists may make *use* of commemorative signs, but they will not be committed to any underlying methodology. Hence even at the level of the basic commemorative sign-inference, Empiricists may distinguish between the *endorsement* of a procedure and the mere *employment* of it.

The dispute within the school: the Empiricism of Menodotus

That is a thumb-nail sketch of an ideologically pure Empiricist who rejects all reasoning (or rather rejects it *as* reasoning). But, as we have seen, not all Empiricists were in agreement about the role of reason; and this impression is corroborated by the last chapters of Galen's *Outline of Empiricism*. Thus in chapter 11 Galen discusses 'the language appropriate to an Empiricist', and takes Empiricists from Serapion onwards (he is particularly severe on Menodotus, of whom more in a moment) to task for failing to live up to the ideal of Pyrrho (who was, as philosophical legend had it, a modest and unassuming man of few words) and throwing themselves instead into heated debate and controversy. Such practices are, Galen thinks, inconsistent with the professed ideals of Empiricist life – they should rest content with being judged on the basis of their deeds alone. Galen indeed charges Menodotus with inconsistently lapsing into Dogmatism, as well as with abandoning rational argument in favour of mere personal abuse. Apparently Menodotus wrote a book which purported to show that all of Asclepiades' views were false, 'in spite of the fact that on innumerable occasions he has said that one should approach everything non-evident as if it perhaps is, and perhaps is not true' (Galen, *Outline*, 11). That is, Menodotus engaged in a species of negative Dogmatism at the same time as advocating a genuine scepticism.

Galen may be misinterpreting Menodotus' intentions in writing against Asclepiades – Asclepiades had, after all, made a serious attack upon the very foundations of the Empirical method, the substance of which we find reproduced in Galen's *On Medical Experience*. It is conceivable that Menodotus' 'refutation' should be taken purely dialectically, not as professing to demonstrate that Asclepiades' views were as a matter of fact false, but rather that the arguments with which he advocated them were vulnerable. Such a procedure is eminently compatible with, indeed distinctive of, Pyrrhonian Scepticism.

On the other hand, it would be surprising if Sextus Empiricus, who is particularly sensitive to the need to distinguish genuine Scepticism from negative dogmatism,[13] were to fail to see the distinction in another author; yet he writes (and presumably with Menodotus principally in mind) that 'Empiricism positively affirms the non-apprehensibility of the non-evident' (*PH*, 1, 236), in sharp contrast with the official Sceptical attitude, which is to reserve judgement over the question of whether anything non-evident is or is not in principle apprehensible (while of course noting that nothing non-evident seems *to him* to have been apprehended).

However, we also know from Sextus (*PH*, 1, 222) that Menodotus and his followers (along with Aenesidemus) were among those who argued that, properly interpreted, Plato himself was a sceptic. Menodotus' interests clearly ranged well beyond the confines of simple Empiricist practice. It then seems plausible to connect this species of Empiricism with Sextus' claim quoted above, making Menodotus hold that certain things really were non-apprehensible, a view derived ultimately from a sceptical reading of Plato's dialogues, in contrast with what Sextus at least recognizes as the proper Pyrrhonian line. Thus, Sextus saw in the Empiricism of Menodotus and his party an unacceptable streak of negative dogmatism, an impression perhaps confirmed by the quotation on page 75, where akatalēpsia is even alleged to be a cause of something, namely undecidable dispute – a claim which on the face of it goes well beyond merely how things appear.

In any event, the Empiricism of Menodotus was at least on occasion more accommodating than that of the hardliners: 'Menodotus frequently introduces a third thing in addition to perception and memory, which he calls "epilogism"; sometimes, however, he does not posit anything in addition to memory except perception' (Galen, *Outline*, 12). Frede takes this to mean that Menodotus accepted both memoristic and epilogistic accounts into Empiricism, but in different ways: memorism, the 'theory'

[13] It lies at the core of his – controversial – account of the difference between Academic and Pyrrhonian scepticisms: *PH*, 1, 229–35; 'negative dogmatism' in this sense amounts to positively denying the existence of something rather than, as the Pyrrhonist at least officially should, suspending judgement about the question either way.

which eschews all reasoning, was elaborated to show that there is an alternative to the Dogmatists' view of the impossibility of abandoning reasoning altogether; while epilogism simply reports, without endorsing, the actual practice of the Empirical doctor.[14]

That account exhibits the close connection between Empiricism and Pyrrhonism, since the latter too consists of a negative component, in which Dogmatic positions are criticized and alternatives offered, and a 'positive' one, in which the Pyrrhonian way of life is laid out, albeit in 'undogmatic' terms. If this is correct, then Galen's criticisms of Menodotus and other Empiricists for engaging in argument at all are as misguided as the claims of those Dogmatists who alleged that the Pyrrhonian position was self-refuting, since they attempted to use argument to destroy the plausibility of argument itself.[15] An unimpeachably sceptical Menodotus thus emerges from the thickets of misinterpretation.

Thus, both Sceptic and Empiricist will make use of commemorative signs; but they will do so undogmatically, that is with no theoretical backdrop, and no *commitment* to the correctness of the procedure. That does not, however, imply that the dispute between Empirical doctors regarding the role of reason which I outlined earlier is merely chimerical, since some Empiricists did indeed allow, in a quasi-Dogmatic manner, the existence and utility of human powers of reason. But they too would draw the epistemological line at indicative sign-inference.

Causes and the medical sects

We have already alluded to the centrality of the debate concerning the status and the allowability of causal explanation among the doctors. And it is not much of an exaggeration to say that the differences between the three principal Medical tendencies of the Roman Empire, Dogmatist (or Rationalist), Empiricist, and Methodist, are to be located precisely in their different attitudes to cause and explanation.

We have already met Dogmatism (a useful umbrella-term covering a variety of distinct and mutually hostile schools, united by the belief that theoretical knowledge is humanly discoverable, rather than a single orthodoxy) and Empiricism. The Methodist school arose early in the first century AD. It appears to have arisen as a result of the development of Asclepiadean corpuscularian physiology, first by Themison of Laodicea at the end of the first century BC, and then by his pupil Thessalus, a contemporary (and perhaps associate) of Nero, the first

[14]   Frede (note 11), pp. 248–50.
[15]   On these charges, and the Sceptical response to them, see *PH*, 2, 185–8.

genuine Methodist. For our purposes what matters is the Methodists' attitude to medical explanation. They rejected as irrelevant and of no therapeutic importance factors in the patient's causal history,

claiming that the indication (endeixis) as to what is beneficial, derived directly from the affections themselves, is enough for them, and not even these taken as specific particulars, but taking them to be common and universal. Thus they also call these affections which pervade all particulars 'commonalities' ... which they call restriction and relaxation, and they say that each disease is either constricted, relaxed, or a mixture of the two. (Galen, *On Sects*, 6)

There are, thus, two basic pathological conditions, loose and tight: in the first 'the bodily fluids flow too freely' and in the second they do not flow freely enough (there is also a third, mixed condition). Nothing else counts in therapy – and the physician's only task is to recognize the existence of these states, which, on the Methodists' account, he should be able, with a little practice, to manage without difficulty.

Sextus actually takes the Methodists to be closer to the Pyrrhonists than the Empiricists are, since 'the Methodist speaks of "commonality" and "pervade" and the like in a non-committal way. Thus also he uses the term "indication" undogmatically to denote the guidance derived from the apparent affections or symptoms, both natural and unnatural, for the discovery of the apparently appropriate remedies' (*PH*, 1, 240). Moreover, the Methodist is guided, as the Sceptic is, by the 'compulsion of the affections' to seek remedies which are opposite in character to them.

But however one interprets Sextus' endorsement of Methodism over Empiricism, it appears that Methodism does not even appeal to the importance of memory. There is no suggestion that one needs to build up an appreciation of the commonalities on the basis of long experience. Rather, one is simply supposed to be able, in some relatively direct sense, to *see* them. So, to the extent to which Empiricism emphasizes the importance of memory, it is perhaps fair to say, with Sextus, that Methodism involves even less theoretical commitment.

Furthermore, although the Methodists explicitly allow for a kind of indication (as in the above quotations), there appears to be no hint of any endorsement of sign-*inference* of any kind in the official Methodist doctrine. Indeed, 'Thessalus and his sect ... argue thus: "if there were sure and inevitable signs of future events, such as the onset of phrenitis, all who manifested them would necessarily develop phrenitis. But some of those who show these symptoms do not develop phrenitis." '[16] And a little later on in the same passage, 'every sign is understood in relation to

[16]   Caelius Aurelianus, *On Acute Diseases*, 1, 22.

what is signified, since signs belong in the category of relations. But can anything be called a sign if the thing signified is not only not present now, but in some cases never will be?'[17]

The connections between these arguments and the general Pyrrhonist attack on signs are obvious. Yet, the Methodists do have some use for the notion of an indication, even if Sextus is right to say that they do so undogmatically. This, Galen thinks, distinguishes them from the Empiricists:

> nor yet are they Empiricists: for however much they occupy themselves with what is apparent, they are distinguished from the Empiricists by their use of indication (endeixis) . . . And the Empiricists, they say, will have nothing to do with anything non-evident, claiming it is unknowable, while they themselves will have nothing to do with anything non-evident since it is useless. Furthermore, the Empiricists derive observation from the apparent, while they derive indication from it. (Galen, *On Sects*, 6)

The precise force of the claim that Methodists 'derive indication' from the apparent is unclear. But it suggests a level of theoretical commitment on the Methodists' part unshared by their Empiricist cousins. However, they too may simply be pointing to what they take to be a piece of psychological compulsion – it is not that the observed facts make an *inference* to some therapy rationally inescapable: rather they simply *cause* it.

But for our purposes, the most important features of Methodist medicine are its simplicity (it could be learned in six months, Galen notes with disdain: ibid., 6), and its utter disregard for the antecedent history of a complaint. The Empiricists were perfectly happy to make use (in a sense) of antecedent causes (ibid., 7): for example, in a case of rabies, the fact that the patient was bitten by a mad dog will form part of their general *sundromē*, or account of the relevant features of the case (ibid., 18) which will guide their therapy. The Empiricist will note that, in general, cases where the dog in question was mad have differed drastically from those in which it was not; and that as such they require urgently different treatment.

By contrast, Galen alleges, Methodists reject as unimportant the dog's condition, and will treat the bite simply as a wound (ibid., 8). Rationalists, while agreeing with the Empiricists in taking note of the antecedent circumstances, will not rely merely on experience, but will proceed to construct an elaborate theory to explain the connection between the madness of the dog and the ensuing hydrophobia in terms

[17] Ibid., 1, 29.

of how the dog's bite can alter the internal, non-evident, but theoretically discoverable constitution of the patient.

Here it becomes important to defuse an apparent inconsistency in our reports of the Empiricist position. Galen says that Empiricists 'do not hesitate to ask for the so-called antecedent cause' (ibid., 4), and the report of their attitude to rabies cases confirms this. Yet, Galen elsewhere remarks that the Empiricists 'doubt whether there are causes or not' (*CP*, xiii, 162), and a little later on writes that 'even those doctors from the Empirical school, who above all others proclaim things in accordance with common sense, were so overcome by the sophism as to be moved to doubt concerning antecedent causes' (ibid., 170). The 'sophism' is Erasistratus' claim that something which is not invariably correlated with some subsequent event cannot be a cause of it. How are we to reconcile these (and other) differing testimonies?

Quite simply, I suggest, by attending to the *way* in which an Empiricist accepts antecedent causes. He does not do so on the basis of any causal *theory*: he has no developed account of how the dog's bite brings about rabies. Nor, strictly speaking, does he even know *if* it does. Rather he knows that bites of that sort are followed by the onset of hydrophobia. That is simply to observe the existence of an empirical connection in best Humean fashion, and not to invoke some arcane, underlying mechanism that produces the result. By contrast, in addition to allowing the causal and therapeutic relevance of the dog's bite, the Rationalist will attempt to elaborate just such a mechanism. Empiricists and Rationalists do not, then, disagree about the facts (construed as sequences of evident events); they differ over their proper interpretation. And that is how an Empiricist can both accept and reject antecedent causes.

Thus both Methodists and Empiricists lay claim to a type of sceptical epistemology; and the case of Empiricism in particular highlights the issue of how far if at all a consistent sceptic can be allowed to make use of inference.

Conclusion: explanation and ontology

Galen, for all his Rationalism and for all his criticisms of particular Empiricists such as Menodotus and their practices, allows that Empiricists can be perfectly respectable doctors. In fact, he says, competent Empiricists and qualified Rationalists will regularly agree on what the appropriate therapy is in a particular case. Indeed, from his Rationalist perspective, he can account for this convergence of practice:

the same things from which the Dogmatists derive the indication of what is beneficial form the basis of the Empiricist's observation. For the collection of symptoms in the case of the person who has a fever, which they are accustomed to call the 'syndrome', suggests evacuation to a Dogmatist, but to an Empiricist the recollection of his observation ... And in general the Dogmatists and the Empiricists draw on the same medicines for the same affections. What they disagree about is the way these remedies are discovered. For, given the same apparent bodily symptoms, the Dogmatists derive from them an indication of the cause, and on the basis of this cause they find a treatment, whereas the Empiricists are reminded by them of what has happened often in the same way. (Galen, *On Sects*, 4)

The only difference between them is that the Dogmatist is led 'by the nature of the matter', i.e., by indicative sign-inference, while the Empiricist is not; and, evidently, the more the Empiricist is prepared to allow the admissibility of analogical procedures such as transition, the closer the convergence will become.

Furthermore, the Dogmatist thinks that the 'nature of the matter' (i.e., the underlying physical structures of things, along with a theory of their interactions), will explain *why* the therapies work in particular cases. The Empiricist on the other hand will have no such explanatory pretensions: or rather his explanations will be epistemic rather than ontological in form. He will be able to explain why he adopts a certain practice and what gives him his (albeit limited, and intrinsically defeasible) confidence in it; but he will have no views as to the underlying structure of reality, if any, in virtue of which his procedures are effective. Indeed, he has no commitment to any ontology at all – and in this too his position resembles that of a Pyrrhonian Sceptic.

Thus, in a manner which precisely parallels present-day disputes between realists and anti-realists, the protagonists can agree absolutely (at a certain level) about the facts, and yet disagree completely about their interpretation. The realist buys a metaphysically satisfying explanation at the expense of an increasingly implausible epistemology, while the anti-realist, or instrumentalist (to whom the Empiricists can, without great anachronistic strain, be assimilated), has a clear and coherent (because unambitious) epistemology – but has no satisfactory metaphysical underpinning for it.

But the lack of a 'satisfactory' metaphysics here amounts simply to the rejection of the belief that a certain class of things requires explanation at all, or that the attempt to explain them can be remotely fruitful. Galileo revolutionized science by focusing attention on the how of things, and simply abandoning the quest for the why. Newton, following in his footsteps, framed no hypotheses. In a sense the groundwork for such a conceptual breakthrough was laid first by Diocles' and Herophilus' denial that everything needed to be set upon a certain type of firm foundation, and later by the Empiricists' insistence that all that mattered for successful therapy was an instrumental science, free of ontological commitment. The disagreements between medical Empiricists and their Rationalist opponents as to the role and discoverability of explanatory theory were the earliest precursors of what has become the hardiest of perennials in the garden of scientific methodological disputation.

ABBREVIATIONS

CP	Galen, *On Antecedent Causes*
DL	Diogenes Laertius, *Lives of the Philosophers*
Loc. Aff.	Galen, *On the Affected Parts*
M	Sextus Empiricus, *Against the Mathematicians*
Med. Exp.	Galen, *On Medical Experience*
MM	Galen, *On the Therapeutic Method*
Nic.Eth.	Aristotle, *Nicomachean Ethics*
Outline	Galen, *Outline of Empiricism*
PH	Sextus Empiricus, *Outlines of Pyrrhonism*
Post. An.	Aristotle, *Posterior Analytics*
Top.	Aristotle, *Topics*

5 Scholarship and social context: a medical case from the eleventh-century Near East

Lawrence I. Conrad

In Jumādā II 441/November 1049, the Nestorian Christian physician al-Mukhtār ibn Buṭlān (d. after 455/1063) arrived in Cairo from Baghdad. Shortly thereafter, he sent an essay on a scientific topic to ᶜAlī ibn Riḍwān (d. 460/1067–8), chief physician to the Fāṭimid caliph al-Mustanṣir (r. 427–87/1036–94), and invited him to comment. Ibn Riḍwān's response was two withering public critiques full of *ad hominem* invective (only one of these now survives), and quite predictably they provoked an equally abusive reply from Ibn Buṭlān. Ibn Riḍwān then countered with five further missives: a follow-up critique in reference to the issues already raised in the debate, a more general open letter to 'the physicians of old and new Cairo' in which he poured scorn and abuse on his adversary with even greater violence, and three other now-lost essays bearing titles suggesting the continuation of similar diatribes against his adversary.[1] Ibn Buṭlān eventually left Cairo defeated and humiliated, but some time after his departure from Egypt he returned to the fray with a last shot of his own entitled *Waqᶜat al-aṭibbā'* ('Battle of the Physicians').[2] This work too is lost.

This controversy was long remembered in medical and scientific circles, and the ten essays comprising its literary side were evidently in widespread circulation in later times.[3] In 1937, the German orientalists Joseph Schacht and Max Meyerhof published the five extant works as 'a contribution to the history of Greek learning among the

[1] On the lost essays by Ibn Riḍwān, see Ibn Abī Uṣaybiᶜa (d. 668/1270), *ᶜUyūn al-anbā' fī ṭabaqāt al-aṭibbā'*, ed. August Müller, 2 vols. (Cairo: Al-Maṭbaᶜa al-wahbīya, 1299/ 1882 – Königsberg: A. Müller, 1884), vol. 2, pp. 104, 105 = nos. 57, 59, 61, 101 in the Schacht/Meyerhof collection (see note 4 below), pp. 45, 46, 48.

[2] Ibn Abī Uṣaybiᶜa (note 1), vol. 1, pp. 242, 243.

[3] See Carl Brockelmann, *Geschichte der arabischen Literatur*, 2 vols., 3 supplemental vols. (Leiden: E.J. Brill, 1937–49), vol. 1, pp. 483$_5$, 484$_{18}$; vol. S1, pp. 885$_{5-6}$, 886$_{25}$; Manfred Ullmann, *Die Medizin im Islam*, Handbuch der Orientalistik, erste Abteilung, Ergänzungsband IV, erster Abschnitt (Leiden: E.J. Brill), p. 158.

Arabs'.[4] The essays have been widely read ever since; and indeed, among historians of Islamic science and medicine the Ibn Riḍwān/Ibn Buṭlān polemic has become one of the best-known episodes in the field. Informative as the debate may be, however, it is problematic to view it as a medico-philosophical controversy,[5] and even more so to suggest that it contributes to our understanding of Greek learning among the Arabs, or to our knowledge of 'Hellenism' in Baghdad and Cairo in the eleventh century.[6] The real issues involved and the genuine significance of the debate must be sought elsewhere, and it is to these matters that my remarks will be directed.[7]

A different interpretation of this controversy of course emerges if one approaches it from a different perspective, but it must also be said that far more relevant material is available – primarily other works by both protagonists – than has previously been brought to bear on this topic. One of the more interesting of these works is Ibn Buṭlān's *Da°wat al-aṭibbā'* ('The Physicians' Dinner Party'), composed in a monastery outside Constantinople in 450/1058.[8] In this literary *tour de force* a young

4   Joseph Schacht and Max Mayerhof, *The Medico-Philosophical Controversy between Ibn Butlan of Baghdad and Ibn Ridwan of Cairo: a Contribution to the History of Greek Learning among the Arabs*, Egyptian University, Faculty of Arts, Publication no. 13 (Cairo: Egyptian University, 1937).

5   That this formulation was Meyerhof's is indicated by the title of his preliminary study, 'Une controverse médico-philosophique au Caire en 441 de l'Hégire (1050 ap. J.-C.), avec un aperçu sur les études grecques dans l'Islam', *Bulletin de l'Institut d'Egypte*, 19 (1937), 29–43.

6   I.e., as Schacht described the debate. See his 'Über den Hellenismus in Baghdad und Cairo im 11. Jahrhundert', *Zeitschrift der Deutschen Morgenländischen Gesellschaft*, 90 (1936), 526–45. Scholars of late antiquity and Byzantium are now more wary of the term 'Hellenism', and some have suggested that it be abandoned altogether. For a thoughtful overview, see Averil Cameron, 'The Eastern Provinces in the 7th Century AD: Hellenism and the Emergence of Islam', in S. Said (ed.), *Hellēnismos: quelques jalons pour une histoire de l'identité grecque* (Leiden: E.J. Brill, 1991), pp. 287–313.

7   A note of caution must unfortunately be expressed as to the state of our knowledge of the dispute, apart from the fact that only five of the ten essays written during the controversy seem to have survived to modern times. Schacht and Meyerhof published only an abbreviated version of the Arabic texts, leaving out numerous passages – often quite long ones – which they apparently considered of no value, and their English translation reflects these same gaps. This problem is quite serious, since only one complete Ms. of the extant essays survived to modern times: Ms. 152 in the Al-Madrasa al-Aḥmadīya in Mosul, listed by Dā'ūd Chalabī in his *Makhṭūṭāt al-Mawṣil* (Baghdad: Maṭba°at al-Furāt, 1346/1927), p. 33. But this collection has since disappeared. It may have been transferred, as collections in other *madrasas* were, to the Awqaf General Library in the 1970s; see Usāma Nāṣir al-Naqshabandī, 'Iraq', in Geoffrey Roper (ed.), *World Survey of Islamic Manuscripts*, 4 vols. (London: Al-Furqān Islamic Heritage Foundation, 1992–4), vol. 2, pp. 34–6. In any case, this writer's efforts to trace Ms. 152 have so far been unsuccessful, and if Ms. 152 is indeed lost, then our only means of access to the full texts of essays 2–4 has been lost along with it.

8   This date is given by Ibn Abī Uṣaybi°a (note 1, vol. 1), p. 243, who cites the colophon of the autograph copy of the text.

doctor is invited to a dinner party by a senior physician, and joins his host, a pharmacist, a phlebotomist, an oculist, and a surgeon for the evening; medical ethics, practice, and other matters are discussed, and as the night wears on the petty faults and shortcomings of the others are gradually revealed to the young guest.[9] The work is clearly an allegory on Ibn Buṭlān's experiences with ᶜAlī ibn Riḍwān, and its autobiographical dimension is of considerable importance.[10]

For our purposes here, the debate provides some valuable insights into the processes which served, on the one hand, to establish structures of authority within the ranks of medieval Arab-Islamic scholars,[11] and on the other, to determine the shape and content of scholarship itself. Where epistemology is concerned, my argument will hopefully serve to focus attention on the fact – widely conceded but often under-estimated – that socio-cultural forces, largely independent of specifically 'scientific' considerations or criteria, play a crucial role in the process by which ideas and propositions established within a scientific tradition gain assent as truth and achieve their relative value or importance in that tradition.

The background to the dispute

A reader expecting a medical or philosophical controversy to emerge in the essays referred to above will find that Ibn Riḍwān and Ibn Buṭlān both stand squarely within the framework of medicine and science formulated by Galen in the former case and Aristotle in the latter. The scientific point supposedly at issue between them is simply this: which is warmer by nature, the chicken or the young of the bird? This springs directly from the question of the relation between warmth and movement, a topic often discussed in Aristotelian natural science,[12] and one

9   Ibn Buṭlān, Daᶜwat al-aṭibbā', ed. Felix Klein-Franke (Wiesbaden: Otto Harrassowitz, 1985). A commentary on difficult passages in this work was compiled by Ibn al-Athardī in 507/1113. See Ullmann (note 3), pp. 224–5; Martin Levey, 'Some Eleventh-Century Medical Questions Posed by Ibn Buṭlān and Later Answered by Ibn Ithirdī', Bulletin of the History of Medicine, 39 (1965), 495–507. Both Ibn Buṭlān's work and Ibn al-Athardī's commentary have been translated into German in Felix Klein-Franke, Das Ärztebankett (Stuttgart: Hippokrates Verlag, 1984).
10   See Klein-Franke's comments on this in Das Ärztebankett (note 9), pp. 14–16. Several examples of this will be considered below.
11   It is of course true that many medical and scientific authors were neither Arabs nor Muslims. The term 'Arab-Islamic' is used here to evoke the cosmopolitan cultural milieu which encouraged contributions from scholars of various ethnic backgrounds and religious convictions. See Lawrence I. Conrad, 'Arab-Islamic Medicine', in W.F. Bynum and Roy Porter (eds.), Companion Encyclopedia of the History of Medicine, 2 vols. (London: Routledge, 1993), vol. 1, pp. 676–7.
12   See, for example, Aristotle, De partibus animalium, III.6; IV.6, 10, 13.

might accordingly wish to concede that weightier matters are at least implicitly involved. But our two antagonists do not, in fact, disagree on this point, and Ibn Buṭlān three times concedes that in pursuing the question in the first place he has sought only to set forth an exercise for experts and a conundrum for the pedagogical benefit of students.[13] As for Greek learning, in this debate it is little more than a foil wielded by the two adversaries in more or less equal degree and to more or less equal effect. No particular scientific case is established or refuted: rather, one finds petulant bickering over tendentious sophistries and minute examination of areas either obvious or irrelevant, as later medieval observers were already quick to notice.[14] Having stated that he now intends to 'exult in the gardens of the intellect and pluck the fruits of learning', for example, Ibn Buṭlān launches into eighty-one questions concerning eggs and brooding, although little of this has any bearing on his subject.[15] In Ibn Riḍwān's response, these questions are not addressed, but simply held up for mockery in brief diatribes which contribute nothing to the (supposed) discussion of whether or not the chicken is of a warmer nature than the young of the bird.[16] Real argument focuses on such matters as which of the two physicians has more shockingly betrayed the heritage of the Ancients,[17] which is uglier,[18] which one produces the more incompetent students,[19] which one's urine flasks the angels will present to God on the Judgement Day

[13] Schacht and Mayerhof (note 4), pp. 70, 72, 76.
[14] See al-Qifṭī (d. 646/1248), Ta'rīkh al-ḥukamā', ed. Julius Lippert (Leipzig: Dieter-ich'sche Verlagsbuchhandlung, 1903), p. 294, where he attributes the dispute to 'controversy for the sake of winning an argument' ('al-mubālagha fī l-munāẓara'). As Ibn Abī Uṣaybiʿa remarks (note 1), vol. 1, p. 241: 'One of them could not write an essay or contrive an opinion without the other refuting the work and reducing the views in it to absurdity.'
[15] Schacht and Mayerhof (note 4), pp. 75–6. The editors drop this discussion from their edition, citing as an example Ibn Buṭlān's question of which black animals lay white eggs from which black young hatch.
[16] Ibid., pp. 80, 112.
[17] Ibid., pp. 78, 79, 88, 90, 94, 101, 103, 105, 108–11, 114, 116–17.
[18] Ibid., pp. 97–100, responding to Ibn Riḍwān's accusations of ugliness in one of the essays now lost, and attacking an earlier essay of his asserting that the perfect physician does not need to have a handsome face: see Ibn Abī Uṣaybiʿa (note 1), vol. 1, p. 242, on this work. Neither man seems to have been very attractive: see al-Qifṭī (note 14), pp. 294, 444; Ibn Abī Uṣaybiʿa (note 1), vol. 1, p. 242. Such matters were potentially very embarrassing, since medieval Muslim physicians, very well aware that the Hippocratic Oath specifically states that a physician should be of pleasing appearance, discussed at great length the pains a physician should take with respect to his appearance. See, for example, al-Ruhāwī, Adab al-ṭabīb (Frankfurt am Main: Institut für Islamwissenschaften, 1986), fols. 57r-58v; trans. (badly) by Martin Levey as Medical Ethics of Medieval Islam, Transactions of the American Philosophical Society, New Series, vol. 57.3 (Philadelphia: American Philosophical Society, 1967), pp. 53–5.
[19] Schacht and Mayerhof (note 4), pp. 90–4.

as proof of his ignorance,[20] and whether it is Baghdad or Cairo where the natural environment is conducive to wisdom or stupidity.[21] At the end of his second essay, Ibn Buṭlān launches into an entirely irrelevant critique of a different work by Ibn Riḍwān, for no reason (or so he says) other than the fact that the sheet of paper he is using still has sufficient space for him to do so.[22]

In large part, the origins of the controversy may be found in the character of Ibn Riḍwān. He had been born the son of a poor baker in Giza, and both of his parents died young. He had no money to finance studies with a teacher, and so had to learn on his own, earning his keep by casting horoscopes and telling fortunes by the roadside. An opportunity to substitute for a physician friend launched him on his medical career, which he pursued with almost obsessive determination. He eventually became chief physician to the caliph, assembled a large library, wrote numerous works of his own, attracted many students, and amassed a considerable fortune from investments in real estate.[23]

Throughout his life, however, his humble origins and early difficulties seem to have haunted him. He was notoriously mean and avaricious, and his overweening vanity manifests itself in his repeated efforts – none particularly subtle – to draw his readers' attention to his gentility, integrity, learning, and solicitude for the progress of scholarship.[24] This progress, however, he defined in terms of two important but ultimately self-serving considerations: first, only those personally familiar with Egyptian conditions – led, of course, by himself – were qualified to speak about medicine and the natural sciences in Egypt,[25] and second, legitimate scholarship in

[20]   Ibid., p. 76.
[21]   Ibid., pp. 89–90. Ibn Buṭlān returns to this theme in Daᶜwat al-aṭibbā' (note 9, 1985), pp. 5–12; trans. Klein-Franke (note 9, 1984), pp. 50–8.
[22]   Schacht and Mayerhof (note 4), p. 103.
[23]   For a useful summary of the life and career of Ibn Riḍwān, see Michael W. Dols's 'Introduction' to his Medieval Islamic Medicine: Ibn Riḍwān's Treatise 'On the Prevention of Bodily Ills in Egypt', trans. Michael W. Dols, Arabic text ed. Adil S. Gamal (Berkeley and Los Angeles: University of California Press, 1984), pp. 54–66.
[24]   Particularly stunning is the statement in his autobiographical sketch, quoted in Ibn Abī Uṣaybiᶜa (note 1), vol. 2, p. 100: 'I keep silent and hold my tongue where people's faults are concerned; I strive to speak only as I should, and I beware of [swearing] oaths and casting blame on the opinions [of others].' Hardly less extraordinary is his admonition in his unpublished Al-Kitāb al-nāfiᶜ fī kayfiyat taᶜlīm ṣināᶜat al-ṭibb ('The Useful Book on How to Teach the Art of Medicine') that knowledge of logic should not be used to gratuitously contradict the opinions of others, a practice which he dismisses as 'nonsensical'. See the extracts from this work translated in M.C. Lyons, 'The Kitāb al-Nāfiᶜ of ᶜAlī ibn Riḍwān', Islamic Quarterly, 6 (1961), 68.
[25]   A completely legitimate starting point for this argument would have been the observation, current from the Hippocratics onward, that since human health is affected by prevailing local conditions, physicians need to be familiar with these conditions in order to treat their patients. ᶜAlī ibn Riḍwān, however, routinely takes this to unreasonable extremes.

medicine and the sciences demanded strict adherence to and mastery of the classical Greek corpus, the dedicated and unaided study of which had been his own route to the medical profession.[26] Jealously guarding his privileged position in Egypt, he was as likely as not to take offence at any work by a non-Egyptian which dared to comment on Ibn Riḍwān's homeland, or any that deviated (in his view) from the wisdom of the ancient Greeks. The great Nestorian Christian translator and scientific author Ḥunayn ibn Isḥāq (d. 260/873) he vilified for allegedly misunderstanding and misrepresenting Galen; in reality, his ire seems to have been aroused by Ḥunayn's efforts to systematize Galenic thinking in original works of his own.[27] Another eminent victim was Muḥammad ibn Zakarīyā al-Rāzī (d. c. 320/923), one of the most important philosophers, scientists, and medical authors of medieval Islamic times, but the target of at least two (and perhaps three) attacks by ᶜAlī ibn Riḍwān: one for his allegedly shallow learning in medicine, logic, astronomy, and the natural sciences, as reflected primarily in his faulty understanding of Galen; another (probably part of the first) for doubting and challenging Galen; and another refuting al-Rāzī's sceptical views on theology, prophecy, and religion in general.[28] Ibn Riḍwān's Fī dafᶜ maḍārr al-abdān bi-arḍ Miṣr ('On the Prevention of Bodily Ills in the Land of Egypt') is a reply to a now-lost work by Aḥmad ibn Abī Khālid Ibn al-Jazzār (d. c. 395/1004) of al-Qayrawān (in modern-day Tunisia) in which the latter discussed epidemic disease in Egypt, the ignorance of its physicians, and recommendations for corrective steps in hygiene and public health – all of which Ibn Riḍwān rejected as not based on personal

[26]   For a physician to be self-taught was not unusual in medieval Islamic times; Ibn Sīnā
       (d. 428/1037), for example, had also studied medicine without the aid of teachers. See
       the autobiographical notice in Ibn Abī Uṣaybiᶜa (note 1), vol. 2, p. 3; trans. William E.
       Gohlman in his *The Life of Ibn Sina* (Albany: State University of New York Press,
       1974), pp. 25–7. More will be said below concerning ᶜAlī ibn Riḍwān's attitude toward
       classical Greek medical texts.
[27]   Ibn Riḍwān's criticisms of Ḥunayn are set forth in his *Al-Kitāb al-nāfiᶜ* (note 24), and
       it may be an extract from this text which is cited as an independent work in Ibn Abī
       Uṣaybiᶜa (note 1), vol. 2, p. 103. For the gist of the case set forth against Ḥunayn, see
       Schacht and Mayerhof (note 4), pp. 26–7. Ibn Buṭlān attacks this critique in Schacht
       and Mayerhof, p. 101; and Ibn Abī Uṣaybiᶜa (note 1), vol. 2, p. 62, refers to another
       refutation of it by Abū l-Ṣalt (d. 529/1134), an Andalusian who must have become
       aware of Ibn Riḍwān's critique during a long sojourn he is known to have had in Egypt.
       See Brockelmann (note 3), vol. 1, p. 486; vol. S2, p. 889; Ullmann (note 3), p. 276.
[28]   The criticisms for doubting Galen survive in Ibn Riḍwān's *Al-Kitāb al-nāfiᶜ*. See the
       summary in Schacht and Mayerhof (note 4), pp. 27–8; also Ibn Abī Uṣaybiᶜa (note 1),
       vol. 2, pp. 104, 105, referring to three separate works. On the criticisms of Galen by al-
       Rāzī and others, especially Ibn Rushd (d. 595/1198), see J. Christoph Bürgel, *Averroes
       'contra Galenum'*, Nachrichten der Akademie der Wissenschaften in Göttingen,
       Philologisch-Historische Klasse, 1967, Nr. 9 (Göttingen: Vandenhoeck und Ruprecht,
       1968), pp. 263–340. See also the summary in Ullmann (note 3), pp. 67–8.

experience in Egypt.[29] To a work by ᶜAbd Allāh Ibn al-Ṭayyib (d. 435/
1043), celebrated philosopher and physician and secretary to the
Nestorian catholicos in Baghdad, he replied with a polemic arguing that
Ibn al-Ṭayyib's sophistries are his prime achievement.[30] Ibn al-Ṭayyib's
real offence was probably the preparation of Arabic paraphrases of
Galenic works:[31] Ibn Riḍwān spent much of his career writing
commentaries and glosses on Galenic texts,[32] but simplified Arabic
versions of such texts of course reduced the need for commentaries and
glosses, and indeed, potentially conflicted with them.

Overall, Ibn Riḍwān was a thoroughly difficult individual. Even in his
own country, his students mocked him behind his back.[33] People spread
tales about his meanness,[34] and his colleagues never allowed him to live
down his early career as a fortuneteller.[35]

Ibn Buṭlān was perfectly well aware of Ibn Riḍwān's vain and
temperamental ways,[36] for his mentor in Baghdad had been none other
than Ibn al-Ṭayyib, an earlier victim of Ibn Riḍwān's abuse.[37] Nevertheless, Ibn Buṭlān set out for Egypt in Ramaḍān 440/January 1049.
One medieval authority states that he went for the specific purpose of
meeting Ibn Riḍwān;[38] his difficult personality notwithstanding, the
latter did enjoy a formidable reputation as an authority on medicine, and
Ibn Buṭlān seems to have made an effort to familiarize himself with his
medical scholarship.[39] Schacht and Meyerhof suggest that Ibn Buṭlān

---

[29]   Dols (note 23), pp. 67–9, 77, 99–103, 121; Aḥmad ibn Mīlād, *Ta'rīkh al-ṭibb al-ᶜarabī
       al-tūnisī* (Tunis, 1980), pp. 48–74. Brockelmann (note 3), vol. S1, p. 886₂₆, refers to a
       manuscript of a 'polemic against Ibn al-Jazzār' as a work independent of the *Fī dafᶜ
       maḍārr al-abdān*, but in fact it is the same text. See Karl Vollers, 'Aus der
       viceköniglichen Bibliothek in Cairo', *Zeitschrift der Deutschen Morgenländischen Ge-
       sellschaft*, 44 (1890), p. 386.
[30]   Ibn Abī Uṣaybiᶜa (note 1), vol. 2, p. 104.
[31]   See Brockelmann (note 3), vol. 1, pp. 482–3.
[32]   Ibn Abī Uṣaybiᶜa (note 1), vol. 2, pp. 103, 104, lists sixteen such works by Ibn
       Riḍwān.
[33]   Al-Qifṭī (note 14), p. 444.
[34]   For a telling example, see Ibn Abī Uṣaybiᶜa (note 1), vol. 2, p. 101.
[35]   Ibid. Ibn Riḍwān's roadside prognostications are said by al-Qifṭī (note 14), p. 443, to
       have been 'not in accordance with critical method' ('lā bi-ṭarīq al-taḥqīq').
[36]   Schacht and Meyerhof (note 4), p. 81, where Ibn Buṭlān expresses his familiarity with
       Ibn Riḍwān's hot-tempered demeanour and his 'inclination to idle uproar'.
[37]   According to al-Qifṭī (note 14), p. 314, Ibn Buṭlān was Ibn al-Ṭayyib's favourite
       student.
[38]   Ibn Abī Uṣaybiᶜa (note 1), vol. 2, p. 241. It must be borne in mind, however, that this
       author sometimes injects into his narrative statements which come from no source, but
       rather represent highly arbitrary conclusions of his own.
[39]   Ibn Buṭlān quotes Ibn Riḍwān in his *Taqwīm al-ṣiḥḥa* ('Regimen of Health'); see
       Hosam Elkhadem (ed. and trans.), *Le Taqwīm al-Ṣiḥḥa (Tacuini Sanitatis) d'Ibn
       Buṭlān: un traité du XIᵉ siècle* (Louvain: Peeters, 1990), pp. 215, 217 (naming him as
       'al-Miṣrī'). As will become clear below, Ibn Buṭlān's comments during the controversy
       reflect a thorough knowledge of Ibn Riḍwān's medical writings.

may have come to Egypt to seek a position at the court of al-Mustanṣir, who was well disposed to non-Muslim physicians.[40] But closer to the truth, perhaps, is the example of the young physician in Ibn Buṭlān's *Da ᶜwat al-aṭibbā*'; beset by financial pressures and the high cost of living in Baghdad, he sets out with hopes of establishing a medical practice in another land where he can afford to live.[41]

Along the way, it became clear that Ibn Buṭlān too had a penchant for disputation with professional colleagues. In Aleppo he became involved in a medical altercation with a Christian secretary and physician and defeated his adversary completely. His humiliated victim, however, proceeded to arouse the Christians of the city against Ibn Buṭlān. Our traveller was hurried into a premature departure,[42] and it may be significant that upon his later retreat from Cairo, he proceeded not to Aleppo, but to Constantinople and then Antioch.

The course and issues of the dispute

The events which transpired when Ibn Buṭlān arrived in Cairo must be viewed against this background, and also in terms of the fluid nature of the scholarly disciplines in medieval Islamic times. There were no prescribed routes of access to particular fields, or specified conditions for recognition of personal status within them. The role of communal assent was crucial, and within that context, so also was one's position among local circles of intellectual and cultural endeavour. This was particularly true for the field of medicine. There were many types of medical practitioners, including humoral physicians trained in the Galenic tradition, purveyors of popular folklore and herbal and magical cures, cuppers, barbers, and phlebotomists, and a goodly measure of outright quacks and frauds. There were no procedures for systematic examinations or verification of qualifications, and structures of authority and sanction were based on personalities rather than institutions.[43] As was the case generally for professional men who travelled in the medieval Islamic world,[44] the fate of a physician arriving in a new city from afar completely depended upon his ability to win acceptance among his local

---

[40] Schacht and Mayerhof (note 4), p. 14.
[41] Ibn Buṭlān (note 9), p. 7; trans. Klein-Franke, pp. 52–3.
[42] Al-Qifṭī (note 14), p. 315.
[43] See Gary Leiser, 'Medical Education in Islamic Lands from the Seventh to the Fourteenth Century', *Journal of the History of Medicine*, 38 (1983), 48–75; Conrad (note 11), pp. 709–14.
[44] A.L. Udovitch, 'Formalism and Informalism in the Social and Economic Institutions of the Medieval Islamic World', in Amin Banani and Speros Vryonis (eds.), *Individualism and Conformity in Classical Islam* (Wiesbaden: Otto Harrassowitz, 1977), pp. 61–81.

peers, and so gain broader assent to his professional credentials and his claims to status in his field.

This is precisely what Ibn Buṭlān sought to achieve in his first weeks, or perhaps months, in Cairo; and if he had set out from Baghdad with fairly modest ambitions, he had revised his goals considerably by the time he reached Egypt ten months later. The fact that he sought contact with Ibn Riḍwān shows that he was aiming for recognition and acceptance at the highest level, a signal which could hardly have been missed by the élite humoral practitioners in Cairo. At first, all seems to have gone well. Ibn Buṭlān was introduced to Ibn Riḍwān in the palace of the *amīr* Jawhar ibn Māḍī, where Ibn Riḍwān praised the newcomer to the assembled company.[45] But before long, Ibn Buṭlān became restless and dissatisfied with Ibn Riḍwān's patronage, and again the autobiographical dimension of the former's dinner party tale is illuminating. Here the young Baghdadi doctor, seeking the company of other medical men in a distant city, is directed to an eminent and elderly physician of imposing reputation and demeanour. This authority warmly welcomes his young colleague and invites him to dinner, and the visitor, pleased at his good fortune, gladly accepts. As they wait for the other guests, however, the newcomer comes to realize that his host is a mean, deceitful, and avaricious opportunist who is concerned for others only if and to the extent that it will redound to his own greater advantage.[46]

Ibn Buṭlān thus decided to strike out on his own. Encouraged by an unnamed *wazīr* at the court,[47] he composed his essay arguing that the chicken is of a warmer nature than the young of the bird, taking as his starting point an essay on this same subject written by Georgius ibn Yūḥannā al-Yabrūdī (d. before 441/1050), a Jacobite Christian physician from Yabrūd, near Damascus.[48] Ibn Buṭlān does not refute this epistle, which he probably came to know on his way through Syria;[49] he rather asserts that al-Yabrūdī had failed to give a proper scientific justification for his position, and so sets out to provide this himself, though not wishing to be understood as accepting al-Yabrūdī's views.[50]

---

[45]   Schacht and Mayerhof (note 4), p. 108. To be rejected, then, is Schacht and Mayerhof's view (ibid., p. 14) that Ibn Buṭlān met with hostility from Ibn Riḍwān from the very beginning.

[46]   Ibn Buṭlān (note 9), pp. 5–29; trans. Klein-Franke, pp. 50–79.

[47]   Schacht and Mayerhof (note 4), p. 82.

[48]   On this personality see Ibn Abī Uṣaybiʿa (note 1), vol. 2, pp. 140–3.

[49]   Based on a passage in Schacht and Mayerhof (note 4), p. 70, where discussion of the essay in Cairo is mentioned, Schacht and Mayerhof (ibid., p. 15) state that Ibn Buṭlān first heard of al-Yabrūdī's work in Cairo. But the text simply shows that the essay was already known in Cairo by the time Ibn Buṭlān arrived; it is likely that the Iraqi traveller was already familiar with it from discussions in medical circles in Damascus.

[50]   Ibid., pp. 72–5.

It was this critique which went to Ibn Riḍwān for comment, but with a higher agenda in mind. Other copies of the essay would have been transcribed and circulated, and served to set before Ibn Buṭlān's Egyptian peers a sample of his rhetorical and dialectical skills, his broad Aristotelian learning, and his general cultural breeding. The topic was probably chosen not only for its innocuous character, but also for its relevance to the situation in Egypt, and especially Cairo, where poultry raising and the artificial incubation of eggs were highly developed and extremely profitable enterprises.[51] In this context, his eighty-one questions on eggs and brooding become very relevant indeed. The topic could not have met with indifference in élite educated circles in Cairo, and his presentation of page upon page of enigmatic questions harked back to the old Greek *problemata* literature, which Arab-Islamic culture had already taken up with manifest relish several centuries earlier.[52]

Nevertheless, it was inevitable that Ibn Riḍwān would react badly to this turn of events. The fact that the essay was written with some official encouragement could only have been taken by Ibn Riḍwān as a threat to his own position, and Ibn Buṭlān himself hints at this when (in his second essay) he reminds Ibn Riḍwān that his master, the Fāṭimid caliph, could at any time mutilate his already ugly face.[53] Likewise, he could not have failed to see that by displaying Ibn Buṭlān's talents and learning for all to see, the public nature of the missive challenged Ibn Riḍwān to concede these qualities. The relevance of the topic to specifically Egyptian concerns also flew in the face of one of Ibn Riḍwān's favourite polemical hobbyhorses: that only local practitioners knew conditions in Egypt well enough to write authoritatively about them.

That the publication of Ibn Buṭlān's essay comprised, overall, a massive affront to Ibn Riḍwān's colossal ego is a factor in play throughout, and perhaps most obviously in his response to his Iraqi colleague's comment in his first essay that his work concerns an enigma

---

51 See, for example, the detailed account of this industry as practised near Cairo in ᶜAbd al-Laṭīf al-Baghdādī (d. 629/1231), *Al-Ifāda wa-l-iᶜtibār*, ed. Aḥmad Ghassān Sabānū (Damascus: Dār Qutayba, 1403/1983), pp. 35–8; trans. Kamal Hafuth Zand and John A. and Ivy E. Videan as *The Eastern Key* (London: George Allen and Unwin, 1965), pp. 79–89.

52 For a text full of such questions, see, for example, al-Jāḥiẓ (d. 255/868), *Al-Tarbīᶜ wa-l-tadwīr*, ed. Charles Pellat (Damascus: Institut Français, 1955); trans. Maurice Adad in *Arabica*, 13 (1966), 268–94; 14 (1967), 32–59, 167–90, 298–317; also Mary Elizabeth Malkhmus, 'Syntax and Epistemology in the *Kitāb al-tarbīᶜ wa-l-tadwīr of al-Jāḥiẓ*', unpublished Ph.D. thesis, School of Oriental and African Studies (1983); Hans Daiber, *Naturwissenschaft bei den Arabern im 10. Jahrhundert n. Chr.: Briefe des Abū l-Faḍl Ibn al-ᶜAmīd (gest. 360/970) an ᶜAḍudaddaula* (Leiden: E.J. Brill, 1993).

53 Schacht and Mayerhof (note 4), p. 98. As Schacht and Mayerhof point out (ibid., n. 37), the allusion is to the criminal punishment of cutting off the nose and/or ears.

that al-Yabrūdī had put to the physicians of Egypt.[54] Ibn Riḍwān finds this impossible to believe, for the simple reason that he himself knows nothing about such a communication: had al-Yabrūdī discussed any medical matter with the physicians of Egypt, he vainly proclaims, he would have discussed it with him first.[55]

But there was more. Ibn Buṭlān complains in his opening statement that in Egypt the learned man cannot even gain *equal* footing with the ignoramus,[56] a slip which must have reduced Ibn Riḍwān to near apoplexy. And the visitor could not have known that al-Yabrūdī, by then deceased, had been an esteemed colleague of Ibn Riḍwān.[57]

Ibn Riḍwān's impassioned response was thus his reaction to a development which he regarded as a personal affront and a threat to his professional status and privileged official position. Ibn Buṭlān sarcastically compares Ibn Riḍwān's attitude to that of the host in his *Daʿwat al-aṭibbāʾ*, who invites his visitor to dinner, and then rages when he picks at the leftovers while the master sleeps.[58] In reality, however, his essay *was* a challenge to Ibn Riḍwān's hegemony, and the ensuing polemic became a battlefield where the issue was largely decided.[59] Evidence that this was the essential matter of contention abounds in the five extant essays, and one example is especially illustrative. In chapter 1 of the third essay, Ibn Buṭlān advances seven reasons why oral instruction from teachers provides an education superior to that gained by him who learns from books. A teacher, for example, can correct copyists' errors in manuscripts, elucidate obscure passages, and correct the student's mistakes.[60] In chapter 2, he argues that without a teacher to rescue him, a student's inevitable mistakes will lead him into doubt and confusion, which will produce further error, which will compound his confusion, and so on, in a vicious circle.[61]

In other words, it is education and connections with teachers that produce the expert physician. Many of Ibn Buṭlān's points are eminently reasonable ones, but his argument is completely self-serving.[62] Ibn Buṭlān had studied with Ibn al-Ṭayyib and other eminent physicians in

[54] Ibid., p. 70.
[55] Ibid., p. 78. On al-Yabrūdī's contacts with Egyptian physicians, see Ibn Abī Uṣaybiʿa (note 1), vol. 2, p. 141.
[56] Schacht and Mayerhof (note 4), p. 70.
[57] Ibid., p. 77.
[58] Ibn Buṭlān (note 9), pp. 12–13, 88–90; trans. Klein-Franke, pp. 58–60, 141–3.
[59] On the basis of his reading of Ibn Buṭlān's *Waqʿat al-aṭibbāʾ*, Ibn Abī Uṣaybiʿa (note 1), vol. 1, p. 242, suggests that there were physical altercations as well, but offers no details.
[60] Schacht and Mayerhof (note 4), pp. 83–6.
[61] Ibid., p. 86.
[62] As Ibn Riḍwān was of course quick to notice: ibid., p. 108.

Baghdad,[63] and so had benefited from opportunities denied to the penniless young ᶜAlī ibn Riḍwān; further, his entire case is clearly intended to refute Ibn Riḍwān's argument – set forth in earlier works unrelated to the polemic – that learning from books is superior to studying with teachers.[64] In this connection it may be significant that in one of these works Ibn Riḍwān relates that in his youth he had wanted to go to Baghdad to study with a medical scholar known to be working there, but could not do so for lack of funds.[65] At that time, the physician in question was probably Ibn al-Ṭayyib, Ibn Buṭlān's mentor. Assuming this to have been the case, Ibn Buṭlān's comments on the importance of teachers must have had, from his opponent's point of view, an especially vicious edge.[66]

Ultimately, then, the controversy was not about Greek learning, much less about the warmth of birds, but rather about whether Ibn Buṭlān would be successful in his bid for recognition – gained in independence from the grudging and unreliable ᶜAlī ibn Riḍwān. Viewed from this perspective, the abuse, accusations, and slander which comprise the bulk of the literary product of the controversy are very much to the point: in what amounted to a conflict over social and professional status, to fail to hold one's own against such attacks – whether real or perceived – was as much as to lose the contest.

A decisive step seems to have been marked by Ibn Riḍwān's last essay – or at least, the final one in the extant series – where he called upon the physicians of Cairo for support. His colleagues, he says, will be astonished to find that although Ibn Buṭlān poses as the consummate physician (*ṭabīb*), he does not deserve even the indulgence of acknowl-edgement as a medical practitioner (*mutaṭabbib*), since in his writings he cannot manage to write a single true word, even by chance. His arguments appear clever, but in reality only reflect a talent for baseless posturing. After elaborating a number of examples, Ibn Riḍwān concludes that Ibn Buṭlān's ideas are worthy only of laughter. The

---

[63]   Al-Qifṭī (note 14), p. 294.
[64]   Ibn Riḍwān advances a detailed defence of this view in his *Al-Kitāb al-nāfiᶜ* (note 24). See Schacht and Mayerhof (note 4), pp. 20–9 (a detailed summary of the contents of the incomplete Cairo Ms.); Lyons (note 24), pp. 66–7, 69. Closely related to this is his argument that in three years a novice can teach himself medicine, and for that will need only the works of Hippocrates and Galen and the *Materia medica* of Dioscorides – all other books can be dispensed with. The quintessential statement of this view is elaborated as his *Al-Taṭurruq bi-l-ṭibb ilā l-saᶜāda*, ed. and trans. Albert Dietrich as *ᶜAlī ibn Riḍwān. Über den Weg zur Glückseligkeit durch den ärztlichen Beruf* (Göttingen: Vandenhoeck und Ruprecht, 1982).
[65]   Ibn Riḍwān, *Kitāb al-nāfiᶜ*, in Lyons (note 24), p. 67.
[66]   See Schacht and Mayerhof (note 4), p. 102, where Ibn Buṭlān joins the ranks of Ibn Riḍwān's other critics in contemptuously pointing to his early career as a fortuneteller.

physicians of Cairo should therefore ignore and avoid him as a babbler subject to confused and evil delusions. His death would not be worth lamenting, nor merit the invocation of God's mercy upon his soul.[67]

Faced with a clear-cut choice between a foreign newcomer and an established local luminary of considerable power and influence, and bombarded with further polemical essays (all now lost) against the former, the physicians of Cairo could hardly have done other than heed Ibn Riḍwān's appeal. That they did so, and that the result was a decisive professional boycott, is confirmed by the fact that later, in Constantinople, Ibn Buṭlān compared his situation back in Cairo to that of the young man at the hypothetical dinner party, whom the host invites in expectation that he will not eat much. But when the old man rises from a post-dinner nap and finds that the bowl of sweets is empty and the bones of the roast are showing, he flies into a vile rage at his guest for picking at his leftovers. The embarrassed youth replies that he was only acting in response to his host's earlier hospitable and welcoming attitude, and protests that compared to what he could have consumed he has actually eaten very little. But then the host declares him fouler than a sycophant and more insufferable than the most burdensome parasite, so the young man rises and leaves. In a chance encounter at the old physician's window a few days later, he politely tries to redeem the situation, but his former host rebuffs him and slams the shutter in his face.[68]

Just as the young man in $Da^c wat\ al\text{-}aṭibbā'$ has no option but to turn from the locked window and leave, never to see the old man again, Ibn Buṭlān left Cairo 'in wrath against ^{c}Alī ibn Riḍwān' in 444/1052 and proceeded eventually to Constantinople. Later he went to Antioch, where he entered a cloister and wrote a work on medical regimen for monks and monasteries.[69] In 455/1063 he was still active, writing a treatise on therapy and supervising the construction of a hospital in Antioch,[70] but beyond this no further information is known about the last years of his life.

Patterns of affirmation and confirmation

The dispute between Ibn Riḍwān and Ibn Buṭlān comprises an unusually clear vignette on the sort of social manoeuvring and negotiating in scholarly circles that was very common in medieval times. More importantly, it illustrates the ways in which literary endeavour

[67]   Ibid., pp. 112–18.
[68]   Ibn Buṭlān (note 9), pp. 12–13, 88–91; trans. Klein-Franke, pp. 58–60, 141–4.
[69]   See Brockelmann (note 3), vol. 1, p. 483$_2$; vol. S1, p. 885$_3$; Ullmann (note 3), p. 158.
[70]   Ibn Abī Uṣaybi^{c}a (note 1), vol. 1, p. 243.

could be used – and indeed, very often was used – for purposes external to the topic under discussion, but contributing to the establishment of both the scholarly status of individuals and the content of the traditions to which they dedicated their studies.

As intimated above, Ibn Buṭlān's first essay represented an exercise in affirmation, a claim to valid status as a scholar worthy of esteem and respect in his field. All literary works may be said to participate in this agenda to some extent; here, however, we have to do in the first instance with texts in which this is the primary purpose, and which thus typify the pattern more broadly than do other works. Ibn Riḍwān, for example, wrote essays with precisely this aim in mind. As we have already seen, his *Al-Kitāb al-nāfiᶜ* and his *Al-Taṭurruq bi-l-ṭibb ilā l-saᶜāda* serve to justify his background as a *medicus autodidactus* and his narrow devotion to booklearning, but numerous other examples exist, among them his *Kifāyat al-ṭabīb* ('The Book Sufficient for the Physician').[71] This is a concise summary of the vast ancient and medieval literature on urine and the pulse, but in fact it serves to affirm Ibn Riḍwān's status as an authority qualified to undertake such a major task; it is very likely that it was for this purpose that he wrote the work.

Perhaps the clearest examples of scholarship as affirmation may be seen in the career of Jalāl al-Dīn al-Suyūṭī (d. 911/1505). Over three hundred of this renowned Egyptian scholar's works have survived to modern times, ranging from complex multi-volume compendia and studies to brief essays of only a few pages.[72] He routinely used his literary work as a vehicle to promote his own status and reputation, and as the year AH 900 (= 1494–5 AD) approached, he produced a number of works which campaigned in one way or another on behalf of his claim to be acknowledged as the *mujaddid*, one of a series of 'renewers' which Muslims believed God sent at the turn of each century to renew and revitalize the Islamic faith and community.[73]

Like Ibn Riḍwān and Ibn Buṭlān, al-Suyūṭī became embroiled in disputes with colleagues,[74] but such altercations were simply extreme

---

[71]   Ibn Ridwān, *Kifāyat al-ṭabīb*, ed. and trans. Jacques Grand'Henry as *Le Livre de la méthode du médicin de ᶜAlī b. Riḍwān (998–1067)*, 2 vols. (Louvain: Université catholique de Louvain, 1979–84).

[72]   See Brockelmann (note 3), vol. 2, pp. 144–59; vol. S2, pp. 178–98.

[73]   The most obvious arguments are in his *Al-Tanbi'a biman yabᶜathuhu llāh ᶜalā rās kull mi'at sana*, Leiden University Library (Leiden), Ms. Ar. 1109; and his *Al-Taḥadduth bi-niᶜmat Allāh*, ed. E.M. Sartain in her *Jalāl al-Dīn al-Suyūṭī*, 2 vols. (Cambridge: Cambridge University Press, 1975), vol. 2, pp. 215–27. For a discussion of al-Suyūṭī's controversial claims, see Sartain, vol. 1, pp. 61–72. On the *mujaddid* more generally, see Ella Landau-Tasseron, 'The "Cyclical Reform": a Study of the *Mujaddid* Tradition', *Studia Islamica*, 70 (1990), 79–117.

[74]   Sartain (note 73), vol. 1, pp. 53–60.

manifestations of a process which usually occurred without incident as a routine aspect of intellectual life, and which made its influence felt in numerous ways. In later medieval times, for example, it became extremely common for authors in all fields to begin a book by stating that they had been asked or prevailed upon by teachers, colleagues, or students to undertake the work. While in some cases this may actually have been the case, it is usually an affirming convention through which the author insinuates: 'I was the one who was asked.' It can also be seen in works with specific objectives in other areas. The eminent Egyptian jurist Abū l-Ikhlāṣ al-Shurunbulālī (d. 1069/1658), for example, wrote many essays on both abstract theological questions and responses to problems which actually arose in Cairo in his day.[75] In these works he often reviewed and critiqued past opinions on the subject, and clearly did so because this was the common procedure; but in all such cases the exercise also served the function of affirming the author's role as the last link in a long and venerable tradition of scholarship.[76]

Processes of affirmation thus served to assert intellectual credentials in a milieu in which, as observed above, the status of individuals within various fields was not definable or subject to verification through such clear-cut means as regular examination, completion of fixed curricula, or official regulation or inspection. As this in itself shows, affirmation was organically linked to parallel processes of confirmation.

In medieval Islamic culture such processes of confirmation not only passed judgement on the claims of individual scholars, but also determined the scope and content of knowledge as living tradition – the body of knowledge actually known to scholars, discussed among them, and used in their own works. Processes of confirmation addressed several major problems which were becoming increasingly troublesome as medieval Islamic culture expanded and flourished. By the time of Ibn Riḍwān and Ibn Buṭlān, scholarship in all fields had proceeded through the initial stages characterized by the writing of monographs on restricted topics (and in the case of such fields as medicine, translation of the relevant ancient texts), to those marked by the appearance of comprehensive compendia.[77] The corpus of available literature in any field – whether medicine, natural science, philosophy, theology, Qur'ānic exegesis, ḥadīth (the traditions ascribed to the

[75] See Brockelmann (note 3), vol. 2, p. 313; vol. S2, pp. 430–1.
[76] A collection of sixty such essays may be found in his Al-Taḥqīqāt al-qudsīya, Khalidi Library (Jerusalem), Ms. Arabic 393.
[77] Conrad (note 11), pp. 698–702.

prophet Muḥammad), history, *belles lettres*, grammar, or philology – was increasing by leaps and bounds, and included works of considerable complexity and difficulty. At the same time, the fact that all books had to be copied by hand, coupled with the limited means for distributing them across the vast extent of the Muslim world, meant that copies of specific texts were routinely scarce and often inaccessible.[78] That is, individual scholars did not have physical access to all the literature relevant to their work, and even if they had, no one would have been able to read it all, much less master it.

In consequence, a work or idea in any given field did not automatically become part of living tradition simply because it had been written down, nor even because it was a good book or idea; this status had to be confirmed in the socio-intellectual context of the ongoing discussions and writings of scholars in the field. The famous *Al-Qānūn fī l-ṭibb* ('Canon of Medicine') by Ibn Sīnā (d. 428/1037), for example, does not yet seem to have enjoyed much renown in Iraq or Egypt in his own lifetime. Ibn Buṭlān takes no account of the *Qānūn* in his works, not even in his *Taqwīm al-ṣiḥḥa*, in the tables of which he refers to numerous works of the Islamic period, including, as mentioned earlier, ᶜAlī ibn Riḍwān.[79] The preparation of commentaries, abridgements, and glosses, and extensive copying of the original text and these secondary aids, do not seem to have begun in earnest until the late sixth/twelfth century,[80] and it was this activity itself – not as decisive moment, but as a pattern of ongoing attention and interest – which confirmed the *Qānūn*, as it were, and accorded it the paramount status it was to enjoy for hundreds of years.

In some cases, confirmation of the importance of a work or idea never came. The commentary by Ibn al-Nafīs (d. 687/1288) on the *Qānūn* contained numerous valuable medical observations, including his

---

[78] Scholars in Islamic Spain, for example, often complained of this problem. See Lawrence I. Conrad, 'Through the Thin Veil: On the Question of Communication and the Socialization of Knowledge in *Ḥayy ibn Yaqẓān*', in Lawrence I. Conrad (ed.), *The World of Ibn Ṭufayl: Interdisciplinary Perspectives on Ḥayy ibn Yaqẓān* (Leiden: E.J. Brill, forthcoming).

[79] See note 39 above.

[80] Brockelmann (note 3), vol. S1, 824$_{82aa}$, refers to a commentary on the *Qānūn* by Ibn Riḍwān, but this attribution is probably false, since the latter never refers to Ibn Sīnā in other works known to be his, and in any case would have been unlikely to make such a major concession of eminence to another medical authority of his own era. The earliest commentary on Ibn Sīnā's work seems to have been that of Ibn Abī l-Khayr (d. 589/1193); see Ekmaleddin Ihsanoglu et al., *Fihris makhṭūṭāt al-ṭibb al-islāmī bi-l-lughāt al-ᶜarabīya wa-l-turkīya wa-l-fārisīya fī maktabāt Turkīyā* (Istanbul: Research Centre for Islamic History, Art and Culture, 1984), p. 66. The first abridgement of the *Qānūn* was an early effort by al-Īlāqī (*c.* 460/1068); see Brockelmann (note 3), vol. S1, p. 826$_{82c}$. But this work was not followed by any other for nearly 150 years.

famous pronouncement on the lesser circulation of the blood,[81] but
these comments were not discussed or further considered in subsequent
medical scholarship – that is, they were never confirmed as part of the
living intellectual tradition of Islamic medicine.

Viewed from this perspective, the controversy between Ibn Riḍwān
and Ibn Buṭlān can be said to have played its part as one moment
among innumerable others, involving scholars all across the Islamic
world, which – taken together – served to determine who would shape
the future of medical scholarship and what the content of living medical
knowledge would be. At one level, the deliverances of both serve in their
own small way to confirm the authority of Aristotelian science and
Galenic medicine. As argued above, it is at other levels that their
essential disagreement must be sought.

Ibn Buṭlān's first essay served to affirm his right to status as a
respected physician, independent of the opinion or patronage of ʿAlī ibn
Riḍwān, and his second essay simply renewed these claims by casting
doubt not only on his opponent's rebuttal, but also on his qualifications
to make such a rebuttal. Ibn Riḍwān's position was more complicated,
but stronger as well. His attacks on Ibn Buṭlān were in essence efforts to
counter his affirmation of status, and as the gap between the two
antagonists widened it must have become clear that eventually other
physicians in Cairo would have to choose sides. Ibn Riḍwān's appeal to
these physicians represented a call for confirmation of his own position,
and for the decisive rejection of Ibn Buṭlān's claims through personal
boycott.

One could hardly ask for a more vivid indication of the power and
importance of these processes than the image of Ibn Buṭlān, in his
monastery on the outskirts of the Byzantine capital, penning his dinner
party tale and contemplating how utterly he had been defeated and
humiliated in Cairo. For him, of course, this was what ultimately
mattered. For us, however, the episode illustrates the complex intertwining of literary endeavour, intellectual life, and social milieu which
served – then, but now as well – to condition the content of knowledge
and define who its exponents were to be.

---

[81]   See Ullmann (note 3), pp. 173–5; Max Meyerhof, 'Ibn an-Nafīs (XIIIth cent.) and his
Theory of the Lesser Circulation', *Isis*, 23 (1935), 100–20; Abdul-Karim Chéhadé, *Ibn
an-Nafis et la découverte de la circulation pulmonaire* (Damascus: Institut franççais de
Damas, 1955). This material has recently been published; see Ibn al-Nafīs, *Sharḥ
tashrīḥ al-Qānūn*, ed. Salmān Qaṭāya (Cairo: Al-Hay'a al-ʿāmma al-miṣrīya li-l-kitāb,
1988).

6 The experience of the book: manuscripts, texts, and the role of epistemology in early medieval medicine

Faith Wallis

The historiographical problem of early medieval medicine

Since the time of Karl Sudhoff and his students, medical historians have been labouring with patience and energy to edit the texts available in the pre-Salernitan period (sixth to eleventh centuries), and to present the manuscripts through which these texts were conveyed.[1] Yet no satisfactory history of early medieval medicine has appeared, nor has any been attempted since MacKinney's slender 1937 survey.[2] This lacuna is all the more curious in that, more than half a century ago, Henry Sigerist set out a cogent plan for how a critical and synthetic history of early medieval medicine, based in the manuscript sources, might be written.[3] Sigerist proposed a survey in three volumes. The first would be a catalogue of manuscripts containing early medieval medical materials, the second an anthology of texts, the third the narrative history.

Sigerist's plan seemed clear and practical, yet it never materialized. To be sure, the intention of the first volume was fulfilled in 1956 with

---

[1]   In citations of medieval manuscripts, I have adopted the abbreviations for shelfmarks listed at the end of the chapter.

[2]   Loren C. MacKinney, *Early Medieval Medicine with Special Reference to France and Chartres*, Publications of the Institute of the History of Medicine, The Johns Hopkins University, Ser. 2, vol. 3 (Baltimore: The Johns Hopkins Press, 1937). Other efforts to survey the entire pre-Salernitan period have been restricted to essays, most of which are, typically, surveys of source materials, e.g. Henry E. Sigerist, 'The Latin Medical Literature of the Early Middle Ages', *Journal of the History of Medicine*, 13 (1958), 127–146; Gerhard Baader, 'Zur Überlieferung der lateinischen medizinischen Literatur des frühen Mittelalters', *Forschung, Praxis, Fortbildung*, 17 (1966), 139–141; Gerhard Baader, 'Die Entwicklung der medizinischen Fachsprache im frühen Mittelalter', in Gerhard Baader and Gundolf Keil (eds.), *Medizin im mittelalterlichen Abendland*, Wege der Forschung 363 (Darmstadt: Wissenschaftliche Buchgesellschaft, 1982), pp. 417–42; Enrico Coturri, 'Libri e cultura dei medici medioevali fino all rinascita carolina', in Innocenzo Mazzini and Franca Fusco (eds.), *I testi di medicina latini antichi. Problemi filologici e storici*, Università di Macerata, Pubb. della Facoltà di lettere e filosofia, 28 (Milan: Giorgio Bretschneider, 1985), pp. 377–82.

[3]   'The Medical Literature of the Early Middle Ages. A Program – and a Report of a Summer of Research in Italy', *Bulletin of the History of Medicine*, 2 (1934), 26–50.

the publication of Augusto Beccaria's repertory of early medieval medical manuscripts, supplemented in 1966 by that of Ernest Wickersheimer.[4] As well, the editing of texts and the provision of studies of individual manuscripts continues apace.[5] Yet despite the wealth of primary materials now accessible, there is no sign of any plans to attempt the third stage, the general history. Was there something wrong with Sigerist's logic? Why is a plethora of sources not leading us inexorably towards a narrative account?

I would suggest that the problem lies in the process of text edition itself, or more precisely, in the often unexamined assumptions about texts that editing reinforces. The method of text edition adopted by medievalists, including the pioneering historians of medieval medicine, is derived from that of classical philology. The paradigm for the philologist is the ancient literary text, the 'classic', for which a critical edition can be prepared by recension, that is, by comparing the readings of the manuscript witnesses, and determining their affiliations. By weighing the merits of variant readings in the manuscripts, the editor can eventually sift out a reading which represents a scientifically defensible reconstruction of the author's autograph, the ultimate archetype of all the manuscript progeny. Recension editing assumes that the text is a stable, objective entity, possessing and retaining a specific and definitive form (save for accidental variants or errors) from manuscript to manuscript. It also assumes that there is a single author whose intentions the editor can intuit. Such a text is 'canonized', and it is with a view to presenting such texts that classical editing methods were developed.

A 'classic' is a canonized text *par excellence*. It might have been commented upon or glossed, but its formal integrity was protected

---

4   Augusto Beccaria, *I codici di medicina del periodo presalernitano (secoli IX, X, e XI)* (Rome: Storia e Letteratura, 1956); Ernest Wickersheimer, *Les Manuscrits latins de médecine du haut moyen âge dans les bibliothèques de France*, Documents, études et répertoires publiés par l'Institut de Recherche et d'Histoire des Textes, 11 (Paris: CNRS, 1966). Sigerist also published some preliminary reports on his manuscript researches: 'A Summer of Research in European Libraries', *Bulletin of the History of Medicine*, 2 (1934), 559–610; 'Early Medieval Medical Texts in Manuscripts of Montpellier', *Bulletin of the History of Medicine*, 10 (1941), 27–47; and 'Early Medieval Medical Texts in the Manuscripts of Vendôme', *Bulletin of the History of Medicine*, 14 (1943), 68–113.

5   For a comprehensive listing of editions, see Guy Sabbah, Pierre-Paul Corsetti and Klaus-Dieter Fischer (eds.), *Bibliographie des textes médicaux latins. Antiquité et haut moyen âge*, Centre Jean-Palerne, Mémoires, no. 6 (Saint-Etienne: Publications de l'Université, 1987). Walter Puhlmann, 'Die lateinische medizinische Literatur des frühen Mittelalters', *Kyklos*, 3 (1930), 396–401, remains a useful overview of the range of textual materials available in the early Middle Ages, particularly when supplemented by Beccaria (note 4), introduction.

by the prestige of its author or presumed author. The scribes who transmitted the classic through manuscript copies intended to convey the text in its specific form, and under its author's name, without introducing changes of their own, though this might happen inadvertently. On the other hand, a text which is deliberately reorganized, interpolated, abbreviated or otherwise altered is often regarded as either unimportant (not a 'classic'), or as evidence of intellectual dishonesty or carelessness on the part of those who transmitted it.

But this is what medical texts in early medieval manuscripts are like, even medical texts originally composed by named authors of classical Antiquity. They are overwhelmingly uncanonized, and this uncanonized character makes it difficult to edit them by the recension method. Editors have been aware of this problem, and have adopted a number of creative strategies for presenting such texts, ranging from diplomatic editions based on a single manuscript or parallel manuscripts, to ingenious experiments in parallel editions. Yet even this ingenuity has not precipitated the long-awaited critical narrative of early medieval history. It may, ironically, be contributing to its delay. It is not enough, it seems, to tinker with editorial tactics. To understand the medical literature of this period, scholars must invert the values of classical philology, and in particular, abandon the assumption that the more important a text is, the more stable it will be, because its value will cause it to be canonized.

Understandably, such a reversal of values is difficult, not only because ancient medical texts tend towards canonization, but because Salernitan and Scholastic ones do as well. The medical text of the High Middle Ages was essentially a vehicle for university-style education. In such a functional context, textual integrity and consistency are valued and necessary. Since Scholastic argumentation was based on authorities, this also reinforced the preference for canonized text forms. But in the early Middle Ages, medicine was not taught through institutions, and while it was a subject of very considerable interest, it was not discussed in terms which privileged arguments from authority.[6] Hence, the importance of a text for an early medieval reader is not necessarily signalled by canonized status. Indeed, quite the opposite is the case. The more important the text was for the early medieval reader, the more it was used, and hence

---

[6]   On the informal, one-on-one training of early medieval physicians, see Gerhard Baader, 'Die Anfänge der medizinischen Ausbildung im Abendland bis 1100', in *La scuola nell'occidente latino dell'alto medioevo*, Settimane di studio del Centro italiano di studi sull'alto medioevo 19, 15–21 aprile 1971 (Spoleto: Centro italiano di studi sull'alto medioevo, 1972), pp. 669–717, esp. p. 683.

the more it was subject to dismemberment, rearrangement, abbreviation, interpolation and so forth.

Bewilderment in the face of these materials has, I would argue, set up an invisible road-block to our effort to describe the medicine of the period comprehensively. It boils down to this: How can one generalize from textual material that resists any general and consistent form? Given the fluid and protean character of early medieval medical sources, how can a historian declare that early medieval practitioners believed this or that, or did this or that?

My purpose in this essay is simply to set out this problem in some detail. My argument is that understanding the quality of early medieval medical knowledge depends on understanding the interactive dynamics of three elements in the process of its communication: the form of the manuscripts, the form of the texts, and the contents of the texts. These manuscripts are characteristically *florilegia* or anthologies. The texts within them are characteristically uncanonized, and the contents of these texts are distinctively non-theoretical. I shall attempt here to show how manuscript form, text form and text content shed light upon one another, and upon the issues of medical knowledge as early medieval people conceived them.

Manuscript vehicles for early medieval medical texts

Manuscript books differ from printed books with respect to the relationship between the text and its material support. Every copy of a printed book issuing from a single print run exactly resembles every other copy, not only with respect to the text itself, where there is word-for-word congruence, but also as to the format and layout of the volume. Every page in every copy of the book matches exactly; every line begins and ends with precisely the same words. In a manuscript situation, on the other hand, neither the text nor its physical presentation is congruent from copy to copy. Even in the unlikely event that two copies of a manuscript text match word for word, they will never match page for page or line for line, because the size of the parchment and the scale of the handwriting are peculiar to each act of copying. In short, medieval readers were accustomed to a situation where each discrete volume presented a unique encounter with the written text. It would not be much of an exaggeration to claim that, for them, the 'text' did not exist as an abstract entity; it was always *this* text, fused to *this* manuscript support. This underlay the distinctive medieval way of reading, digesting and remembering texts. Students were encouraged to learn a text from one particular manuscript volume, in order that its physical aspect –

layout, rubrication and even decoration – could assist them in imprinting and recalling the material.[7]

Second, printed books adopted at a very early stage a convention whereby each physical volume normally contains only one textual unit, or if it contains more than one, the texts are transparently related to each other by common authorship or subject. In the Middle Ages, however, a book in the textual sense (*liber*) was distinguished from a book in the physical sense (*volumen, codex*), because a physical volume more often than not contained more than one text. Moreover, in medieval manuscripts the cohabitation of texts within the same covers was not always governed by transparent criteria. Some manuscripts are composite, that is, the codex is formed of two or more originally independent manuscripts, bound together for convenience. Others, however, contain a number of texts, some evidently related, others much less evidently, copied at one time into a single volume. Such anthologies, whose contents are culled from a variety of sources, and then chosen and arranged by the compiler, are so characteristic of medieval book production that they have a distinctive generic name, florilegia (literally, 'nosegays of readings').

Florilegia of every dimension and on every topic are extraordinarily numerous, and notoriously challenging to study. To begin with, some florilegia circulate as canonized anthologies, while others, probably most, are assembled *ad hoc* by the compiler of the volume. Second, even within genre patterns, choice and above all arrangement of materials can vary widely. This process of selection and ordering is not mechanical or random; choice and arrangement almost invariably mean something. As Jaroslav Pelikan has expressed it, in a striking analogy,

a florilegium is, I have come to think, like a ransom note sent by a kidnapper. The identification of the newspapers from which the individual words and letters have been clipped may become a clue to the date of the note and to the whereabouts and habits of the kidnapper, but it is in the arrangement of the clippings, whatever their sources, that the meaning of the document lies.[8]

One of the most striking characteristics of medical manuscripts in the pre-Salernitan era is their predilection for florilegial form. The scholar who knew these manuscripts best, Augusto Beccaria, was also the first to observe that groups of texts tended to travel together; such manuscripts were not infrequently canonized anthologies. Beccaria

---

[7] For a detailed and magisterial discussion of this phenomenon, see Mary J. Carruthers, *The Book of Memory* (Cambridge: Cambridge University Press, 1990), particularly ch. 7, 'Memory and the Book'.

[8] *The Vindication of Tradition* (New Haven and London: Yale University Press, 1984), p. 74.

was mainly interested in clusters of texts by Galen and Hippocrates, which he saw as distant echoes of Alexandrian syllabi.[9] Gerhard Baader has signalled other canonized groupings, such as the 'herbal corpus' formed of the pseudo-Hippocratic *Epistula ad Maecenatem*, the herbals of pseudo-Apuleius and Antonius Musa, the *De taxone liber*, and pseudo-Dioscorides' *De herbis femininis*.[10] The preface of one of the more popular texts of early medieval medicine, Marcellus of Bordeaux's *De medicamentis*, is itself an anthology comprising texts on weights and measures, as well as the letters of pseudo-Hippocrates to Antiochus and Maecenas, and of Pliny, Cornelius Celsus and Vindicianus.

Moreover, the compilation or *ad hoc* florilegium is the preferred formal arrangement of early medieval medical manuscripts. Transmission of texts through florilegia is associated with the unsystematized, apprentice-style medical training of the early Middle Ages, which put a premium on personally significant and practical arrangements of material. Scholastic education, on the other hand, favoured the uniform and impersonal grouping of texts for formal, collective study, such as the *articella*.[11]

Yet it is precisely this florilegial form which presents serious interpretative difficulties for the historian, difficulties which are well illustrated by Peter Murray Jones's chapter on 'Medical Books Before the Invention of Printing' in the new edition of *Thornton's Medical Books*.[12] What is intriguing about this conspectus is that, in discussing Salernitan and Scholastic manuscripts, Jones concentrates on *texts*, but when he turns to pre-Salernitan and late medieval vernacular manuscripts, he focuses on *manuscript forms*. From reading Jones, it would be difficult to learn what a Scholastic medical manuscript looks like, but easy to discover what texts it contains: translations from Greek and Arabic writers, commentaries of these texts, compendia based upon them, and so forth.

On the other hand, he describes the contents of pre-Salernitan and vernacular manuscripts only generically, but their form in much detail. Describing one pre-Salernitan manuscript, Jones observes that its

[9] 'Sulle tracce di un antico canone latino di Ippocrate e di Galeno', part 1, *Italia medioevale e umanistica*, 2 (1959), 1–56; part 2, ibid., 4 (1962), 1–75; and part 3, ibid., 14 (1971), 1–21.
[10] 'Handschrift und Inkunabel in der Überlieferung der medizinischen Literatur', in Baader and Keil (note 2), pp. 363–4.
[11] See Gerhard Baader, 'Handschrift und Frühdruck als Überlieferungsinstrumente der Wissenschaften', *Berichte zur Wissenschaftsgeschichte*, 3 (1980), pp. 7–22, esp. pp. 8–13.
[12] Alain Besson (ed.), *Thornton's Medical Books, Libraries and Collectors. A Study of Bibliography and the Book Trade in Relation to the Medical Sciences*, 3rd edn (London: Gower, 1990), pp. 1–29.

florilegial form ignores textual integrity and textual boundaries by stitching together a wide variety of unascribed materials, apparently fragments of ancient medical treatises and encyclopaedias, to form a handbook of practical medicine (basic humoral physiology, blood-letting prescriptives, herbal pharmacy). In short, this is a 'ransom note' type of manuscript. However, Jones reads no message in the cut-out letters. For him, the early medieval indifference to canonized texts is evidence of cultural decline and mental confusion. In short, the dominance of florilegia over the canonized text is a symptom of decadence or low intellectual status.

Texts uncanonized and decanonized

Turning from the manuscripts to the texts they contain, we encounter a similarly fluid and unsettled situation. These texts display two salient characteristics: they are, to all appearances, deliberately decanonized; second, they are (again, apparently deliberately) stripped of theoretical elements. I shall discuss each of these characteristics separately, and then suggest ways in which decanonization and elimination of theory functioned synergetically.

In early medieval medical manuscripts, reverence for ancient authority coincides with extraordinary indifference to textual authenticity. Almost all the texts actually ascribed to Galen, for example, are pseudepigrapha; on the other hand, virtually all the genuine Galenic texts appear as fragments in anthologies, stripped of the author's name. This process of decanonizing ancient texts took a number of forms. The parent text might be dismembered into excerpts presented in isolation, or else creatively reassembled into new composite texts. Very frequently, the text was 'de-authorized' in the excerpting process. For example, in Beccaria's repertory, Galen's *Ad Glauconem de medendi methodo* appears in seventeen manuscripts. Of the eleven manuscripts of the full text, only three are unascribed, and one is mis-ascribed to Hippocrates. In the six manuscripts containing extracts, however, the text appears anonymously in four cases. Sometimes extracts took on a separate, but anonymous, textual existence: Alexander of Tralles' *Therapeutica* 2. 235–70, for example, circulated on its own as *De podagra*.[13] Indeed, Sigerist advised that, since so many chapters or groups of chapters from the works of Oribasius were transmitted independently and anonymously, 'whenever one finds unidentified short treatises, one should remember Oribasius'.[14]

Revision and re-working also entailed 'de-authorization'. When the

---

[13] See Sabbah et al. (note 5), p. 135.
[14] Sigerist (note 4, 1934), p. 567.

Latin translation of the *Therapeutica* of Alexander of Tralles was re-edited in the early Middle Ages, it emerged as the anonymous *Liber diaetarum diversorum medicorum*, and then rather later as book 5 of one of the many recensions of the *Physica Plinii*, the 'Florentino-Pragensis'.[15] But the licence to strip texts of their authorship could extend even to integral treatises. Of the nine manuscripts containing the full text of Sextus Placitus' *Liber medicinae ex animalibus* listed by Beccaria, five are unascribed; of the eleven of Vindicianus Afer's *Gynaecia*, only two contain the author's correct name.

It might be thought that decanonizing the text of a pagan author was a way of disparaging or disinfecting secular learning so that it could be safely used by Christians, but even a Church father like Isidore of Seville lost his authorial rights over his medical texts when they were anthologized. Extracts from his *Etymologiae* were frequently included in early medieval medical manuscripts, but in an overwhelming number of cases Isidore's name does not appear.[16] Moreover, de-authorizing seems to have occurred only when the manuscript context was medical in character. The one ancient medical text which never appears in an early medieval manuscript without its author's name is Quintus Serenus' *Liber medicinalis*. However, it is an exception which proves the rule, for the *Liber medicinalis* is a poem, and six of its seventeen surviving copies are in literary miscellanies, not medical books.[17]

Conversely, anonymous texts might be ascribed to an ancient authority, either by a sort of scholarly reflex (if it is medicine, it must be by Galen or Hippocrates) or because the text in question bore a generic resemblance to a genuine ancient text by that author. For example, because the *Liber medicinae ex herbis femininis* was inspired by Dioscorides, it was ascribed to him,[18] and when an early medieval compiler decided to reorganize and condense the herbals of Antonius Musa and pseudo-Apuleius, he reissued it under the name of Dioscorides.[19]

[15] The *Liber diaetarum diversorum medicorum* has not been edited: see Sabbah et al. (note 5), p. 111. For the various versions of the *Physica Plinii*, and its relationship to its earlier medieval antecedent, the *Medicina Plinii*, see Sabbah et al. (note 5), pp. 127–9.

[16] Of the thirteen manuscripts containing excerpts from *Etymologiae* book 4 (on medicine) in Beccaria's repertory, eleven are anonymous, and one (apparently) is ascribed to Hippocrates. There is one manuscript each of excerpts from books 13 (climate), 15 (ages of man), and 17 (agriculture), five of excerpts from book 16 (measures), and two of excerpts from book 20 (food and drink), all unascribed.

[17] These literary anthologies are described in Beccaria (note 4), pp. 17, 20, 30, 32 and 141. On Quintus Serenus, see Sabbah et al. (note 5), pp. 142–4.

[18] See John Riddle, 'Pseudo-Dioscorides' *Ex herbis femininis* and Early Medieval Medical Botany', *Journal of the History of Biology*, 14 (1981), 43–81. For editions, see Sabbah et al. (note 5), pp. 70–1.

[19] Herten, Bibliothek des Grafen Nesselrode-Reichenstein 192 (s. IX fin. and s. XI/XII), fols. 1r–15v; for a description, see Beccaria (note 4), p. 55.

It is here, indeed, that we can best observe what truly interested early medieval medical readers, for the more interested they were in a subject, the more they tinkered with its texts. Pharmacology, materia medica and recipe literature are by far the best represented subject areas in the manuscripts. Consequently, probably the most disturbed textual traditions are found in herbal pharmacology.

A telling example is furnished by the *Dynamidia Hippocratis*. Its sixth-century compiler reworked the Latin translation of book 2 of the pseudo-Hippocratic *Regimen*, and supplemented it with borrowings from other sources, especially the *Medicinae ex oleribus et pomis* of Gargilius Martialis. It has been argued that the compilation was originally in four books, covering cereals and vegetables, bitter vegetables and wild herbs, fruits, and finally, animal food and drinks. However, it was seldom transmitted in exactly this arrangement in the manuscripts,[20] and as we shall see shortly, the assumption that there was any such 'original' may be an artefact of editorial canon-mindedness.

What is striking about many of these 'artificial' texts is the care with which they are presented in textual format, that is, ordered into chapters and books.[21] To cite but one outstanding example, Bamberg Staatsbibliothek cod. med. 1 (s. IX[1]), the renowned *Lorscher Arzneibuch*, advertises itself in its rubrics as a rationally organized anthology, arranged in formal chapters.[22] Clearly, the impulse to deconstruct canonized texts and reassemble them was deliberate and meaningful: manuscripts are 'ransom notes' with coded messages about the medical preoccupations of early medieval readers.

Even when they conveyed an ancient medical text intact, and under its author's name, early medieval medical manuscripts reveal how unwilling their creators were to leave the text alone. Interpolation was one way of improving a text, abbreviation another. A particularly striking example of both is the medieval version of Galen's *Ad*

---

[20] See Sabbah et al. (note 5), p. 73, and Loren C. MacKinney, ' "Dynamidia" in *Medieval Medical Literature*', *Isis*, 24 (1936), 400–14. Significantly, the book on bitter vegetables and wild herbs circulated separately as *De herbis Galieni Apollonii et Ciceronis*.

[21] This effort at coherence in such 'consolidated' texts has been remarked on in the case of some St Gall Manuscripts, by MacKinney (note 2), p. 54, and with respect to Berlin Staatsbibliothek, Phillipps 1790, by Beccaria (note 4), Introduction, pp. 38–9.

[22] For a brief description, see Beccaria (note 4), p. 48. The *Lorscher Arzneibuch* has been fully transcribed, annotated and translated (into German) by Ulrich Stoll, *Das 'Lorscher Arzneibuch'. Ein medizinisches Kompendium des 8. Jahrhunderts (Codex Bambergensis medicinalis 1). Text, Übersetzung und Fachglossar*, Sudhoffs Archiv, Beiheft 28 (Stuttgart: Franz Steiner, 1992). See also Gundolf Keil and Paul Schnitzer (eds.), *Das Lorscher Arzneibuch und die frühmittelalterliche Medizin. Verhandlungen des medizinhistorischen Symposiums im September 1989 in Lorsch* (Lorsch: Verlag Laurissa, 1991).

Glauconem de medendi methodo. The work which circulated in the early Middle Ages under this title is not exactly a translation of Galen's authentic work. There are numerous omissions (particularly of theoretical material) as well as interpolations, notoriously of an entire spurious third book.[23] Again, alphabetization of medical texts, particularly those concerned with drugs, made reference easier. Oribasius, for instance, was reworked to group his materia medica into alphabetical sections.[24] Other forms of creative and useful reorganization were also possible: Modena Archivio capitolare cod. O.I.11 (s. VIII ex. or IX in.) has a version of the *Herbarium* of pseudo-Apuleius reorganized according to therapeutic indications, i.e., the ailment for which the herb is prescribed.[25] Finally, recasting material into poetic form was a way of making a text easy to assimilate and recall.

However, the situation presented by these texts poses serious problems for the student of early medieval medicine. Modern editions of the texts that were available to early medieval readers, while both interesting and important, can ultimately yield an impression of early medieval medical knowledge that is misleading, because they present the texts in a manner almost diametrically opposed to the way in which a medieval reader would have encountered them. While it is true, for example, that Alexander of Tralles' *Therapeutica* was known in the early Middle Ages, the historian who wishes to claim that this or that statement of Alexander's was the basis for any particular early medieval text or practice would be unwise to rely on any version of his text other than those found in the early medieval manuscripts. First of all, the Latin translation is an adaptation which condenses the twelve books of the Greek original into three, inserts additional material from Alexander's treatise on fevers, and interpolates into book 2 considerable material from other sources.[26] Second, of the five surviving early medieval manuscripts, only three contain the whole Latin adaptation; the other two contain fragments and extracts.[27] Third, as I mentioned earlier, Alexander's treatise appeared in a number of adapted and anonymous forms. In short, Alexander of

[23]   See Sabbah et al. (note 5), p. 85.
[24]   Two separate alphabetical reworkings appear in Laon, Bibliothèque publique 424 (s. IX med.) (see Wickersheimer (note 4), p. 36), and Copenhagen, Kgl. Bibliotek, Gamle Kgl. Samling 1653 (s. XI) fols. 189r–215v (Beccaria (note 4), p. 8).
[25]   For description, see Beccaria (note 4), p. 93.
[26]   There is no critical edition of the Latin translation. See Sabbah et al. (note 5), pp. 32–3, for Renaissance editions.
[27]   For the integral text see Beccaria (note 4), pp. 9, 95, and 31; for fragments and extracts, see Beccaria (note 4), pp. 45 and 106.

Tralles' work can be said to be 'available' in the early Middle Ages only in a strictly qualified way.

But the effects of text edition can be even more insidious. It can literally create 'texts' which do not exist, for example the *Sapientia artis medicinae*.[28] This 'text' comprises a survey of humoral physiology, a brief tract on ophthalmology, and finally an inventory of diseases and their causes. Wlaschky found the three sections grouped together, and titled *Sapientia artis medicinae*, in two manuscripts, Glasgow, Hunter T.4.13 (s. IX/X) and St Gall 751. The other two manuscripts used for his edition, St Gall 44 (s. X) and Rome, Biblioteca Angelica N 1502 (s. XIII/XIV) were not so titled, and do not contain the third section. Wlaschky therefore designated these two manuscripts as 'incomplete' versions of the 'full' text, represented by the Glasgow and St Gall 751 codices, and laid out a *stemma* accordingly, in the orthodox manner of a classically trained recensionist editor. But we cannot assume that the 'full' text version of the *Sapientia* is in any way the 'original'. In BN lat. 11219, for example, parts 1 and 2 appear together, but part 3 is copied elsewhere in the volume, and in another hand. In BN nouv. acq. lat. 229, only part 1 appears; in Montecassino 97 and in St Gall 759, only part 3. The rubric for the text group in Montecassino V 225 is not *Sapientia artis medicinae*, which bespeaks a formal compendium, but rather 'Epistole Ypocratis et aliorum', which suggests an anthology of discrete texts. In short, the text which Wlaschky presented as the canonized form of a 'frühmittelalterliche Kompendium' may be only one of several ways in which one or more of its three component parts might be 'packaged'. It would be a distortion to describe the manuscripts which do not contain all three sections as 'fragments', or to label the Montecassino and Vatican versions as 'mis-ascribed'. But the effect of Wlaschky's edition has been to reify one form of packaging as *the* text, and reduce all others to variants.[29]

Medicine without theory

Early medieval people seem to have been extremely interested in healing, but only minimally aware of the possibility of a system which

[28]   M. Wlaschky, '*Sapientia artis medicinae*. Ein frühmittelalterliche Kompendium der Medizin', *Kyklos*, 1 (1928), 103–13.

[29]   These strictures concerning the *Sapientia artis medicinae*, as well as other editions of early medieval texts, are articulated by Beccaria (note 4), Introduction, pp. 42–3. For a more sensible approach to editing a similar text-group, see Rudolf Laux, 'Ars medicinae. Ein frühmittelalterliches Kompendium der Medizin', *Kyklos*, 3 (1930), 417–34.

explains disease and relates this explanation to the coherent picture of the human body. If we look at the subject-matter of the texts available in the pre-Salernitan period, and compare the frequency of various themes, this disinterest in theoretical issues becomes very evident. Basic humoral physiology, preventive medicine and, above all, herbal pharmacy were the topics in which early medieval readers showed the keenest interest.[30]

In places where one might expect to find medical theory, there is little or none. Of the handful of texts which might be characterized as 'philosophy', the *Problemata* ascribed to Aristotle is probably the only text which directly concerns issues of medical philosophy. However, the *Problemata* is not a systematic treatise setting out a coherent medical world-view, but a collection of questions and responses on diverse subjects in physiology. Likewise the *Disputatio Platonis et Aristotelis*, though often found in medical manuscripts, discusses the nature of the soul, not the body.[31]

Similarly, the texts on humoral physiology and pathology, on diseases and remedies, and on diagnosis and semeiotics are heavily weighted towards description and practical applications. In the case of semeiotics, the single most ubiquitous category of texts concerns prognosis; but almost all these texts are either bald lists of signs and significations, unrelated to any underlying explanation of what is occurring in the body (e.g. pseudo-Democritus' *Prognostica*, or the pseudo-Hippocratic *Capsula eburnea*), or else divinatory devices (e.g. the Egyptian Days). Pathology tends towards the descriptive, and often has only a tenuous

---

[30] My observations on the subject-matter of texts contained in early medieval medical manuscripts are based on a tabulation by topic of the incidence of texts in the manuscripts listed in Beccaria (note 4). I have counted the number of manuscripts in which a text occurs, not the number of times it occurs. In most cases there is no difference, but in the case of glossaries, dietary calendars, receptaria, and materials of this nature, many manuscripts contain two or more texts. I have not distinguished between integral texts and fragments or excerpts. My findings may be summarized as follows: medicine 151 (introductions 25; compendia 93; aphorisms 18; medical philosophy 15); history of medicine 11; medical deontology 21; medical glossaries 30; humoral physiology and pathology 54; environmental medicine 8; ages of man 2; hygiene and preventive medicine 96 (hygiene in general 2; balneology and hydrotherapy 2; dietetics 28; seasonal regimen 64); diagnosis and medical semeiotics 112 (general 40; prognosis and prognostica 72); diseases and cures 65; obstetrics, gynaecology and embryology 44; ophthalmology 1; surgery 58 (general 12; phlebotomy 46); pharmacology 324 (materia medica 163; receptaria 137; weights and measures 24).

[31] This text survives in two versions: a presumably older one, and a more recent one demonstrating clear Christian influences. It has been edited by Herbert Normann, 'Disputatio Platonis et Aristotelis. Ein apokrypher Dialog aus dem frühen Mittelalter', *Sudhoffs Archiv*, 23 (1930), 68–86.

connection with humoral theory.[32] Humoral physiology and pathology, where found, are also tilted towards the practical. The *Epistula de ratione ventris vel viscerum*, for example, is an essay in applied humoral theory, concerned with digestion and the genesis of disease.[33] Finally, little attention is given to anatomy, though there are discussions of diseases arranged by affected organ.[34] Nor did the introductions to medicine or the medical compendia offer much theory; indeed, the medieval *Ad Glauconem de medendi methodo*, as I pointed out earlier, omitted the theoretical material in the original. On the other hand, where theoretical or philosophical reflections on the nature of medicine do appear, they often do so as unascribed, adventitious extracts.[35]

The dynamic relationship between the elimination of theory and the decanonization of texts is aptly illustrated by the early medieval fortunes of a distinctive and prestigious corpus, namely the texts by or ascribed to Hippocrates.[36] During the fifth to seventh centuries, Latin translations were prepared or revised of Hippocrates' *Prognosticon, De victus ratione, De aëris, aquis et locis, Aphorismi, De hebdomadibus* and *De mulierum affectibus*,[37]

[32] A good example is the section on diseases and cures (part 3) in the *Sapientia artis medicinae*. The author leads off each section by asking what humour causes each disease, but the response does not address the role of the humours at all. For instance, 'What humour causes frenzy? It is caused by too much wine and cold water. First, they catch a semitertian fever from the cold; due to this disorder, the veins emit a morbid discharge, and the brain is cut off (*suspenditur*), and people suffer from insomnia and become insane' (p. 108). 'Humour' seems to mean everything from ingested liquid (wine and water) to distillation; the only traditional humour mentioned is melancholy, to which, indeed, virtually all the diseases are ascribed.

[33] Edited by Veit Scherer, 'Die *Epistula de ratione ventris vel viscerum*. Ein Beitrag zur Geschichte des Galenismus im frühen Mittelalter', Zahnmed. Diss., Freie Universität Berlin (1976).

[34] E.g. in St Gall 44 (II) (s. IX²) (Beccaria (note 4), p. 129).

[35] For example in B.N. lat. 6882A (I) (s. IX¹) (Beccaria (note 4), p. 26), in the margins of fol. 6r appears a text with the rubric 'Quot naturis constat medicina', and incipit, 'Medicina decem causis constat...'

[36] On the late antique Latin translations of the Hippocratic and pseudo-Hippocratic works in general, see Innocenzo Mazzini, 'Caratteri comuni a tutto l'Ippocrate latino tardo-antico e conseguenti considerazioni su alcuni emendamenti al testo', in Mazzini and Fusco (note 2), pp. 65–74; and his 'Le traduzioni latine di Ippocrate esequite nei secoli V e VI: limiti e caratteristiche della sopravvivenza del corpus ippocratico fra tardo antico ed alto medioevo', in Françcois Laserre and Philippe Mudry (eds.), *Formes de pensée dans la Collection hippocratique. Actes du IVe colloque international hippocratique (Lausanne, 21–26 septembre 1981)*, Université de Lausanne, Publications de la Faculté des lettres, 26 (Geneva: Droz, 1983), pp. 483–92; Jole Agrimi, 'L'Hippocrates latinus nella tradizione manoscritta e nella cultura altomedievali', in Mazzini and Fusco (note 2), pp. 388–98.

[37] For editions of the early medieval Latin translations, see Beccaria (note 4), *s.v.* 'Hippocrate'. On the early medieval fortunes of *De mulierum affectibus*, see the outstanding study by Monica Green, 'The Transmission of Ancient Theories of Female Physiology and Disease through the Early Middle Ages', unpublished Ph.D. thesis, Princeton University (1985).

as well as of other works comprising the syllabus for medical instruction in Alexandria.

The centre of much of this translation activity was Ravenna, headquarters of the Byzantine exarchate or provincial administration in Italy until 752, and from 489 to 552 the capital of the Ostrogothic kingdom of Theodoric. When Theodoric's secretary of state Cassiodorus retired to his estates in Calabria to found the monastery of Vivarium, he took with him a library which included a number of translated medical classics. In the section of his *Institutes of Divine and Human Letters* devoted to medicine, Cassiodorus exhorts the brethren responsible for the care of the sick to learn the nature of herbs and the mixing of drugs, and recommends some books in which those who know no Greek can learn these things: Dioscorides, 'Hippocrates and Galen (that is, the *Therapeutics* of Galen, addressed to the philosopher Glauco) and a certain anonymous work, which has been compiled from various authors', Caelius Aurelianus, and 'Hippocrates on herbs and cures, and various other works on the art of medicine, [which] with God's help I have left you ... stored away in the recesses of our library'.[38]

While manuscript evidence indicates that there were teachers (*iatrosophistae*) at Ravenna[39] giving public instruction based on these same texts and producing commentaries on them, it was nonetheless Vivarium's approach which was destined to dominate the early medieval West. Vivarium's medicine is exclusively clinical and therapeutic, without the theoretical and philosophical elements so characteristic of Alexandria, and especially of Galenism. The involvement of clergy and monks in medical care (albeit never to the exclusion of the lay physician) reinforced an already noticeable tendency in the Latin-speaking world to prefer practical texts, and to confine medicine to a constellation of interests in materia medica, pharmacology, medical semeiotics and fairly unsophisticated humoral physiology.

The Latin canon of Hippocrates provides an excellent laboratory for determining what ancient texts early medieval people wanted translated, and what they did with the translations once they got them. The *Prognosticon*, the classic manual of medical semeiotics and special pathology, was indeed 'available', but only one manuscript of the complete translation survives, along with two fragmentary and much less

---

[38] *Institutiones*, 1.31.2, trans. Leslie Webber Jones, in *An Introduction to Divine and Human Readings* (New York: W.W. Norton, 1946, 1969), p. 136.

[39] The most significant manuscript witnesses are discussed by Beccaria (note 9, part 1), and by Sigerist (note 2), pp. 39–40. Compare Owsei Temkin, 'Byzantine Medicine: Tradition and Empiricism', *Dumbarton Oaks Papers*, 16 (1962), 102–3.

successful translation attempts.[40] In stark contrast to the rarity of the authentic text is the wide diffusion of pseudo-Hippocratic prognostica, a clan of heterogeneous texts ranging in quality from the fairly respectable *Indicia valetudinum* to iatromathematical schemes for predicting the outcome of disease on the basis of the day of the lunar or solar month on which the patient fell ill, such as the *Epitomum Ypocratis de infirmis*.

The fate of the *Prognosticon* reveals, first, that authentic ancient writings were relatively neglected in favour of pseudepigrapha. Second, while semeiotics is a popular subject, it is not oriented towards aetiology or diagnosis, but rather towards prognosis. Indeed, this predilection, so markedly characteristic of the pseudo-Hippocratic prognostica, may in fact be the reason why the authentic text was less popular. Rejection of theory and decanonization go hand in hand.

De aëris, aquis et locis likewise did not fare well in the early medieval period, possibly because its translation was awkwardly literal.[41] *De salubri dieta* and *De victus ratione*, on the other hand, led long and vigorous textual lives. Both were essentially treatises on hygiene, offering a straightforward humoralism which related the constitution of the body to the seasons and explained differences due to age and sex, while surveying the properties of various kinds of food and drink, climates, baths and forms of exercise.

The fortunes of these two works, however, show that early medieval readers could not resist tampering with a text which they valued. 'Pure' copies of *De victus ratione*, for instance, are rather uncommon, and even when they can be found, they have invariably been worked over, with some chapters omitted and new ones inserted, generally to 'update' the work, or to adapt it to transalpine conditions.[42] In fact, where *De victus ratione* found its major diffusion was as the chief source of another, similar work, the *Dynamidia*, which in its turn was subjected to a variety of prunings and interpolations.

De victus ratione was also recycled into individual manuscript

---

[40] The complete version is in Milan Ambrosiana G.108 inf. (s. IX²). The fragmentary version in St Gall, Stiftsbibliothek 44.II, has been edited by Henry E. Sigerist, 'Fragment einer unbekannten lateinischen Übersetzung des hippokratischen Prognosticon', *Archiv für Geschichte der Medizin*, 23 (1930), 87–90. On other fragmentary versions, see Beccaria (note 9, part 1), p. 11.

[41] Beccaria (note 9, part 1), p. 19.

[42] Ibid., p. 28.

compilations,[43] and reworked into one of the most popular of early medieval Latin medical texts, the *Dieta Theodori*, a concise, well-organized little treatise which, among other things, updates for medieval Western readers the list of wines in the original Hippocratic text. Revisions and reworkings such as were perpetrated upon *De victus ratione* suggest a lively and sustained interest in medical matters, fundamentally empirical or practical in character, but withal confident and intelligent.

Perhaps the most popular item of the early medieval Hippocratic canon was the pseudonymous *Epistola ad Maecenatem*, also known as the *Liber de natura generis humani*. This work is a Latin translation of Hippocrates' *De mulierum affectibus*, joined together with the section of the *Gynaecia* of the fourth-century African physician Vindicianus Afer devoted to the anatomy and physiology of the internal organs. A prefatory letter, purportedly from Hippocrates to Maecenas, announces a work divided into three parts: a treatise on conception, one on internal organs, and finally a philosophical and moral conclusion. Beccaria suggests that the treatise was confected to answer the promise contained in the letter; if so, it is rather significant that a philosophical and moral conclusion was never found to make up the third book.[44]

Finally, even when they were translating the canonized works of Hippocrates into Latin, early medieval physicians manifested their interest in the text by changing and 'improving' it, in the interests of scientific clarity (e.g. additions of detail to instructions for preparing a medicament), or of didactic effectiveness (e.g. internal references, glossing of terminology, suppression of repetitions).[45]

But the translators of ancient medical texts introduced other, more problematic kinds of modifications. For some time, these modifications went unnoticed, because they looked like simple mistranslations. However, Innocenzo Mazzini has pointed out that in some cases the 'mistranslation' is a deliberate attempt to censor some philosophical or ethical point of the Hippocratic text. In *De victus ratione*, for example, modifications were introduced which effaced allusions in the original to the divinity of the material cosmos. In the Ravenna translation of

---

[43]   It appears as the first and fourth books of a compendium on the properties of plants found in St Gall ‹762 (Paris, 1st quarter of s. IX). The first book of the St Gall compilation is an abbreviation of the *Dynamidia*, the second the herbal of pseudo-Apuleius, the third an extract in Latin from Galen's *De simplicium medicamentorum temperamentis et facultatibus* (here without ascription), and book 4 is the sections of *De victus ratione* not already included in the *Dynamidia*: Beccaria (note 9, part 1), pp. 30–1. The St Gall compilation was edited by Valentine Rose, *Anecdota graeca et graecolatina*, vol. 2 (Berlin: Dümmler, 1870), pp. 131–50.

[44]   Beccaria (note 9, part 1), pp. 53–4.

[45]   Mazzini (note 36, 1983), pp. 487–9.

De mulierum affectibus, references to the necessary role of woman's sexual desire in conception are deleted. Monogamy is subtly stressed by the gratuitous addition of *suus* in any reference to the man with whom the woman consorts.[46] In short, Hippocratic texts were valuable enough to translate, but their translators were under no illusions about their total compatibility with Christian ways of thinking. We must ask, then, whether the early medieval avoidance of medical theory was deliberate.

A deliberate elimination of theory

Until recently, this disconcerting lack of theory seemed relatively simple to explain. It was argued that Christian ascetics and Church leaders were hostile to ancient medicine as a rational and essentially pagan rival to religious healing. Christian religious healing, based on relics, prayers and miracles, was radically set over against natural or scientific medicine, grounded in reason and experience. The issue for ordinary Christians was: To whom should they resort when ill, the saint or the physician?[47] The conflict was therefore between rival practices; theory did not really enter into it. A corollary of this position is that the absence of theory in early medieval medicine was an accident of history, the result of the cultural disruption of late Antiquity and the intellectual poverty of the early Middle Ages. The implication is that ancient medical theory was something which medieval people would have welcomed had they known about it, or had they the intelligence and leisure to appreciate it.

The major challenges which have been posed to this model suggest, however, that the cleavage between Hippocratic-style medicine and Christian medicine was not, in fact, along lines of practice. The religious elements within ancient Hippocratic and Galenic medicine, and the phenomenon of pagan religious healing in late Antiquity are attracting more concerted attention.[48] It is evident as well that in the early Middle

---

[46] 'Cristianesimo e scienza pagana: tracce di un conflitto nelle traduzioni latine di Ippocrate eseguite nei secoli V e VI', in *Saggi di storia del pensiero scientifico dedicati a V. Tonini* (Rome: Jouvence, 1983), pp. 69–77.

[47] This is the interpretation favoured, e.g., by MacKinney (note 2), pp. 23ff.

[48] See Owsei Temkin, *Hippocrates in a World of Pagans and Christians* (Baltimore: Johns Hopkins University Press, 1991), ch. 14, 'Was there a Hippocratic religion?' On the generalized interest in miracles and religious healing in late Antiquity, see Robert M. Grant, *Miracle and Natural Law in Greco-Roman and Early Christian Thought* (Amsterdam: North-Holland, 1952); Howard Clark Kee, *Miracle in the Early Christian World* (New Haven: Yale University Press, 1983), esp. ch. 3, 'Asklepios the Healer'; and Aline Rouselle, *Croire et guérir. La Foi en Gaule dans l'Antiquité tardive* (Paris: Fayard, 1990).

Ages, non-religious medicine not only never died out, but was used without scruple by bishops, abbots and popes. Fiercely ascetic desert hermits consulted doctors and counselled others to do so; monks like St Basil of Caesarea were instrumental in founding the first Christian public hospitals, one of whose functions was to dispense conventional medicine.[49] Moreover, as time passed, non-religious medicine came more and more to be practised by monks and clergy. Plainly the 'two medicines' were not seen as inherently incompatible kinds of practice. On the other hand, the subtle and precise manner in which the translators censored Hippocrates bespeaks a clear understanding of the *ideological* tensions between the world-view of ancient medicine, and that of Christianity.

Two recent studies have clarified the subtleties of this ideological strife. Gundolf Keil's essay 'Möglichkeiten und Grenzen frühmittelalterlicher Medizin'[50] argues that monasticism was self-consciously hostile to the naturalism and to the covert philosophical assumptions of ancient medicine. The monks' specific response, significantly, was to *dismember* the ancient medical texts, salvaging the practical material while dismantling the larger structures and arguments that might convey, or at least imply, potentially offensive modes of explanation. Since the originals were almost all in Greek, and since the West was increasingly unilingual, and without the material or political incentives available in the Islamic world to promote translations, the fundamental arguments of ancient medicine – its nosology, aetiology, pathology – were simply rendered invisible. In Keil's view, this had a determining effect on the form of the early medieval medical manuscript as a florilegium of uncanonized or decanonized texts.[51]

Keil also perspicaciously notes the 'functional ambivalence' of the epistolary form in which early medieval anonymous or pseudonymous texts are often cast.[52] Gerhard Baader has likewise observed that short treatises and letters are the favoured forms of early medieval medical literature, and stand in sharp contrast to the formal compendia and encyclopaedias of Arabic and Scholastic medicine. Such short treatises are by their nature unconducive to extended argument or abstraction, and philosophically unpretentious. Baader points out that this demotion of medical texts, combined with their uncanonized status, effectively excluded medicine from consideration as a branch of the

---

[49] Temkin (note 48), ch. 12.
[50] Keil and Schnitzer (note 22), pp. 219–52.
[51] Ibid., pp. 229–30.
[52] Ibid., p. 223.

Liberal Arts.[53] It should be noted that Cassiodorus discussed medicine in the 'divine readings' section of his *Institutiones*, as part of monastic praxis, not in the 'human readings' section, with the Liberal Arts. As Baader indicates, the emergence of medicine into the Salernitan era is marked not only by the arrival of fresh texts, but by the conceptualization of a distinction between medical knowledge and medical practice.

But in the pre-Salernitan centuries, medicine was treated as a craft, not a branch of knowledge; it could not make knowledge claims in its own right, nor be pursued for its own sake, nor aspire to the status of 'wisdom'. The freedom with which its textual materials were treated is of a piece with the absence of theory within the texts themselves. And there is every evidence that this is exactly what earnest Christians wanted medicine to be.

Owsei Temkin, in his study of *Hippocrates in a World of Pagans and Christians*, demonstrates clearly that while Christians held a variety of opinions about the legitimacy of resorting to secular medicine, they were consistent and united in their insistence that this secular medicine renounce three claims: the global naturalistic explanation of disease, the belief in the corporeality of the soul, and the conception of the physician as autonomous healer. Christians could no more do without an idea of nature than pagans could, but they differed from pagans in insisting that nature was neither divine nor the exclusive ruler of the human body. Hence the physician was obliged to acknowledge that some diseases – perhaps most – were caused by God rather than nature. The corollary was that resorting to medicine would not be in every case effective, or even ethical. Second, the soul, for Christians, was an immaterial substance with a separate destiny from the body. This had implications both for interpreting disorders (e.g., 'possession'), and for the value placed upon bodily medicine as a whole. Finally, physicians were at best the agents of God, the true healer; they should not presume to claim the power to heal themselves.[54]

Temkin points out that these issues remained lively ones in the East,

---

[53] 'Lehrbrief und Kurztraktat in der medizinischen Wissensvermittlung des Früh- und Hochmittelalters', in Norbert Richard Wolf (ed.), *Wissenorganisierende und wissensver-mittelnde Literatur im Mittelalter*, Wissensliteratur im Mittelalter, 1 (Wiesbaden: Dr Ludwig Reichert Verlag, 1987), pp. 246–54, esp. pp. 253–4. See also Joan Cadden, *The Meaning of Sex Difference in the Middle Ages* (Cambridge: Cambridge University Press, 1993), pp. 39–53; I became aware of Cadden's work after the final version of this essay was submitted. Many of her conclusions about the relationship between text form and lack of theory in early medieval medical treatises coincide with those presented here, though she uses different sources and different arguments.

[54] See the illuminating comparison of Marcellus of Bordeaux's medical writings to contemporary hagiographical texts in Peter Brown's *The Cult of the Saints* (Chicago: University of Chicago Press, 1981), pp. 113–27.

because the ancient medical texts were always around to be read, and in the common language of learning. In the West, on the other hand, the challenge of Hippocratism was quickly extinguished, because only a handful of texts were available in bowdlerized translation.[55] What is not acknowledged, even by Temkin, is that the triumph of 'monastic medicine' went beyond the amputation of medical theory, especially theory about how diseases are caused, and the agency by which they are cured. Christian medicine substituted its own form of medical theory, a theory which can be detected in the texts of the early medieval period.

This substitution theory is less a coherent medical world-view than a constellation of concepts, some derived from ancient medicine itself, which reinforced the Christian ideology of disease and healing outlined by Temkin. The first of these involved prognosis. As we have seen, prognosis and prognostics occupy a very important position in the medical literature of this period. In a telling passage, Cassiodorus characterizes medical knowledge as a whole in terms of prognosis: 'By his art [the physician] finds out things about a man about which he himself is ignorant; and his prognosis of a case, though founded on reason, seems to the ignorant like a prophecy.'[56]

The link of prognosis and prophecy is a significant one for Christians. Stephanus, a late Alexandrian professor of medicine and a Christian, sees prognosis as a divine attribute which assimilates the physician, like the prophet, to God.[57] In the abbey of St Gall in the tenth century, the expertise of the monk-physician Notker was described not in relation to his ability to explain or even cure disease, but in terms of his almost preternatural powers of prognosis.[58] What is significant about prognosis is that it sidesteps the whole issue of cause and cure. The physician's skill, perhaps one ought to say his gift, was to foresee what God would do to the patient, not to discern the cause of his ailment, nor yet to lay claim to a cure. He had insight into time, not power over the body.

This emphasis on time is a particularly Christian response to ancient

[55] Temkin (note 48), p. 241. He also suggests (pp. 214–16) that the medical profession in the Greek East remained dominated by pagans for much longer than was the case in the West; see also Keil and Schnitzer (note 22), p. 228.
[56] Cassiodorus, *Variae*, 6.19, in A. Fridh (ed.), *Corpus Christianorum series latina*, vol. 96 (Turnhout: Brepols, 1973). This translation is from MacKinney (note 2), p. 47.
[57] Temkin (note 48), p. 192.
[58] In the *Casus Sancti Galli*, Ekkehard IV relates a number of stories of Notker's almost divinatory prowess, e.g. how he predicted, on the basis of the smell of the blood emanating from a patient's nosebleed, that the patient would fall ill with smallpox: Hans F. Haefele (ed.), *Ekkehard IV. St. Galler Klostergeschichte*, Ausgewählte Quellen zur deutschen Geschichte des Mittelalters, no. 10 (Darmstadt: Wissenschaftliche Buchgesellschaft, 1980), p. 240. Significantly, Ekkehard never suggests that there was some logical train of reasoning behind Notker's prognoses.

philosophical and medical naturalism. Nature, in the Christian world-view, does not disappear, but is stripped of its divinity and its identity with fate or necessity. It is God's creation and tool, and only His will has true necessity. For an early medieval historian like Gregory of Tours, for instance, chronological coincidence becomes a mode of causation. Nature itself becomes simply the wonted pattern of events in time, and God's intervention is signalled by ruptures in this pattern: roses blooming in January become a sign of divine communication.[59]

Early medieval people saw time as a crucial element in the physician's expertise. Isidore of Seville, commenting on how medicine uses all the seven Liberal Arts, says that the medical man should know arithmetic, so as to calculate the times and periods of the day. 'Finally also, he ought to know astronomy by which he should study the motions of the stars and the changes of seasons, for as a certain physician said, our bodies are also changed with their courses.'[60] Time also assumed the explanatory functions once enjoyed by nature or necessity. I will illustrate this by examining the time-themes in the *Sapientia artis medicinae*.

As I explained earlier, this 'text' is really a mosaic of quasi-independent tractates, but this in itself suits it to our purposes, for it shows how widely such themes are scattered across the spectrum of early medieval medical thought. The first section of the *Sapientia* is a summary of humoral physiology and pathology. Interestingly, the humours are not connected with either the elements or the primal qualities of hot, cold, moist and dry, but they are associated with the four seasons, as are the various diseases connected with them. They are also associated with the four ages of human life in a passage evidently derived from Vindicianus Afer's *Epistula ad Pentadium*. Most curious, however, is the passage which closes this initial segment of the *Sapientia*: 'The human head is positioned at four angles, but it rests at a fifth. There are eight bones in the face; however, we distinguish the [two]

<hr>

[59]   Giselle de Nie presents a sensitive and original reading of Gregory's understanding of nature and causality in *Views from a Many-Windowed Tower: Studies of Imagination in the Works of Gregory of Tours* (Amsterdam: Rodopi, 1987), and in 'Roses in January', *Journal of Medieval History*, 5 (1979), 258–89. There is surprisingly little historical analysis of the concept of nature in the period between the Patristic age and the twelfth century 'renaissance', apart from studies of rare figures like Scottus Eriugena. Charles Radding's *A World Made by Men. Cognition and Society, 400–1200* (Chapel Hill and London: University of North Carolina Press, 1985), attempts to characterize the early medieval understanding of natural causality, but its application of Piaget's models of cognitive development to historical cultures, especially cultures based on written texts, is not convincing.

[60]   W.W. Lindsay (ed.), *Etymologiae*, 4.13 (Oxford: Clarendon Press, 1911). The translation is by William D. Sharpe, *Isidore of Seville: The Medical Writings*, Transactions of the American Philosophical Society, n.s. 54 (Philadelphia: American Philosophical Society, 1964), p. 64.

jaws. There are 228 bones in the human body, but in women, 226, and in *frigiscis*[61] 227. There are 32 teeth, and in women, 30.'[62]

The editor of the *Sapientia*, Wlaschky, sees this curious calculus as a kind of anatomical numerology, since all the numbers (setting aside those applicable to women) are divisible by four, corresponding to the *quaternitas* of the elements, qualities, seasons etc.[63] In part 2, on ophthalmology, the accent on enumeration becomes even more pronounced. There are not only seven tunics to the eye,[64] but seven cataracts, and each cataract should be couched at a specific time following its onset. Here, the text has broken free of its ancient models, for the classical texts distinguish cataracts by colour, not by number, and none of them make mention of time-constraints on couching.[65] Closer to ancient sources is the next piece of advice, namely that cataracts should be cured in spring, summer and autumn, but not operated on in winter. Our author adds new details, however: the treatment is to unfold over nine days, on each of which there is a specific medical ritual, such as special diet, phlebotomy, etc.

In the third part, on diseases and cures, the zeal for enumeration reaches new heights. The text opens with a list of the *number* of cures for each kind of disease. We are not told *what* the cures are, but simply *how many* of them there are: twenty-four for the head, twelve for the eye, twenty-five for the thorax and so on. Though the figures understandably vary amongst the manuscript witnesses, the total number of cures for the whole body, in the Glasgow manuscript at least, totals 365, the number of days in the year – a point which the editor rightly thought significant.

This predilection for counting, numbering and measuring might at first sight seem oddly primitive, some bleedthrough from Germanic or Celtic folklore, with its penchant for organizing knowledge into numbered lists or triads. But an alternative explanation lies much closer to hand in the form of the medieval science of calendar construction, the *computus*.[66]

---

61   Wlaschky (note 28) does not know what to make of this term, and neither do I. Though the passage as a whole is dependent on Vindicianus, *Epistula altera*, this term does not occur there.

62   Wlaschky (note 28), p. 106, lines 12–15.

63   Ibid., p. 112.

64   The source of this number is uncertain. Ancient ophthalmological texts list only four tunics, though Arabic texts also list seven: ibid.

65   See Wlaschky (note 28), p. 112. Colour, for instance, was used by Paulus of Aegina to distinguish cataracts (6.20).

66   On the medieval computus in general, and for orientation to the vast, but scattered bibliography on this subject, see my articles, 'The Church, the World, and the Time', in Marie-Claude Deprez-Masson (ed.), *Normes et pouvoirs à la fin du moyen âge* (Montreal: Ceres, 1990), pp. 15–29, and 'Chronology and Systems of Dating', in George Rigg and Frank A. C. Mantello (eds.), *Medieval Latin Studies: an Introduction and Bibliographic Guide* (Washington: Catholic University of America Press, forthcoming).

Unlike any ancient calendar, the Christian calendar had to be projected into the future in order to determine upcoming dates of important movable feasts, particularly Easter. It also had to be controlled by a mathematical cycle, since the far-flung churches needed to assume local responsibility for the calendar in the absence of any effective central institution. The computus was one of the few scientific enterprises of the early medieval period which elicited lively and broad-based interest; indeed, the development, testing and eventual generalization of a reliable Paschal cycle was a major cultural and communications achievement in this troubled and disrupted age. What is significant about this early medieval calendar science is that it diagrammed time mathematically, and generalized that mathematical vision of time for an entire culture.

It is not widely appreciated how dominant a role computus played in the shaping of the early medieval view of nature and science, nor is the intimate connection between computus and medicine often recognized. Computus manuscripts very frequently contain medical materials which resonate with calendar themes: treatises on the four humours, and their relationship to the seasons and the ages of man; dietary and hygiene advice for each month of the year; prescriptives on the correct phase of the moon for blood-letting or other interventions; or prognostica, such as the 'Egyptian Days'.[67] And computus also shows an affinity for enumeration: counting and measuring link the computist's task of bringing time beneath the sway of mathematics to the work of the Creator who 'ordered all things according to measure, number and weight'.[68] In short, medicine's embeddedness in time brought it into the orbit of the dominant science of the age, computus, and coloured it with computus' characteristic interest in numbering and mensuration.

Another element in the constellation of substitutes for theory is deontology, that is, texts about the education, ethics and etiquette of the physician. These early medieval texts have been edited and studied extensively, but withal somewhat naïvely interpreted as 'the persistence of Hippocratic ideals'.[69] But, as Temkin points out, Christians were

---

[67] I enlarge upon this subject in my article 'Medicine in Medieval Computus Manuscripts', in Margaret Schleissner (ed.), *Manuscript Sources of Medieval Medicine* (New York: Garland, 1994), 105–43.

[68] The phrase 'Thou has ordered all things according to measure, number and weight', from *Wisdom*, 11.20, was extensively quoted by the computists, a subject which is explored in my article, 'Images of Order in the Medieval Computus', in Warren Ginsberg (ed.), *ACTA XIV: Ideas of Order in the Middle Ages* (Binghamton: State University of New York Press, 1990), pp. 45–67.

[69] Loren C. MacKinney, 'Medical Ethics and Etiquette in the Early Middle Ages: the Persistence of Hippocratic Ideals', *Bulletin of the History of Medicine*, 26 (1952), 1–31. For editions, see Ernst Hirschfeld, 'Deontologische Texte des frühen Mittelalters', *Sudhoffs Archiv*, 20 (1928), 353–71.

interested in deontological texts for anything but antiquarian reasons. These texts could be made to serve, in fact, as models for the behaviour of the true 'physician of the soul', namely the priest.[70] Co-opting them was also part of a concerted campaign to wrest the Hippocratic ideals of selfless service and sacrifice away from secular doctors, and bestow them on the clergy and the saints. Indeed, as St Basil of Caesarea declared, one of God's main reasons for giving medicine to man in the first place is so that it could provide a model for the therapy of the soul.[71]

The continuous diffusion of these deontological texts – which were, after all, largely collected and copied by monks – is due in no small measure to the Christians' need to argue out a new, religious interpretation of medicine. An important witness to this quest for a Christian medical philosophy, or at least a Christian medical *policy*, is the apology for medicine which prefaces the *Lorscher Arzneibuch*.[72] Though it justifies the study of human medicine by Christians, it does so by defining 'human medicine' as any kind of therapeutic activity mediated through a human being, including religious healing and miracle:

> In all this, it is evident that human relief and human medicine are not to be rejected out of hand, because if they deserved to be condemned, the Lord would never have commanded Paul to receive his sight back by the imposition of the hands of Ananias, nor would He have commanded His disciples to lay their hands upon the sick, that they might get better. Nor would He have cured Tobias through his son, by means of the medicine which the angel indicated.[73]

This text, far from being a straightforward invitation to study medicine, is really a controversial prologue to the *Arzneibuch* as a whole, and an important expression of monastic hostility to an independent and naturalistic medical philosophy. It is, in Keil's words, a piece of medical politics, carefully juxtaposed to the *vita* of Saints Cosmas and Damian which follows it, and deliberately congruent with the practical contents of the entire florilegium.[74]

Conclusion

Henry Sigerist's instincts and logic in sketching out his tripartite history of early medieval medicine were evidently sound: we must examine the manuscripts through which medical learning was conveyed, study the

---

[70]   Temkin (note 48), p. 142. See also Fridolf Kudlein, 'Der Arzt des Körpers und der Arzt der Seele', *Clio medica*, 3 (1968), 1–20.
[71]   *Regulae fusius tractatae*, in J.-P. Migne, *Patrologia Graeca*, 31, 1044C; cited in Temkin (note 48), p. 172.
[72]   Stoll (note 22), pp. 48–63.
[73]   Ibid., pp. 50–2. My translation.
[74]   Keil and Schnitzer (note 22), pp. 235–6.

textual materials within them, and on the basis of these, fashion a synthesis that sheds light not only on what early medieval medical practitioners knew, but on what they expected to do with what they knew. If Sigerist, and the two generations of medical historians who followed him, failed to realize this programme, it was, I would argue, because their training – their admirably rigorous philological training, the likes of which can hardly be had today – conditioned them to expect that the texts would simply cascade out of the manuscripts, and in turn unveil their contents before the analytical gaze of the historian.

Instead, we find that the texts stubbornly refuse to come unstuck from their florilegial matrices, and that they yield up their theoretical agendas only when they are read obliquely, in the context of strong but barely articulated ascetic and theological concerns, and in the light of other related cultural enterprises, such as computus. If our hopes for completing the third part of Sigerist's project are ever to bear fruit, we must surrender to the early medieval medical texts as they are, where they are, and let them tell us, between the lines if need be, what makes medicine work, and what gives it meaning.

But the questions explored in this essay, raw as they are, might also alert us to some provocative comparative perspectives. It would seem that texts come in three species: scripture, or sacred texts; classics, or authoritative (though not sacred) texts; and plain texts. Āyurveda is based on scriptures, to be absorbed in reverent memorization; Chinese traditional medicine is based on classics, to be commented, glossed and edited; Western medicine, at least after the end of Antiquity, was based on plain texts. The medical texts of Antiquity could not be revered by a Christian reader, for they fell into the category of secular literature, and were derived from an alien religious and cultural milieu. Hence they could with impunity be subjected to radical and unabashed reworking, dismemberment and de-authorization.

Although the great translation movement of the eleventh and twelfth centuries was motivated by a quest for the important texts of Antiquity, even these texts, and *a fortiori* the Arabic works that came in their wake, could never rise higher than the rank of plain texts in the value system of the medieval West. This phenomenon, so plainly demonstrated by the fate of medical texts in the early medieval centuries, merits our close attention. Might not the crucial difference between early Western medicine, on the one hand, and Indian or Chinese medicine on the other, lie in their respective attitudes towards text? When Vesalius, however deferentially and ambiguously, contradicted Galen, did he not do so on the unspoken grounds that, in the end, what he rejected was *only* a text, neither divinely inspired nor culturally canonized? To what extent are the contemporary dynamics of biomedical knowledge based on the assumption that its textual formulations (monographs, journal articles) are provisional and disposable? And to what degree does Western medicine owe the liberty it takes with its texts to the self-consciously anti-theoretical and anti-canonical textual practices of the early medieval centuries?

ABBREVIATIONS

BN	Paris, Bibliothèque nationale
Montecassino	Montecassino, Archivio della Badia
St Gall	St Gall, Stiftsbibliothek

7   *Artifex factivus sanitatis*: health and medical care in medieval Latin Galenism

Luis García-Ballester

Introduction

In his commentary on Aristotle's *De sensu et sensato*, written in 1269, Thomas Aquinas did not hesitate to define the physician to his students as the *artifex factivus sanitatis*, the maker of health.[1] The context in which this attractive definition arose was the relationship between natural philosophy and medicine, a problem that greatly concerned medieval scholars, whether they were physicians or not, in the period between the twelfth and fourteenth centuries. For this reason, Latin European students were confronted with a question that was by no means trivial and in no sense abstract: what was the difference, in intellectual and practical terms, between two activities that had emerged from the newly founded universities of the time. I refer, on the one hand, to the new, university-trained physicians, educated according to the Galenic paradigm following an intellectual model that was increasingly clearly defined in the Latin West in the twelfth century, and, on the other, to the natural philosophers, who had become firmly established in the already influential Schools of Arts. Neither of these two groups of 'professionals'[2] could remain detached from such important human phenomena as health and illness, at both the individual and collective level. In case of the physicians, this was for obvious reasons; in the case of the natural philosophers, their intellectual discipline could not remain detached from anything connected with the human being.[3] 'It is the task of the natural philosopher', commented Thomas Aquinas,

to investigate the primary and universal principles that govern health and illness; it is the physician's to put these principles into practice, in keeping with the idea

---

[1]   TA, *De sensu*, p. 128*. (For a list of bibliographical abbreviations, please see the end of this chapter.)

[2]   About the concept of 'professional' in the medieval context, see V.L. Bullough, 'Achievement, Professionalization, and the University', in J. Ijsewijn and J. Paquet (eds.), *The Universities in the Late Middle Ages* (Louvain, 1978), pp. 497–510, especially pp. 508–9.

[3]   TA, *De sensu*, p. 9.292–5.

that he is the maker of health ... The physician should not limit himself to making use of medicines, but he should also be able to reflect upon the causes [of health and illness]. To this purpose, the good physician begins his training [with the study of] natural philosophy.[4]

Two activities which were an innovation of the period were thus delimited. Naturally, the variety of natural philosophy to which Thomas Aquinas was alluding was the Aristotelian form. Aristotle himself spoke of the physician when he used medicine to illustrate how an *artifex* carried out something; in the physician's case, to achieve health.[5] There can be no doubt that the universities of the thirteenth century proved to be the most efficient instrument for the Aristotelianization of the Western intellectual world, including, of course, the field of medicine.[6]

The fact that Thomas Aquinas' opinion was expounded in the open and relatively informal surroundings of a class with his students reflects the high degree to which the new model of university-trained physicians (i.e. those who based their practice on a knowledge of natural philosophy), had already been accepted among the intellectual minority in Europe who were most open to new developments. On the other hand, full social acceptance of this new way, and of the new type of physician trained within it, took longer, and was achieved only after heated debate. It was a lengthy process, lasting almost a hundred and fifty years, from the early twelfth century onwards.

In the course of this century, it began in the southern part of Latin Christendom (Sicily, the south of Italy, and Salerno in particular) where practical medicine was being based on the natural part of philosophy, in particular of Aristotle's philosophy.[7] Naturally, this did not happen by chance. New physicians did not begin to be socially accepted until they were able to offer specific solutions for the maintenance of health and for its recovery when it had been lost, both at an individual and at a collective level, and until the European social system opened new markets for these 'professionals' in the field of health. The founding of universities, which included the study of medicine among the subjects

---

[4]   ad naturalem philosophum pertinet inuenire prima et universalia principia sanitatis et infirmitatis; particularia autem principia considerare pertinet ad medicum, qui est artifex factiuus sanitatis ... [medici] non solum experimentis utentes sed causas [sanitatis et egritudinis] inquirentes ... et hec est ratio quare medici bene artem prosequentes a naturalibus incipiunt. (TA, *De sensu*, pp. 8.277–9.316)
[5]   A, *Metaph.*, 1032b.13–14.
[6]   See Hilde de Ridder-Symoens (ed.), *A History of the University in Europe*, vol. 1: *Universities in the Middle Ages* (Cambridge, 1992).
[7]   L. García-Ballester, in L. García-Ballester, R.K. French, J. Arrizabalaga and A. Cunningham (eds.), *Practical Medicine from Salerno to the Black Death* (Cambridge, 1993), pp. 1–29.

taught, was a factor that was intimately associated with this process. We shall return to this point.

On the concept of health in thirteenth-century university circles

The definition of the physician as the *artifex factivus sanitatis* makes it necessary to consider the concept of health, which was extremely sensitive to a wide range of influences of an intellectual and social nature. What did health mean to Thomas Aquinas and his students, a small group of non-medical intellectuals in Paris in the 1260s? In the first place, and in view of the context in which he was speaking, it was the health of the body, the primary object of the physician's attention, that was being referred to.[8] 'Health, illness, body and medicine' were clearly bound together by Aristotle's *Metaphysics*, the influential work in the training of the medieval intellectual.[9] I shall not consider the so-called 'physician of the soul', whether a natural philosopher or a priest, nor the problem of their competition and 'professional' relationships with the physicians in an age in which the frontier between the two activities was not well defined, either at an intellectual or doctrinal level, or, above all, in everyday practice.[10]

Second, health was understood, both by Thomas Aquinas and by his Arts students, according to the intellectual criteria formulated by Aristotle in his *libri naturales*, upon one of which Aquinas was commenting. As is well known, Albert the Great's intellectual scheme ('making the natural works of Aristotle known to the Latins') reached its most developed phase during these years and culminated a process that had been initiated in the Latin West some one hundred years before.[11] In one of the parts making up the collection known to the medieval world by the name of *De animalibus*, Aristotle defined health in terms of a balance of the basic qualities (heat, cold, dampness and dryness). Thus, bodily health would be displayed when the body as a whole (and each one of its parts) achieved and maintained a suitable balance among its qualities.[12]

8 TA, *De sensu*, p. 9.289–90.
9 'Sanitas, infirmitas, corpus; movens, medicativa', (A, *Metaph.*, 1070b.28); 'nam medicativa est quodammodo sanitas' (ibid., 1075b.10).
10 TA, *Summa*, vol. 11, quaestio 44, 3, 3um, and vol. 12, quaestio 86, 5, 1um.
11 Albertus Magnus, *Physica*, book 1, tr. 1, ch. 1, vol. 3, p. 3. See J.A. Weisheipl, 'Appendix: Albert's Works on Natural Science [*libri naturales*] in Probable Chronological Order', in J.A. Weisheipl (ed.), *Albertus Magnus and the Sciences* (Toronto, 1980), p. 565.
12 A, *De partibus animalium*, 648b.4ff.

The world of medieval medicine – and in general the intellectual
world of the Latin West – underwent a major upheaval when it was
persuaded that the intellectual key for distinguishing the frontier
between life and death, between health and illness, between the basic
vital everyday process such as growth and ageing, was none other than
the theory of the elements and the qualities.[13]

The initial discovery was indirect, through Arabic medical texts
translated into Latin, in which the Aristotelian doctrines had already
been developed and integrated into a doctrinal system with practical
medical implications (Galenism).[14] It suffices to glance through the first
few pages of Constantine's *Pantegni*, one of the best-organized medical
encyclopaedias of the Arab world, written by al-Magusi, which began to
circulate in medical circles in the first decades of the twelfth century.[15]

Neither should we forget the role played by the early personal contacts
among physicians from other areas of southern Europe (e.g., the Ebro
valley), physicians who were in contact with highly developed forms of
Arab medicine and natural philosophy in this process of discovery of the
Aristotelian world. Such contacts can be detected at the end of the first
decade of the twelfth century. The clearest example is represented by the
physician and astronomer known as Petrus Alfonsi, an Aragonese Jew
belonging to the court circle in Muslim-controlled Zaragoza, who
converted to Christianity in 1106. He had contacts with England and
the north of France at precisely this time.[16]

This gave rise to a whole new class of Latin medical terms.
Constantine, who was obviously in possession of a solid base of medical
learning (at least if we understand medicine as knowledge referring to
the natural world and not just as the specific procedure to follow in

[13] 'It seems evident that [these four primary qualities] are practically the causes of death
and of life, as also of sleep and waking, of maturity and old age, and of disease and
health': A, *De partibus animalium*, 648b.4ff; A, *De gen. et corr.*, 732b.28–733b.16.
[14] As an example, see PH, *De animalibus*, written probably after 1230 and before 1246,
fol. 23ra. The most recent study on Petrus Hispanus is Miguel de Asúa, 'The
Commentaries on "De animalibus" by Peter of Spain and Albert the Great's
"Quaestiones super de animalibus"', unpublished Ph.D. thesis, University of Notre-
Dame, Indiana (1992). Other examples are: Albert the Great, in his commentary on
Aristotle's *Metaphysics*, written between 1264 and 1267, AM, *Metaph.*, book 7, tr. 2,
chs. 5.55–8; a few years later, Thomas of Aquinas, commenting on Aristotle's work,
insists on the same: A, *Metaph.*, lect. 6, ch. 7, num. 1406, p. 345a. Probably the source
is the *Pantegni*, *Lib. theorice*, book 1, ch. 25 [De humoribus]. On Galenism, see O.
Temkin, *Galenism. Rise and Decline of a Medical Philosophy* (Ithaca and London, 1973).
[15] *Pantegni*, *Lib. theorice*, book 1, ch. 7 (on the concept of *complexio*), fol. 2rb. See the
recent book by D. Jacquart and F. Micheau, *La Médecine et l'occident médiéval* (Paris,
1990), pp. 104ff.
[16] On Petrus Alfonsi, see J.H. Reuter, 'Petrus Alfonsi: An Examination of his Works,
their Scientific Content and their Background', unpublished Ph.D. thesis, University
of Oxford (1975). The medical contents are not specifically analysed.

order to cure), knew how to identify terms in medieval Latin which would translate these new conceptual realities that were already clearly defined in Arab medicine. Through this means the most developed form of Galenism entered the Latin West.

The quantitative and qualitative balance of the body as a whole, and of each of its parts, was to receive the name of *complexio*, or the more precisely expressed form of *equalis complexio*, balanced complexion, so as to distinguish it from the *inequalis* form. The latter indicated the presence of an illness because the above-mentioned balance had been broken.[17] The *medicus* (whether *physicus* or *cirurgicus*) was the person who was qualified to diagnose the body's state of health, identified on the basis of the complexio.

What is being described here was no mere theoretical pedantry or a game with words. It had important practical repercussions of a social and economic nature. For example, the slave trade – which was so dynamic and significant in the Christian-controlled regions of the western Mediterranean in the thirteenth and fourteenth centuries – was strengthened with the diffusion of the *Pantegni* and the physician's participation as a guarantor of the good or bad complexio of this human merchandise.[18] All the legal documentation (contracts of sale, lawsuits concerning 'damaged merchandise') to which this trade gave rise relied on the active participation of physicians as experts in the recognition of the state of physical health.[19]

Health considered as a state of balance of bodily qualities (*temperantia*) in accordance with which all the natural functions can be carried out in a perfect way (*perfectae*) is no more than an ideal. And it was thus perceived by physicians and non-medical intellectuals of the mid-thirteenth century. With the help of the *Pantegni* the physician and the intellectual came to discover that the concept of health is somewhat relative. It could be preached with the same level of acceptance in three different circumstances: in the first place, the circumstances of those who perform their vital functions completely and who are in the age of adulthood; second, of those who need some form of help or reinforcement to carry out these functions, a group made up of children, the

---

[17] D. Jacquart, 'De *crasis* à *complexio*: Note sur le vocabulaire du tempérament en latin médiéval', in G. Sabbah (ed.), *Textes médicaux latins antiques* (Saint-Etienne, 1984), pp. 71–6.

[18] *Pantegni, Lib. theorice*, book 1, ch. 24, fol. 4ra. See also *Rhazes*, book 2, ch. 25, pp. 47–8, where he very carefully describes the physical examination of the slaves by the doctor.

[19] The archives of the kingdoms of the Crown of Aragon are very rich in this kind of documentation, especially that of Majorca where the trade of slaves was an important source of income.

elderly and convalescents; third, of those who are especially prone to illness or who are suspected to be heading towards being ill. The physician's intervention – particularly decisive in the third situation – would be very different according to which of the three sets of circumstances he or she was faced with. Be that as it may, the *Pantegni* provided those who made health the subject of intellectual reflection and 'professional' activity with an ample conceptual basis upon which to develop their ideas and activities.[20]

The world of the elements and the qualities requires a certain level of abstraction and is not particularly close to the physician's specific field of activity. As a result, health is also defined in terms of the humours, although always in accordance with the doctrine of balance (temperantia). The need to possess practical, visible criteria led physicians to interpret the concept of health in terms of the humour blood and of the two qualities that it possessed that are most obvious to the senses, namely heat and dampness.[21] It was Rhazes' work (in particular his *Liber ad regem Almansorem*), available in Latin from the end of the twelfth century and more attentive to clinical practice, which allowed for a better understanding and management of the concept of health in everyday practice. Nor did this feature pass unnoticed to non-medical intellectuals of the mid-thirteenth century, people such as Vincent of Beauvais.[22]

Health was also defined with the help of other concepts that were introduced by means of translations of Arabic works including those of Galen's own writings. We are here referring especially to the concept of 'radical moisture' (*humiditas substanciale*), which was developed to explain the nature of life and both natural processes (e.g., ageing) and pathological ones (e.g., that of fevers).[23] Life is possible, from the formation of the embryo onwards, only by means of the maintenance of a certain level of moisture (*humiditas*) compatible with the necessary vital heat, a principle whose roots go back to the Galenic and Hippocratic medical tradition. Both radical moisture and innate heat vary in the course of each individual's life. Leaving aside the possibility of a sudden cause of death, variation in innate heat is an inevitable process as a consequence, at least, of the natural process of the drying-up of the radical moisture. However, this radical moisture can be corrupted or destroyed. Although physicians cannot avoid the ageing process and

[20] *Pantegni, Lib. practice*, book 1, chs. 1ff.; VB, *Speculum doc.*, book 12, ch. 1, col. 1073.7.
[21] *Pantegni, Lib. theorice*, book 1, ch. 25.
[22] See the general preface to VB, *Speculum maius*, vol. 1, ch. 18, col. 15, where the author summarizes the medical authorities he uses.
[23] There is a good survey in M.R. McVaugh, 'The "Humidum radicale" in Thirteenth-century Medicine', *Traditio*, 30 (1974), 259–83.

death, they can at least delay or slow down the process of drying or desiccation.[24] The concepts of innate heat, dryness and radical moisture could be used by physicians to develop a doctrine of an eminently practical nature (*ars quidem sanitatem custodiendi*), in the service of health (*custodiendi sanitatem scientia*).[25]

The medieval physician found abundant material for this purpose in those works translated from the late eleventh century onwards and throughout the twelfth century by Constantine, Gerald of Cremona, and Burgundio of Pisa among others.[26] Nevertheless, it was in Avicenna's *Canon* that the practising physician found the association between the concept of radical moisture and that of the *complexio*, and thus the key to individualizing care in the maintenance of his or her patient's health.

Avicenna seems to express a certain predetermined view of the individual vital process (each would have its own life span) according to its primal complexion (*prima complexio*). This had its origins in the embryonic process, and was defined in accordance with the double parameter of radical moisture and innate heat. Physicians thus opened up a new perspective for such basic concepts as their patient's health and life expectancy. It became a matter of finding the signs by means of which they might identify 'the time of each individual according to his primal complexion'[27] and of being able to 'measure' (in a qualitative way of course) 'the strength of the radical moisture and innate heat of each one, since in this matter each body is different'.[28]

Once this primal complexion was identified, the physician could elaborate a *regimen* for the well-being and protection (*custodiam et tutelam*) of his or her patient's health. This was made possible, as will be seen, by means of knowledge and skilful management of what medieval Galenism knew as the 'non-natural things'. The metaphor of oil, already used by Galen, and which Avicenna employed as an analogous explanation of the life/health/ageing/death process, would be extremely useful for medieval physicians in order to explain to their patients not only this doctrine (*scientia*) of health, but also the reasons for the specific measures to be put into practice in their particular case (*operationes secundum artem*) to delay, as far as possible, the inevitable process of ageing and its final outcome, death.

These problems were of great concern to Latin physicians about the

24 I am summarizing *Canon*, book 1, fen. 3, ch. 1, pp. 162–3.
25 Ibid., pp. 162a and 163a.
26 M.-T. d'Alverny, 'Translations and Translators', in R.L. Benson, G. Constable and G.D. Lanham (eds.), *Renaissance and Renewal in the Twelfth Century* (Oxford, 1982), pp. 421–62.
27 *Canon*, book 1, fen. 3, ch. 1, p. 163a.
28 Ibid.

middle of the thirteenth century. For example, in the list of *quaestiones* discussed by Petrus Hispanus in his commentary *In techne Galieni*, we find questions as significant as 'whether natural death could be postponed by means of medicine', 'whether a man could live free of illnesses', or 'what is the cause of a long continuance or shortness of life'.[29]

Nevertheless, a person's bodily health was not fully dealt with only by considering the balance of the body, or of each of its parts, nor through knowledge of one's primal complexion 'measured' according to the degree of innate heat and radical moisture. For a medieval intellectual (a natural philosopher), and especially for a physician educated according to the Galenic paradigm, a human body is conceivable only in relation to its physical, social and moral surroundings. This is what medieval physicians – and also natural philosophers – expressed under the heading of the 'non-natural things' (*res non naturales*). This expression gains its fullest sense when it is placed alongside the other two categories of 'natural things' (*res naturales*) and 'pathological things' (*res praeter naturam*). Medieval Galenism, initially in its Islamic form and subsequently in that found in the Latin West, was structured around them.[30]

Under the name of the 'natural things' were included all those things that the human body is composed of and which enable it to exist as a living being (elements, qualities, complexion, humours, spirits, virtues or powers, morphological constituents, etc.). The 'pathological things' included everything that is altered during the state of illness and were fundamentally three in number: the illness with respect to the immediate alteration of the 'natural things'; the cause of the illness; and the symptoms or the specific manner in which the illness expressed itself or made itself apparent. The 'non-natural things', even though they were not a constituent part of the body, made up the physical, social and even moral surroundings of the living being that closely interacted with it, whether in a normal or a pathological way. Connected as they were in six groups (five of them being linked in pairs) – air and environment, food and drink, sleep and wakefulness, motion and rest, evacuation and repletion, and passions of the mind – they came to form one of the principal ideas of the doctrine of Galenism. In fact, a substantial part of the causal and therapeutic system of Galenic pathology was based on them, while, at the same time, all the doctrine for the preservation and

---

[29] 'Utrum mors naturalis per beneficium medicine possit retardari'; 'Utrum homo possit vivere absque egritudine'; and 'Queritur quod sit causa brevitatis et duracionis vite': PH, *In techne*, fols. 3va and 92ra–93vb.

[30] *Pantegni, Lib. theorice*, book 1, ch. 3, fol. 1vb. See Temkin (note 14), pp. 105–6.

maintenance of health was built on them. The line between what was normal and what was pathological lay in the correct, or incorrect, quantitative and/or qualitative management of each of these 'six non-natural things' on the part of the physician, together with the active participation of the client. The latter may or may not have been ill, but always needed to maintain a suitable standard of health. By means of this concept, Galenism endeavoured to regulate human life from the standpoint of medicine. By virtue of this, it aimed to guarantee the maintenance of the health of particular persons, health here being regarded as a balance between the individual's body and the environment – in the widest sense of the word – in which he or she moved on a daily basis.[31]

The works which were initially responsible for converting these concepts into 'normal knowledge' among the contemporary European learned community – not restricted to medical circles – were the *Pantegni* of al-Magusi (Ali Habbas) and, in particular, the *Isagoge* of Johannicius, both of which were translated into Latin by Constantine at the Benedictine Abbey of Monte Cassino around the late 1070s. These works were known by physicians and intellectuals in the Latin West, at least since the second decade of the twelfth century.[32]

The popularity of the *Pantegni* in French and British intellectual circles in the first half of the thirteenth century is demonstrated by the fact that it constituted the principal medical source for the popular scientific encyclopaedia 'On the properties of things' (*De proprietatibus rerum*) written by Bartholomaeus Anglicus and by the fact that it was the only one to warrant the praise of Vincent of Beauvais in his *Speculum Naturale*.[33] The *Isagoge* was the first medical text in the *Articella*,[34] a

---

[31] See L. García-Ballester, 'On the Origin of the "Six Non-Natural Things" in Galen', in G. Harig and J. Harig-Kollesch (eds.), *Galen und die hellenistische Erbe* (Wiesbaden, 1993), pp. 105–15.

[32] See Jacquart and Micheau (note 15), pp. 118ff.

[33] Ibid., p. 157.

[34] See P.O. Kristeller, 'The School of Salerno: Its Development and Its Contribution to the History of Learning', in his *Studies in Renaissance Thought and Letters* (Rome, 1956), pp. 495–551; 'Bartholomaeus, Musandinus, and Maurus of Salerno and Other Early Commentators of the "Articella", with a Tentative List of Texts and Manuscripts', *Italia Medioevale e Umanistica*, 19 (1976), 57–87. Both articles have been translated into Italian with new material and published together in a volume, *Studi sulla Scuola medica salernitana* (Naples, 1986). The most recent approach to the origins of the collection is T. Pesenti, '"Articella" dagli incunabuli ai manoscritti: origini e vicende di un titolo', in M. Cochetti (ed.), *Mercurius in Trivio. Studi di Bibliografia e di Biblioteconomia per Alfredo Serrai nel 60° compleanno* (Rome, 1993), pp. 129–45.

collection of writings upon which medical teaching focused in Paris,[35] as well as in Montpellier[36] and Bologna,[37] in the mid-thirteenth century.

From the latter part of the twelfth century onwards, the *Canon* of Avicenna also exerted an increasing influence.[38] It soon became the standard treatise, to the extent that it was identified with medical knowledge even by such a non-medical intellectual as Vincent of Beauvais, who, in about the year 1250, did not hesitate to state that 'among the natural philosophers, I pick out Aristotle for dealing with animals, Avicenna for medicine and Pliny for natural history'.[39] Other general medical treatises, similar in structure to the great Arab manuals, but which were written in the 1230s and 1240s by Christian physicians in environments dominated by a transformed Aristotle and Galen, contributed towards maintaining these concepts of Galenism for wide sectors of the lay public who were not necessarily physicians. We might cite, by way of example, the *Compendium medicine* (*c.* 1240) by Gilbertus de Aquila (Anglicus).[40] This medical treatise, together with the above-mentioned *Canon* of Avicenna, were the principal medical sources for the scientific encyclopaedia (*Historia naturalis*) drawn up by the Castilian Franciscan friar, Juan Gil of Zamora (Johannes Aegidius Zamorensis), in the 1280s.[41]

It should be pointed out that these works, especially the *Pantegni*, together with their medieval medical tradition, made the physician's

35   There is a useful table with the medical teaching books and programme in Paris (1270–74), in Jacquart and Micheau (note 15), p. 172. See also E. Seidler, *Die Heilkunde des Ausgehenden Mittelalters in Paris. Studien zur Struktur der Spätscholastischen Medizin* (Wiesbaden, 1967).

36   See M.R. McVaugh (note 23), and 'An Early Discussion on Medicinal Degrees at Montpellier by Henry of Winchester', *Bulletin of the History of Medicine*, 49 (1975), 57–71.

37   N. Siraisi, *Taddeo Alderotti and his Pupils. Two Generations of Italian Medical Learning* (Princeton, 1981), pp. 98–9.

38   The *Canon* was probably used in the north of Italy in the 1180s. See K. Goehl, *Guido d'Arezzo der Jüngere und sein 'Liber mitis'* (Pattensen, 1984), pp. 23–7 (Würzburger medizinhistorische Forschungen, 32); D. Jacquart, 'La Réception du Canon d'Avicenne: comparaison entre Montpellier et Paris aux XIIIe et XIVe siècles', *Histoire de l'Ecole médicale de Montpellier*, *Actes du 110e Congrès national des sociétés savantes* (Paris, 1985), pp. 69–77.

39   *Speculum maius*, vol. 1, Prologus, ch. 4, col. 4.

40   We do not yet have a critical edition of the *Compendium*. See M. Kurdzialek, 'Gilbertus Anglicus und die psychologischen Erörterungen in seinem *Compendium Medicinae*', *Sudhoffs Archiv*, 47 (1963), 106–26; C. Talbot and E.A. Hammond, *The Medical Practitioners in Medieval England. A Biographical Register* (London, 1965), pp. 58–60; D. Jacquart, *Supplément* to E. Wickersheimer, *Dictionnaire biographique des médecins en France au Moyen Age* (Geneva, 1979), pp. 88–9.

41   *Johannes Aegidius Zamorensis. Historia naturalis*, introduction, critical edition, Spanish translation and indexes by A. Domínguez and L. García Ballester, 3 vols. (Valladolid, 1994).

functions turn on the concept of health, and that they did not restrict 'health' to its negative definition, 'absence of illness'. On the contrary, Aristotle explained that 'illness is the absence of health'.[42] Health is the natural state of man and the physician should contribute to its maintenance.[43] Three objectives related to this were indicated. In the first place is the maintenance of control over the individual's internal factors ('natural things' centring on the concept of complexion and of humour) and over the external ones ('non-natural things'), the alteration of which might be a danger for the maintenance of the existing level of health.[44]

Second is the stimulation or encouragement of those aspects of the individual's way of life that are most suitable for attaining the optimum level of health, in other words, those that enable the body to carry out its natural functions in better conditions. This was achieved by means of the management of each and every one of the six 'non-natural things', with special emphasis on diet.[45] Such measures were put into practice only in the case of the minority that formed part of the highest-ranking sectors of society.[46] Nevertheless, both physicians and those who held responsibility for government (especially the town councils) warned that the alteration of physical surroundings – both their improvement and their deterioration – had repercussions for the health of individuals and also for that of human communities.[47]

The third aim was to achieve a return to an acceptable level of health when this had been lost through illness ('praeternatural things'). Whenever possible, it was best to undertake the latter process in the

---

[42] A, *Metaph.*, 1030b.4–5.

[43] *Pantegni, Lib. practice*, book 1, ch. 1, fol. 58rb.

[44] Ibid., fols. 58–65.

[45] For example, Bernard de Gordon in his *Regimina sanitatis* says, 'regimen sanitatis consistit in debita applicatione sex rerum non naturalium': *De conservatione 4: regimen sanitatis*, Vatican MS Pal. lat. 1174, fol. 72v. Cited by L.E. Demaitre, *Doctor Bernard de Gordon: Professor and Practitioner* (Toronto, 1980), p. 69, n. 166.

[46] H. Schipperges, *Lebendige Heilkunde* (Olten and Freiburg i. Br., 1962); L. Garcia-Ballester, 'Dietetic and Pharmacological Therapy: A Dilemma Among Fourteenth-Century Jewish Practitioners in the Montpellier Area', in W.F. Bynum and V. Nutton (eds.), *Essays in the History of Therapeutics* (Amsterdam and Atlanta, 1991), pp. 23–37 (*Clio Medica*, 22 (1991)).

[47] Changes in the air were considered as a cause of illnesses. According to the *Pantegni* one of the origins of such changes were, following Aristotelian ideas, smoke from organic putrefaction: *Pantegni, Lib. theorice*, book 5, ch. 11, fol. 20rb. In this work, translated into Latin at the end of the eleventh century, the smoke produced by craft industry was not considered. In an urban milieu (e.g., Barcelona, Paris), at the beginning of the fourteenth century at least, smoke produced by artisan industry (e.g., the manufacture of vermilion – a bright red powder used as a pigment – or coal smoke) was considered by lay people as a cause of illnesses, and physicians were consulted with regard to it. See L. Garcia-Ballester, 'The Construction of a New Form of Learning and Practising Medicine in Medieval Latin Europe', in H. Heyd et al. (eds.), *Medicine as a Cultural System* (Cambridge, 1995).

intermediate phase between health and illness, before the latter had fully gained hold, that is to say, in the period that medieval physicians called *neutralitas*. According to them, it was easier to return to health from that stage than to seek to do so when health had been definitively lost.[48]

This active, triple dimension of the physician's role, in connection with the health of clients, is what was being emphasized by Thomas Aquinas' definition when he spoke of the practitioner as the *artifex factivus*.

However, this tripartite activity was not restricted to the application of a few recipes that were the consequence of accumulated experience (either of a personal or historical nature).[49] Experience was not despised (hence all the wide range of prescription literature, and the great prestige of the so-called *experimenta*),[50] but it was not sufficient, as the above-mentioned text of Thomas Aquinas' commentary points out: 'the physician should not restrict himself to making use of medicines, but he should be capable of enquiring about the causes [of health and illness]'.[51]

In this way, we reach a new intellectual frontier, that defined by Aristotelian causality. Aristotle established very clearly that the difference between an empiricist (*expertus*) and a technician (artifex) is the following: 'the first knows what he is doing but not why he does it; however, the artifex knows why he is doing something [e.g., giving a drug or a surgical treatment, in the case of a medical practitioner] and the cause of it'.[52] Precisely because of that the latter is on a higher intellectual plane.[53] This was the explicit message that was introduced into Latin, European, intellectual circles by the *Pantegni* at the beginning of its second part, the part dedicated to *practica*; a message strengthened, as we have already seen, by the *Canon*.

It was thus stressed that the physician's activity was based on a rational knowledge of what was happening to patients' bodies (whether they were ill or not) as a natural phenomenon. In accordance with Aristotelian philosophy, this form of knowledge aimed to include within its scope the whole range of natural movements of the living being by reason of their causes (material, formal, efficient and final). Such a form of knowledge – in the case of subjects related to health and illness – was supplied by the works of Hippocrates and Galen (and in the main by those of the latter),

---

48 *Pantegni, Lib. practice*, book 1, ch. 1, fol. 58rb.
49 'Experimentum fit ex memoria. Nam sicut ex multis memoriis fit una experimentalis scientia': A, *Metaph.*, p. 9.
50 M.R. McVaugh, 'Two Montpellier Recipe Collections', *Manuscripta*, 20 (1976), 175–80.
51 See note 4.
52 'Experti quidem enim ipsum sciunt quia, sed propter quid nesciunt; hi autem propter quid, et causam cognoscunt': A, *Metaph.*, 981a.28–30.
53 A, *Metaph.*, 981a.26.

whose intellectual argument was unintelligible without a knowledge of Aristotelian natural philosophy.

This was in many ways a transformed Galen which had little to do with the historical Galen. That is to say, it was a reading of Galen (or rather of those of his works that were available) in line with the intellectual keys that defined medieval medicine, both in its scholastic form (i.e., the version that was expounded in university circles) and in its non-scholastic form (the mixed bag that is known by the name of 'Fachliteratur'). This process made no attempt to exclude observation, which physicians exercised in the course of their daily practice, and which was stimulated by Aristotle himself and by Galen. Causal knowledge of the reasons behind a process (in this case a natural process) was a part of what was known as scientia in the medieval world.[54]

To define health in terms of Aristotelian causality was the great conceptual development offered by Avicenna in his *Canon*. 'Medicine deals with the health of the human body ... we must know the causes of health and of illness if we wish to make it a scientia ... The causes are but four: material, efficient, formal and final.'[55] The material causes coincide in part with the already-mentioned res naturales (spirits, humours, limbs); the efficient causes with the contents of the res non naturales; the formal causes with the remaining of res naturales that are more closely associated with the elements (complexion, virtues and compositions); the final causes with the physician's specific actions (the so-called *operationes*) that have health as their objective.[56] This work was translated into Latin in Toledo in about the 1180s by Gerardo de Cremona.[57]

Even though the *Canon* was widely used by non-medical intellectuals, especially by those belonging to the new mendicant orders, it still did not enjoy the same popularity as the *Pantegni* in the 1250s. But the manner of its approach to medicine finally won the day, if we bear in mind Thomas Aquinas' commentary, produced at the end of the 1260s.[58] As can be

---

[54] See the recent general survey by N. Siraisi, *Medieval and Early Renaissance Medicine. An Introduction to Knowledge and Practice* (Chicago and London, 1990); F. Salmón, 'The Many Galens of the Medieval Commentators on Vision', *Revue d'Historie des Sciences* (1994) (in press).

[55] *Canon*, book 1, fen. 1, doc. 1, ch. 1, p. 7b.

[56] Ibid., pp. 7–8.

[57] M.-T. d'Alverny (note 26).

[58] The most important medical source of Bartholomaeus Anglicus' *De proprietatibus rerum* (written c. 1245) was still the *Pantegni*: see R.J. Long (ed.), *Bartholomaeus Anglicus. On the Properties of Soul and Body. The Proprietatibus rerum libri III and IV* (Toronto, 1979), p. 9 and the critical notes, *passim*, and M.C. Seymour et al., *Bartholomaeus Anglicus and his Encyclopedia* (Cambridge and London, 1992). A few years later the *Canon* was an important medical source for Albert the Great: see N. Siraisi, 'The Medical Learning of Albertus Magnus', in J.A. Weisheipl (note 11), pp. 379–404.

observed, Avicenna's definition of health in terms of Aristotelian causality also included the elements that had been contributed by Constantine (in the *Pantegni* and *Isagoge*) and endowed them with a conceptual precision more in line with the new university form of Scholasticism.

Yet Avicenna went even further in the topic we are discussing. First, the identification of the final causes of the state of health of human nature with the physician's specific action (*operatio*) represented a novelty with regard to the Aristotelian idea of nature. For Aristotle, human nature included the individual's goal (*tēlos*), the good she or he fulfilled or brought about.[59] As far as the subject under discussion is concerned, this means that nature tends to favour health. That is its aim. The physician's actions (the so-called operationes) can be explained – and make sense – only insofar as they are capable of recognizing this purpose and coincide with it. The physician is an assistant to nature, or the 'oarsman of nature' in the words of the Hippocratic metaphor, which in this context is not so much a figure of speech but a true expression of the real Aristotelian concept of nature and of the physician's relationship with human nature.

Avicenna (or at least the Latin Avicenna) did not reject this attitude as regards the physician-human nature relationship, which was supposed to maintain good health or recover it if it had been lost. However, he went a step further when he introduced the physician's actions (his opera-tiones) into the structure of human nature itself when the physician sought health. First, the *Canon* offered the late medieval physician a new intellectual tool which provided (or was in a position to provide) the possibility of a greater initiative in his or her relationship with patients, whether they were healthy or sick. Success in achieving good health was not *only* a matter of the patient's human nature, but physicians also played an active role, inasmuch as they worked according to nature. A new horizon, both intellectual and social, opened up before learned physicians who, in the same way as had been done for human nature, defined their activity in terms of the goal: to maintain or to recover the health of those who sought their services while maintaining a certain decisive role.

Second, Avicenna did what is even more important for our purposes: he contributed to delimiting the fields of the two university disciplines, that of the physician and that of the natural philosopher, when he clarified that it was possible to approach the contents of the different causes both from the physician's perspective ('in quantum est medicus') and from the natural philosopher's standpoint ('in quantum est

---

[59]   G.E.R. Lloyd, 'The Invention of Nature', *Methods and Problems in Greek Science* (Cambridge, 1991), pp. 417–34, especially p. 430.

philosophus').[60] Within the causal system that has been described, and without renouncing it, as we will now see, the scholastic physician eventually came to emphasize more strongly the final cause, which takes operationes into account.

Third, Avicenna helped to confirm the increasing social presence of the physician trained in natural philosophy over everything associated with health. In practice, at the beginning of the first book of the *Canon*, in which he integrates natural philosophy within the conceptual framework of medical doctrine and practice, he places special emphasis on the idea that the field of physical health is the exclusive responsibility of the physician.[61]

Be that as it may, as physicians based their knowledge of health on the Aristotelian causes that defined it, they established themselves in the field of *scientia*. When this knowledge was oriented towards direct intervention (in this case, stimulating, maintaining or recovering health) it defined that activity as an *ars* (and whoever practised it as an *artifex*), an action that had to be carried out in order to be fit and suitable. It could not be claimed that the physician's functions were simply of an intellectual nature. The physician was an artifex factivus, a maker.

Drawing the line between the activity of the university physician (and that of anybody who was active in the field of medicine) and that of the natural philosopher in all those matters pertaining to health and illness was something that was discussed in university circles from the 1240s onwards at least. This discussion became particularly intense in the last few decades of the century. We have already noted how such a non-medical intellectual as Thomas Aquinas separated the areas of activity of each of these two 'professionals' at the end of the 1260s. We shall see that the natural philosopher was to move on the level of *veritas*, whereas the physician would act on the plane of *utilitas*. In practice, both activities were to be defined more by their social functions (operationes, i.e., the so-called final cause according to medieval Aristotelianism) than by reasons of a theoretical nature, although the latter did not cease to be present. It was not a matter of renouncing the doctrinal rigour upon which both activities were based.

The result was that medicine did not have to renounce its status as a scientia. Rather, the aim was to establish criteria which would allow the physician's own area of activity to be recognized – both in intellectual,

---

[60]   *Canon*, book 1, fen. 1, doc. 1, ch. 1, p. 8b. This point was reinforced at the end of the thirteenth century by the reading of new Galenic works such as *De interioribus*; see my introduction to Arnald's commentary on the first Hippocratic aphorism, 'Vita brevis', in M.R. McVaugh (ed.), *Arnaldi de Villanova Repetitio super canonem 'Vita brevis'* (Barcelona, in press) (Arnaldi de Villanova Opera Medica Omnia, vol. 16).

[61]   *Canon*, book 1, fen. 1, doc. 1, ch. 1, p. 8a.

and, above all, social terms – without renouncing the benefits (among them economic) that were derived from practising something described as and socially recognized as a scientia in the thirteenth and fourteenth centuries in the medieval West.

One of the first solutions to this problem provided by a Christian medieval physician dates from about 1240. We are referring to what Gilbertus de Aquila (Anglicus) expounded in his *Compendium medicine*, one of the most popular medical treatises of the thirteenth century.[62] His words were provoked by the need to reply to the inevitable intellectual uneasiness that any medieval physician felt when faced with the conflicting opinions of Aristotle (the true representative of the natural philosophers) and Galen (the undeniable spokesman of the physicians) on such an important topic as the role of the heart and the liver in the working of the body. These were his words:

The heart is at the middle, like the spider in its web, so that, as it is equidistant from all the extremes, it is the starting point and the source for diffusing all the virtues throughout the body ... The liver is nothing but a way towards the heart ... The reasons that demonstrate that the heart is the source of blood, not the liver, are three in number. The first is that the heart is the starting point of all things. The second is that the liver is a route through which things pass before terminating in the heart ... The third is that the deficiencies of the liver are made good by the heart. Therefore, the liver, by itself, serves the heart as a preparatory and purgative virtue. The error [that physicians make] is due to the fact that when the humours are neither cleansed nor prepared, this is taken to be a defect of the liver, with the result that the physician attributes this failure to the liver, because this is what seems to be the case to the senses ... This opinion [that the heart is the origin of blood] is far from being shared by physicians ... Aristotle speaks according to the truth, while physicians do so in accordance with what is evident to the senses. The better way, of course, would be the two together. However, concealing the truth in no way prejudices the physician, since what is open to the senses is sufficient for healing.[63]

The physician as such does not aim to seek the truth, in the sense of discovering reality as it actually is. That was the function of the natural philosopher. Let us leave, for a moment, the inevitable conflicts that this could give rise to in a Christian society which identified the truth with God, the exclusive domain of the theologian. Let us put aside also the desire for reconciling both opinions, something perhaps to be expected in the process of cross-cultural fertilization in which Christian intellectuals had been living since the twelfth century.[64] Physicians aimed at

[62] See notes 40 and 41.
[63] *Compendium*, fols. 248ra–b.
[64] See P. Dronke (ed.), *A History of Twelfth-Century Western Philosophy* (Cambridge, 1988).

(and this was expected of them) establishing the state of health of a particular person and/or the healing of one sick person or another. For this purpose, it sufficed that they should have been trained to discover and interpret the symptomatic indications (*signa, manifestationes*) that were obtained by means of the senses ('propter manifestationem in sensu').

The truth, knowledge of the essence of things, was the proper domain of the natural philosopher. He alone, as long as he exercised the intellectual function for which he had been trained, had at his disposition the exclusively intellectual resources that enabled him to attain the very plane of the substance (*essentia*) of the human being. In this respect, the human being's state of health or illness was not irrelevant to him. However, the specific state of health or illness, that of this or that man or woman, boy or girl, old man or woman, belonged to another level of the human condition, a plane that could be seen, touched and questioned, and to which access could be gained by means of the senses of the person who was trained for this purpose, the physician (*artifex sanitatis*). This is the plane of utilitas.[65]

A younger contemporary of Gilbertus de Aquila, Cardinalis, professor at the Montpellier school of medicine around the year 1250, summarized this double plane when he distinguished between 'the [natural] philosophers who dedicate their time to getting to know the causes and essences of things', and 'the physician, who pays more attention to usefulness than to the truth'.[66] Some forty years afterwards in the 1290s, another Montpellier university physician, Arnald de Villanova, did not hesitate to state that 'the natural philosopher does not orient his intellectual activity toward practice but toward a full understanding of the nature of the moving body'.[67] These words seem to be an echo of those of Aristotle: '[Natural] philosophy is neither practical nor profitable but purely theoretical in its nature.'[68]

The aim of physicians – their social justification as a last resort – was not to discover the truth, but to treat the individual patient; in brief, to be able, when they were so required, to respond with a certain degree of coherence to the health expectations put forward by the individuals

[65] The problem is analysed by M.R. McVaugh with respect to the medical circle of Montpellier, and especially Arnald de Villanova. See his article, 'The Nature and Limits of Medical Certitude at Early Fourteenth-Century Montpellier', *Osiris*, 2nd series, 6 (1990), 62–84.

[66] *Commentary to Ysagoge*, Kues, Hospital 222, fols. 40va. Cited by M.R. McVaugh (note 23), p. 278, n. 52.

[67] 'Naturalis autem philosophus suam considerationem et cognitionem ad opus non ordinat sed ad plenariam considerationem vere corporis mobilis': *De intentione medicorum*, AV, fol. 52rb.

[68] A, *Metaph.*, 1064a.16–18.

belonging to different social groupings. The social collectives as such (the municipal councils among others) also had these same expectations of the medieval physician.[69] The intellectual detonator that set off these reflections and expectations, which were to occupy a great part of the thirteenth century, were Avicenna's *Canon*, the 'new Galen', and the 'Latin Aristotle', among others. In fact, both Gilbertus de Aquila's reflections and the commentaries of Cardinalis and of Arnald himself, were directly inspired by specific passages of the *Canon*, in which Avicenna himself was stimulated by the problem of reconciling the conflicting opinions about the heart:

> The physician as such need not be concerned about which of these two opinions [on the function of the heart] is true; that is the business of the natural philosopher. The physician, once the existence of the principles of the above-mentioned virtues or powers [the heart, the liver, the brain and the testicles] has been taken for granted, does not question them. When it comes to providing treatment, he does not worry about which is the first of them.[70]

Later on, when considering the role of male and female semen in the formation of the embryo, he did not hesitate to say, 'Knowledge of the truth of the two opinions [expounded] is for the natural philosopher and in no way does it prejudice the physician not to take them into account.'[71] Despite the massive influx of Galen's writings, together with those of Arab medical authors, that occurred in intellectual circles in the Latin West in the 1270s and 1280s, a movement which provoked a real intellectual upheaval in the approach to medical subjects, it was not lost from sight that the physician's mission was to preserve health and to return it when it had been lost, to be an *artifex factivus*. Furthermore, this movement, which has been called the 'new Galen', reinforced the trends we are talking about through the reading and translation of new Galenic works such as *De interioribus*, one of the masterpieces in the approach to clinical problems.[72] The figure of the physician as a 'professional' who carries out something specific (*factibilis*) was to be

---

[69]   See García-Ballester et al. (note 78); V. Nutton, 'Continuity or Rediscovery? The City Physician in Classical Antiquity and Medieval Italy', in A. W. Russel (ed.), *The Town and State Physician in Europe from the Middle Ages to the Enlightenment* (Wolfenbuttel, 1981), pp. 9–46; and M.R. McVaugh, *Medicine Before the Plague. Practitioners and Their Patients in the Crown of Aragon, 1285–1345* (Cambridge, 1993).

[70]   *Canon*, book 1, fen. 1, doc. 6, ch. 1, pp. 70b–71a.

[71]   *Canon*, book 3, fen. 2, treat. 1, ch. 3, p. 901a.

[72]   L. García-Ballester, 'Arnau de Vilanova (*ca.* 1240–1311) y la reforma de los estudios médicos en Montpellier (1309): El Hipócrates latino y la introducción del nuevo Galeno', *Dynamis*, 2 (1982), 97–158. See also my introductory study to R. Durling (ed.), *Arnaldi de Villanova Commentum libri Galieni de interioribus* (Barcelona, 1985), pp. 31–3 (Arnaldi de Villanova Opera Medica Omnia, vol. 15, pp. 297–351).

used in the medical circles of Montpellier again around 1300. Bernard de Angrarra, in one of the quaestiones that he posed concerning Hippocrates' *Aphorisms*, said: 'Medicine considers the naturals and the non-naturals only insofar as they matter in practice (*opus*), namely to the conservation or restoration of health; hence its nature is not purely theoretical (*speculabilis*) but practically oriented (*factibilis*).'[73]

Again Aristotle is in the background of this sequence of assertions: 'And the physician continues reasoning until he arrives at what he himself finally can do; then the process from this point onwards, i.e., the process towards health, is called "production".'[74] Consciously or unconsciously the Montpellier university physicians made a meaningful reading of the Latin Aristotle. Medical speculation on the subjects of health and illness was unjustifiable unless it had as its aim the clarification of a procedure to make it efficient. The physician saw health as the objective in the human body.[75]

The concept of usefulness (utilitas) was closely linked to the justification of the physician's presence in society, both among non-academic social groupings – by demonstrating the efficacy of his knowledge through practice – and in the academic community itself. The presence of physicians in the latter was justified only as long as they were able to train *artifices* (*phisici*, *cirurgici*) who might solve the problems of health arising in the community that the university served. I do not believe that the references to this last point in the foundational statutes of new *Studia Generalia* or universities in frontier regions of western Christendom (for example, the *Studium Generale* of Lleida in 1300) were unrelated to the debates that were taking place in academic circles, such as those of Montpellier or Paris, on the demarcation of the functions of the *phisici* with respect to the *philosophi naturales*.[76]

One of the great developments of the medieval Latin West at an intellectual level was the conviction that this utilitas – whatever its degree of efficiency, and always measured according to the contemporary system of values, rather than our own present-day standards – would be achieved when physicians' actions and all their operations (from the writing of the humblest prescription to the cauterization of haemorrhoids) were

---

[73] Erfurt, Wissenschaftliche Allgemeinbibl., manuscript F 290, fol. 40va. Trans. by McVaugh, slightly modified, in his article (note 65), p. 80.

[74] A, *Metaph.*, 1032b.6–10; 981a.18–20.

[75] For example, Arnald de Villanova: 'In arte medicine in qua sanitas primo': *De intentione medicorum*; see AV, fol. 51b; *Speculum medicine*, AV, fol. 1ra.

[76] 1 September 1300. Published by A. Rubió i Lluch, *Documents per l'histyoria de la cultura catalana mig-eval*, 2 vols. (Barcelona, 1908), vol. 1, pp. 14–16, doc. 15. See M.R. McVaugh and L. García-Ballester, 'The Medical Faculty at Early Fourteenth-Century Lérida', *History of Universities*, 6 (1989), 1–27.

endowed with intellectual rigour. This could be attained – in the opinion
of intellectualized physicians from the twelfth century onwards – only by
means of Aristotelian natural philosophy, from its logic to its embryology,
from its ideas on man and on social organization to its opinions on basic
vital processes such as putrefaction, growth or death.

This intellectual thoroughness was attained by medicine in the
medieval world only when it achieved the status of a scientia. Although in
historical terms such a status was achieved and had a social impact with
the advent of universities from the first third of the thirteenth century, it
cannot be forgotten that medicine as scientia had been considered and
debated in certain circles in the Latin West as much as a century before
(although it is not possible, at the moment, to be more precise about an
initial date). This is reflected in the first commentaries on the *Articella*
produced by the so-called Salernitan masters.[77] Moreover, such a
conviction was transferred to those healers who were not in direct contact
with the university world, and was shared by many of them; not only by
physicians and surgeons, but also by apothecaries and barbers.[78]

Although everything that is here being described had social implications we should not forget the fact that we are describing an intellectual
process. And it is here that the efficacy of Aristotelian methodology,
which we can centre on his *Posterior Analytics* and on the tradition of the
Problemata, was demonstrated. Aristotle provided not only a particular
method of reasoning (which can be described schematically as deductive
syllogism), but at least two further points as well. First, there was a
starting point for a particular form of carrying it out, something that was
characteristic of the most developed form of medieval medical thought
(the isolation of medical problems in order to handle them on
intellectual grounds in the form of quaestiones), and, second, a basic
doctrinal nucleus which enabled rational accounts to be given of natural
processes such as those of health and illness, with their different forms of
manifesting themselves among human beings.[79]

[77] See Kristeller (note 34); T. Pesenti, 'Arti e medicina: la formazione del curriculum
medico', in L. Gargan-Oronzo Limone (ed.), *Luoghi e metodi di insegnamento nell'Italia
medioevale, secoli XII–XIV* (Galatina, 1989), pp. 155–77; and M.D. Jordan, 'The
Construction of a Philosophical Medicine. Exegesis and Argument in Salernitan
Teaching on the Soul', *Osiris*, 2nd series, 6 (1990), 42–61.
[78] L. García-Ballester, M.R. McVaugh and A. Rubio, *Medical Licensing and Learning in
Fourteenth-Century Valencia*, Transactions of the American Philosophical Society, vol.
79, part 6 (Philadelphia, 1989), and the literature cited there.
[79] See D. Jacquart, 'Aristotelian Thought in Salerno' in P. Dronke (note 64), pp. 407–
28; B. Lawn, *The Salernitan Questions: An Introduction to the History of Medieval and
Renaissance Problem Literature* (Oxford, 1963); L. García-Ballester, L. Ferre and
E. Feliu, 'Jewish Appreciation of Fourteenth-Century Scholastic Medicine', *Osiris*,
2nd series, 6 (1990), 85–117.

What is here being expounded is the relationship between a rational knowledge of nature, on the one hand, and the efficient management of nature, on the other, all in connection with the subject of health and illness. This was a matter for debate among, and of considerable concern to, intellectuals in the Latin West throughout the twelfth and thirteenth centuries and even beyond. The debates took the form of a discussion on whether medicine was or was not a mechanical art, on whether it should or should not be included among the so-called Liberal Arts, on whether it should be considered as a scientia, and at the same time as an ars, or the latter alone.

By the middle of the thirteenth century the argument that had occupied the previous years about the overall position of medicine within knowledge as a whole no longer made much sense. Words such as the following, uttered by someone from outside the medical world (Albert the Great in 1246), are a clear indication that the fields of natural philosophy and medicine were by then perfectly demarcated, once medicine had adopted Aristotelian assumptions:

I must point out that should problems arise concerning faith and custom, I am more inclined towards Augustine than towards the [natural] philosophers. If the problems are expounded in the field of medicine (*medicina*), I shall be inclined towards Galen and Hippocrates; and should we be dealing with things concerning nature (*de naturis rerum*), I shall follow Aristotle more than any other.[80]

In the early fourteenth century, both the university physician and surgeon considered both their practice and intellectual terrain as the most highly regarded among the range of fields of learning available at that time. This can be deduced from Arnald de Villanova's evidence as a physician, and from Henri de Mondeville's as a surgeon. The author of the *Antidotarium* was to say, 'Medicine is the most highly esteemed of the present-day sciences.'[81] Henri de Mondeville was to proclaim that 'Surgery should be considered the most highly valued of all the arts, whether liberal or mechanical, and the most highly appreciated of all the sciences.'[82] I believe that the considerable effort dedicated to making the plane of utilitas as respectable as that of veritas on the part of university-trained physicians and surgeons had much to do with the growing status

80 AM, *Super II Sententiarum*, vol. 27, p. 247. The date 1246 is given in one of the arguments in book 2 of the *Sentences*: see Weisheipl (note 11), p. 22.
81 'ac ipsa [medicina] preciosior scientis cunctis existens': *Antidotarium*, in AV, fol. 310vb.
82 'Quod chirurgia super omnes artes et scientias tam liberales quam mechanicas debet beatissima reputari': Henri de Mondeville, *Chirurgia*, J. Pagel (ed.), (Berlin, 1892), p. 134.

of physicians who constituted one of the most influential groups in late medieval Latin society.

Medicine, inasmuch as it was a form of attending and treating a patient, had immediate practical implications, both at an individual and collective level – unlike natural philosophy, which had no apparent practical repercussions outside the academic world (let us remember Arnald's opinion, 'the natural philosopher does not orient his thought toward practice'). We are far from Aristotle's idea of knowledge as a matter of 'intellectual curiosity',[83] even though his doctrines were the intellectual force which took medieval medicine from empirical praxis to a socially and intellectually respected scientia, albeit a science which should be useful in the sense that it involves health as a part of material welfare. In spite of their different objectives, natural philosophy and medicine were closely associated in the Latin West from the twelfth century onwards, and especially when university institutions started to prevail from the first third of the thirteenth century onwards. As already remarked, these institutions endowed medicine with intellectual respectability. But insofar as a wide and relatively rapid geographical spread of physicians and surgeons who based their practice on the new form of medical Galenism can be documented, to such an extent can we also say that it was socially respectable.[84]

These professionals were even sought out by small rural municipalities which included in their annual budgets a sum to cover their medical welfare requirements, in which the basic feature was a contract with a medical practitioner (physician and/or surgeon), if possible, one with university training[85] – the 'maker of health', to return to Thomas Aquinas' attractive, new expression, an expression which demonstrates more of an intellectual innovation and an ideal to stimulate others than a true reflection of a social situation which the medieval Latin world was far from attaining.

ACKNOWLEDGEMENTS

Funding for this research was provided by CICYT grants nos. PB\89–0066 and PB\92–0910–01 from the Spanish Ministry of Education and Science (Dirección General de Investigación Científica y Técnica).

[83]   A, *Metaph.*, 982b.11ff.: 'It was their curiosity that first led men to philosophize ... It is evident that they learned in the pursuit of knowledge, and not for some useful end': *Aristotle's Metaphysics*, trans. by R. Hope (New York, 1952), p. 7.
[84]   M.R. McVaugh (note 69).
[85]   Ibid.

ABBREVIATIONS

A, *De gen. et corr.*	Aristotle, *De generatione et corruptione*, translatio vetus, J. Judycka (ed.), *Aristoteles latinus*, vol. 9, part 1 (Leiden, 1986).
A, *De partibus animalium*	Aristotle, *Parts of Animals*, with an English translation by A.L. Peck (ed.), Loeb Classical Library (Cambridge, Mass. and London, 1983). Treatises of Aristotle cited according to the Greek edition by E. Bekker (Berlin, 1931; repr. Berlin, 1960, 1970) as follows: page, column (a, b), line number(s).
A, *Metaph.*	Aristotle, *Metaphisica*, in Thomas Aquinas, *In duodecim libros Metaphisicorum Aristotelis expositio*, cura et studio R. M. Spiazzi (Turin, 1971). This edition reproduces the thirteenth-century Latin text, translated from Greek by William de Moerbeke, and used by Thomas Aquinas.
AM	Albert the Great, *Opera omnia*, A. Borgnet (ed.), 38 vols. (Paris, 1890–9).
AM, *Metaph.*	Albert the Great, *Metaphysica*, B. Geyer (ed.), vol. 16 (books 6–13), *Opera omnia*, Institutum Alberti Magni Coloniense (ed.) (Münster i. Westf., 1964).
AV	*Opera Arnaldi de Villanova* (Lyon, 1608).
Canon	Avicenna, *Canon medicinae* (Venice, 1608). Fragments cited according to books (five), 'fen', doctrines or treatises and chapters.
Compendium	Gilbertus de Aquila (Anglicus), *Compendium medicine . . . tam morborum universalium quam particularium nondum medicis sed cyrurgicis utilissimum* (Lyon, 1510).
Pantegni	*Liber Pantegni*, in *Omnia Opera Ysaac* (Lyon, 1515). The work is divided into two parts (*Liber theorice* and *Liber practice*) with different books and chapters.
PH, *In techne* or *De animalibus*	Peter of Spain (Petrus Hispanus), *Commentum in techne Galieni, Questiones de animalibus*, Madrid, Biblioteca Nacional, manuscript 1877.
Rhazes	*Abubetri Rhazae Liber ad regem Mansorem* (Basel, 1544; repr. Brussels, 1973). Divided into books (10) and chapters.

TA, *De sensu*   Thomas Aquinas, *Sancti Thomae de Aquino Sententia libri De sensu et sensato, cuius secundus tractatus est De memoria et reminiscentia*, cura et studio Fratrum Praedicatorum, *Opera omnia*, Commissio Leonina (ed.), vol. 45, 2 (Rome and Paris, 1985). Cited according to line number(s). An asterisk refers to the introduction.

TA, *Summa*   Thomas Aquinas, *Summa Theologica*, Tertia pars, cura et studio Fratrum Praedicatorum, *Opera omnia*, Commissio Leonina (ed.), vols. 11 and 12 (Rome, 1903–6).

VB, *Speculum nat.* or *Speculum doc.* or *Speculum maius*   Vincent de Beauvais, *Speculum maius*, 4 vols. (Dvaci, 1624; repr. Graz, 1964–5), vol. 1: *Speculum naturale*; vol. 2: *Speculum doctrinale*. A general prologue is printed in the first volume. Each part is divided into books and chapters. The printed edition is divided into columns instead of pages.

8   Epistemology and learned medicine in early modern England

Andrew Wear

Preface

This paper poses the question as to whether and how far it is possible to talk of epistemology in relation to a learned tradition in medicine, when that tradition is well established and is concerned to emphasize the unchanging nature of its knowledge in the struggles against its competitors in the medical market place. Some of the discussion bears upon the question of why learned medicine came to die out in England, but this issue is not the main focus of the paper.

I have not spelled out modern-day historiographic categories (for instance, epistemic or sociological, or to use more old-fashioned terms from the history of science and medicine, internal or external). They express dichotomies which for the sixteenth and seventeenth centuries are not historically grounded. (For instance, a sixteenth-century divine or politician would not have agreed that a point of religious doctrine was a matter either of epistemology or sociology – even if the latter could have been recognized at the time – though it might be seen as a blend of both. Our modern scholarly traditions and disciplinary rivalries mean that one or the other tend to be given priority.)

Introduction

The epistemology of Western learned or scholarly medicine was not completely successful; it did not produce knowledge of such certainty as to kill off all other rivals in the medical market place. It is also doubtful if in early modern Europe learned medicine was using epistemology in any heuristic sense to create new knowledge. Nevertheless, it is perhaps possible to see a kind of epistemology at work when patients' symptoms were being related to already established explanatory categories, and epistemology was certainly part of the rhetoric used by learned physicians to do down the opposition – they claimed that they possessed the correct epistemology whilst empirics and others did not.

In this paper I want to try to bridge the gap that usually exists between philosophers and historians. Discussion of epistemology is often carried out in terms of the discrete categories of philosophers, such as 'observation', 'reason', etc. and their various amplifications in which everyone, it is assumed, is a rational being, or at least possessing an equal amount of reason. Historians, well aware of the diversity of people and of the uses to which appeals to reason can be put, tend to ignore such epistemological discussions; at least they ignore their details and look only to their effects. I have a sympathy with this latter approach, but in the case of learned medicine consideration of epistemology is at the heart of its claims to be the best form of medicine and the nature of its epistemology cannot be ignored. First, the connection between epistemology and the wider world is worth considering in the broadest of terms.

Learned or scholarly medicine in Europe was born in classical times without any protection or privilege, except insofar as it shared in the power and status of literate culture. Despite the claims of this type of medicine to possess the most certain form of knowledge, neither Greek states nor Roman governments recognized any such claims, for instance, by instituting a system of licensing of medical practitioners or any other measure of protection for learned medicine. In the Middle Ages and Renaissance learned medicine did become more culturally defined and perhaps its epistemological claims came to be more recognized. It was taught in the universities and given some special status by limited local licensing by city colleges of medicine or by Spain's Protomedicato.[1] Epistemology did not play a totally successful role in the career of learned medicine. If epistemology is concerned with how certain knowledge is acquired then it is clear that not everyone from the classical period to the end of the sixteenth century was convinced that medicine had acquired such knowledge. Other systems of healing and other epistemologies managed to compete

---

[1]   See, for instance, Nancy Siraisi, *Medieval and Early Renaissance Medicine* (Chicago: Chicago University Press, 1990); Katharine Park, *Doctors and Medicine in Early Renaissance Florence* (Princeton: Princeton University Press, 1985); Richard Palmer, *The Studio of Venice and its Graduates in the Sixteenth Century* (Padua: Edizioni Lint, 1983); Andrew W. Russell (ed.), *The Town and State Physician in Europe from the Middle Ages to the Enlightenment* (Wolfenbüttel: Wolfenbütteler Forschungen, 1981), vol. 17; Luis García-Ballester, Michael R. McVaugh and Augustin Rubio-Vela, *Medical Licensing and Learning in Fourteenth-Century Valencia*, Transactions of the American Philosophical Society, vol. 79 (Philadelphia: American Philosophical Society, 1989), part 6; J.T. Lanning, *The Royal Protomedicato: The Regulation of the Medical Profession in the Spanish Empire* (Durham: Duke University Press, 1985); Sir George Clark, *A History of the Royal College of Physicians of London*, 2 vols. (Oxford: Clarendon Press, 1964), vol. 1.

successfully with learned medicine, with the medicine of Galen and his followers.[2]

At this point I want to argue, slightly pedantically, that one reading of epistemology, the art of acquiring certain knowledge, is that there is a necessary connection between certainty and the assent of people to that certainty. The acid test of certain knowledge was, as Aristotle argued, that once it was demonstrated or laid out to view then everyone would immediately agree with it.[3] What I am doing here, of course, is trying to show that on philosophical grounds there is a connection between *epistēmē*, certain knowledge, and people or the world at large – rather than imposing the connection.

Of course, not everyone is a philosopher, and Galen for instance could, and did, blame his patients and his medical rivals for not being as educated as he was and thus failing to be convinced by his arguments and conclusions.[4] In other words, despite the belief by some philosophers that *a priori* everyone should be able to recognize and agree to certain knowledge, it might be, as Plato would argue, that most people's minds were too clouded and only the few could achieve such recognition.

Here it seems to me we have two positions. First, it is in the nature of certain knowledge that it is certain only if it is acceded to by all, and if this immediate perception, whether by the mind or eye, does not occur, then it is not certain knowledge (this latter, converse, view, although it logically follows, for obvious reasons was not popular with many philosophers). Second, that failure to agree to what someone puts forward as certain knowledge may not necessarily invalidate such knowledge, but may be the result of the ignorance, obtuseness and blindness of the general population – this view was popular with philosophers (and medical, legal and religious writers), even if by holding this opinion the universal power, to produce assent, inherent in certain knowledge was adversely affected. I suspect that many learned

---

2   On the diversity of the medical market place see Siraisi and Park (note 1); Roy Porter (ed.), *Patients and Practitioners. Lay Perceptions of Medicine in Pre-industrial Society* (Cambridge: Cambridge University Press, 1985); Lucinda McCray Beier, *Sufferers and Healers. The Experience of Illness in Seventeenth-century England* (London: Routledge, 1987); Vivian Nutton, 'Healers in the Medical Market Place: Towards a Social History of Graeco-Roman Medicine', and Katharine Park, 'Medicine and Society in Medieval Europe', in Andrew Wear (ed.), *Medicine in Society. Historical Essays* (Cambridge: Cambridge University Press, 1992), pp. 15–58 and 59–90.

3   See Aristotle, *Posterior Analytics* 71b17–72b4.

4   For example in Galen, *On Examinations by which the Best Physicians are Recognised*, edition of the Arabic version with English translation and commentary by Albert Z. Iskendar (Berlin: Medicorum Graecorum Supplementum Orientale, Academie-Verlag Berlin, 1988).

traditions in many different societies exhibit this tension between the belief that their knowledge is so certain that everyone should agree with it and the realization that in practice not everyone does. Institutionally, the result is that learned traditions make universalistic claims but also have a sense of being an exclusive group with everyone within them sharing and agreeing to a set of accepted propositions, whilst the rest of the world outside has yet to be convinced (as in the case of the learned physicians of sixteenth- and early seventeenth-century England). At different times such groups might feel beleaguered or they might derive a sense of power from their exclusiveness as does, for instance, the medical profession in the twentieth century.

I hope I have made the point that there is a reasonably natural connection between epistemology and people. Other chapters explore in detail the epistemological bases of Western learned medicine. But for the purposes of my chapter I want to point out that classical medicine did not make as strong claims as did classical philosophy to certainty. The perennial debate as to whether medicine was a science, that is concerned with knowledge, or an art or *technē* is one sign of this. Another is the Hippocratic recognition, echoed throughout the centuries, that there is a multiplicity of experience in medicine, some of it fallacious.

Learned medicine did, however, have an epistemological standpoint. Galen's epistemology was a blend of the empirical and the rational, for Galen believed that one without the other led to the excesses of the empiricists and the methodists. I leave it to others to discuss Galen's heuristic use of experience and reason. For learned medicine in the sixteenth century, that is Galenic medicine, there is no doubt that what was crucial was accepting Galen's doctrines rather than developing new fundamental theories by experience or reason.[5] The humanist revival of the *prisca medicina* of the Greeks brought with it a great emphasis on orthodoxy (one can also find the same with the arrival of the 'new Galen' in the Middle Ages).[6] Innovation within learned medicine did occur, but only in one or two areas such as anatomy, where new observational knowledge contradicted Galen's observations but not his physiological

[5]   Walter Pagel, 'Medical Humanism – a Historical Necessity in the Era of the Renaissance', in F. Maddison, M. Pelling and C. Webster (eds.), *Essays on the Life and Work of Thomas Linacre* c. *1460–1524* (Oxford: Oxford University Press, 1977), pp. 375–86; Vivian Nutton, 'John Caius and the Linacre Tradition', *Medical History*, 23 (1979), 373–91; Andrew Wear, 'Galen in the Renaissance', in V. Nutton (ed.), *Galen: Problems and Prospects* (London: Wellcome Institute for the History of Medicine, 1981), pp. 229–56.

[6]   See Luis García-Ballester, 'Arnau de Vilanova (c. 1240–1311) y la reforma de los estudios médicos en Montpellier (1309): el Hippócrates latino y la introducción del nuevo Galeno', *Dynamis*, 2 (1982), 97–158.

theories of the body, or in relation to diseases such as syphilis and plague.

The great effort of the learned physicians lay in trying to get rid of uncertainty in the application of Galen's medicine to the myriad differences that existed among patients. Their different environments and life-styles all had to be taken into account together with their ill conditions or ill constitutions when aetiology and therapy were being considered. Da Monte at Padua, especially, was concerned with the enterprise of making Galenic medicine more methodical.[7] The popularity of tables setting out aspects of Galenic medicine (with the most general categories on the left of the page and then moving by inclusive brackets to more detailed headings on the right of the page) is a sign of this interest in reducing learned medicine to method and hence to greater certainty. But such tables are also to be found at this time in other learned traditions such as law and were not confined only to medicine.[8]

In a sense, the learned traditions of the Renaissance were at a stage where new fundamental knowledge was not the issue. Rather the emphasis lay in being true to the past and in ordering past knowledge in the best possible way. (Here, comparisons with other learned traditions would be interesting.) However, within learned medicine there was some room for creativity and for personally acquiring knowledge, and this is discussed below.

Early modern England

A discussion of epistemology and learned medicine in sixteenth-century England could also apply to much of Europe. However, compared to Italy England was a backwater; it was not a major centre for the renaissance of medicine. It did possess a few good humanist scholars like John Caius though much of medical knowledge was transmitted in English and not in Latin books, and in the seventeenth century William Harvey gave England a reputation in anatomy.

[7]   See A. Wear, 'Contingency and Logic in Renaissance Anatomy and Physiology', unpublished Ph.D. thesis, London University (1973), pp. 175–243; Donald G. Bates, 'Sydenham and the Medical Meaning of "Method" ', *Bulletin of the History of Medicine*, 51 (1977), 324–38; A. Wear (note 5), pp. 238–45; Jerome Bylebyl, 'Teaching *Methodus Medendi* in the Renaissance', in F. Kudlein and Richard J. Durling (eds.), *Galen's Method of Healing* (Leiden: E.J. Brill, 1991), pp. 157–89.

[8]   K.J. Höltgen, 'Synoptische Tabellen in der Medizinischen Literatur und die Logik Agricolas und Ramus', *Sudhoffs Archiv*, 49 (1965), 371–90; more generally N.W. Gilbert, *Renaissance Concepts of Method* (New York: Columbia University Press, 1960); W.J. Ong, *Ramus' Method and the Decay of Dialogue* (Cambridge, Mass.: Harvard University Press, 1958).

It also had the College of Physicians of London, founded on the model of the Italian city college of medicine, which had limited and not very effective powers of overseeing medical practice in London and seven miles around. The College often seemed beleaguered. In the sixteenth century politicians like the Secretary of State Francis Walsingham and at times Elizabeth herself interfered with the College's policing of unlicensed practice in London. In the seventeenth century its powers to prosecute illicit practice began to be circumscribed by the courts and by the beginning of the eighteenth century the apothecaries had acquired the right to practise.[9] Essentially, there was an open medical market place in early modern England, and learned medicine was one amongst many groups which offered medical services.

This was a context in which claims to exclusiveness of knowledge, to having the right answers, was balanced by the fact that the medical culture of the time encouraged an eclectic mix of views. What I want to do is to analyse some of the ways in which epistemology was used by the learned physicians in their war against their medical opponents. But first it is worth considering in a general way the use or otherwise of epistemology in medicine at this time.

Authority, reason and experience

In 1628 the Bath physician Tobias Venner produced one of the many health advice books. His *Via Recta ad Vitam Longam* was:

a plaine Philosophicall demonstration of the Nature, faculties and effects of all such things as by way of nourishment make for the preservation of health, with divers necessary dieticall; as also of the true use and effects of sleepe, exercise, excretions and pertubations, with just applications to every age, constitution of body and time of yeare.[10]

Venner was offering advice on hygiene or the preservation of health, something which the learned physicians took pride in claiming was lacking in their opponents, the empirics, who treated patients only when they became ill.[11]

Venner was a good Galenist, but he had his own opinions. The learned physicians did not have to follow authority slavishly. Galen had

---

[9]   See Sir George Clark (note 1), and especially Harold J. Cook, *The Decline of the Old Medical Regime in Stuart London* (Ithaca and London: Cornell University Press, 1986).

[10]   Tobias Venner, *Via Recta ad Vitam Longam* (London, 1628), title page.

[11]   On the views of learned physicians on empirics and their stress on regimen see Harold J. Cook, 'The New Philosophy and Medicine in Seventeenth-Century England', in David Lindberg and Robert Westman (eds.), *Reappraisals of the Scientific Revolution* (Cambridge: Cambridge University Press, 1990), pp. 396–436.

commended pig's flesh, but Venner disagreed and set up his own criteria of what made for good nourishment:

Swines flesh, because of the strong and abundant nourishment that it yeeldeth, as also of the likenesse that it hath unto mans flesh both in savour and taste, is of Galen and other of the ancient Physicians, commended above all other kindes of flesh in nourishing the body. But in my opinion, the choice of flesh is rather to be taken, from an odoriferous pleasantnesse of the same, laudable substance, good temperature, easie concoction, and goodnesse of iuyce that it breedeth, then from the strongnesses of nourishment that it giveth, or the aforesaid. In respect of all which, Veale, Mutton, Steere or Heyfer Beefe are to be preferred before Porke. (p. 50)

All the criteria here are subjective ones. This, of course, fits the subjective basis of Western learned medicine – its four humours were made up of the different combinations of the qualities hot, cold, dry and wet which are all perceived by the senses. Galen judged pig's meat to be like man's flesh 'both in savour and taste' (the epistemology of cannibalism). Likewise, Venner's criteria were also subjective and based on the senses: 'odoriferous pleasantnesse' is clear enough whilst 'laudable substance', 'good temperature', 'easie concoction' and 'goodnesse of iuyce' are assessments dependent on personal judgement or experience, even if they had some theoretical grounding, for instance, on what 'good temperature' or temperament might be. The subjective experiential element that lay at the heart of Galenic medicine allowed different subjective criteria of, in this case, the goodness of pig's flesh, to be easily substituted. It also meant that, using such criteria, everyone could judge of the goodness of pig meat. An expert like Venner declared what sort of meat was good, but he used language which was held in common with his readers. After all, the goodness of meat, fish, water and so on was something that everyone had to decide daily for themselves. There were no water boards to guarantee the purity of water, and the inspection of markets was not very effective.

But what Venner did was to use this language and also more specialized terminology in areas which his readership would not normally have entered. He was able, as an expert, to make statements about what happened inside the body when particular foods were eaten. He wrote:

But seeing that Porke is of hard digestion, and in substance more grosse than convenient, it is not good for them that be aged, that are grosse, that have weake stomackes, that live at ease, or are any wayes unsound of body. For in such it causeth obstructions of the mesaraicke veines, liver and reines, the Gowte and Dropsie, especially if they shall be cold and moyst by constitution; for unto them is Porke very greatly hurtfull, because in them it is wholly converted into crude and phlegmaticke humors. Wherefore let such as are phelegmaticke, aged or subject unto obstructions, that leade a studious life or have queasie stomackes, altogether abstaine from the use of Porke. (pp. 50–1)

From the possibly common experience that pork is difficult to digest Venner then proceeded to hidden events taking place within the body. He imagines what pork does inside the body: his story is shaped by Galen's theory of digestion (food is concocted in the stomach into chyle which then travels through the mesenteric veins to the liver to be altered into blood) and his conclusions about the effect of pork on phlegmatic constitutions and upon the aged are conditioned by Galenic humoral theories. Yet the reader is given the sense that Venner has really seen what is happening in the body. The anatomical references help to do this for they signify observable structures. In a sense, here we have authority and pre-established theories being used in a reasonably creative and lively way to give the impression that the author has actual (experienced?) knowledge of what he is stating is going on in the body.

Paradoxically, Venner is using Galenic epistemology, the mix of the empirical and the rational, to describe the effect of pork in the body; but he is doing so not in the way we normally think of epistemology being used, that is to discover and establish new knowledge. Instead, Venner is creating knowledge but from old knowledge. And I suspect that this applied to most of learned medicine at this time – inevitably so.

What is striking about Venner's account of the healthiness of pig meat is how his judgement of what is the case appears authoritative. The experiential-subjective basis of the qualitative system in natural philosophy and medicine meant that ultimately each individual had through their senses the capacity to judge the nature of the world and of all living things in it (obviously keeping within the broad theoretical framework of qualities, elements and humours).

Perhaps there is also, as well as the mix of the personal and the Galenic, another aspect to Venner's account. Aphoristic, declaratory, knowledge had a long history going back to the Hippocratics. This type of knowledge is often expressed without any hints as to its origin. Here is Venner on birds:

The Black-bird or Owle that is fat, is greatly commended for pleasantnesse of taste, lightnesse of digestion and goodnesse of nourishment. The Thrush that is of a darke reddish colour, is of the same nature: they are best in the winter, and are convenient for every age and constitution of the body, especially for the phlegmaticke. (p. 60)

Common experience, oral tradition, personal experience and learned authority could be involved in such aphoristic knowledge. Some of this knowledge we tend to call received wisdom, for instance the often repeated view that marshy ground was unhealthy which now has the support of modern historical demographers.[12] However, what is significant is that these pieces of discrete knowledge do not usually disclose how they were arrived at. Their epistemic origins lie hidden.

William Vaughan, an unsuccessful colonizer of Newfoundland and a writer on health matters, wrote in his *Directions for Health* (1617) of the healthiness of water and asked, 'What is the nature of Fountaine-Water?' He answered:

Fountaine-water is the best water for preservation of health: But you must observe, of what side it springs, for if it comes from the East, it excels the rest as well in moysture and thinnesse of substance, as in pleasant smel, and it doth moderately comfort the spirits: Contrariwise those fountaines which spring out of rockes, towards the North, and which have the Sunne backward, are of a hard digestion, and nothing so pure as the other.[13]

Vaughan gave some rationalizations or explanations: fountain waters from the east are thinner and of pleasanter smell, whilst from the north are hard to digest and not so pure. But on the basic points of why fountain water was healthiest and of why the east was better than the north there was no real explanation of how these conclusions were arrived at. This type of declaratory knowledge was very common in learned medicine in the early modern period. It can be found at the centre of curative medicine, in its remedies. The lists of remedies in books on practical medicine are usually presented baldly, as a list of ingredients without any rationale for their use. What was important was the recipe itself, but how it came about, or how it was known that it was successful, was often not discussed. At a popular level there were a large number of books published which gave the remedies collected by the nobility, by royalty or by famous doctors. Again, there was no explanation of why they worked in particular diseases. All one has is the name of the condition and a number of remedies for it. Leonard Sowerby in *The Ladies Dispensatory* (1652), which was concerned to list simples rather than medicines 'compounded by a hodge podge of sophisticated Drugs',[14] advised 'for those which spit and vomite Bloud' one or other of the following simple remedies:

[12] See Mary Dobson, ' "Marsh Fever": A Geography of Malaria in England', *Journal of Historical Geography*, 6 (1980), 359–89; also see Mary Dobson, 'The Last Hiccup of the Old Demographic Regime: Population Stagnation and Decline in Late Seventeenth and Early Eighteenth-Century England', *Continuity and Change*, 4 (1989), 395–428.
[13] William Vaughan, *Directions for Health*, 5th edition (London, 1617), p. 24.
[14] Leonard Sowerby, *The Ladies Dispensatory* (London, 1652), 'To the Reader', p. A4r.

Reere Eggs supped
Ashes of Harts – horne washed, and drunk with Gum Dragant
Water Betony drunk
Juyce of wild Time the weight of two drachms drunk in vinegar
Dung of a wild she goate mingled with wine, or water, drunk
Purslaine well boyled eaten. (p. 62)

Or, of special concern to Ladies, 'to cause standing of the yard' one had the choice of:

Costus drunk in honied wine
Saffron drunk
Lin-Seed taken with hony and peper
Boyled Turnips eaten
Rocket much eaten
Seed of Rocket eaten. (p. 19)

Sowerby wrote that he had followed Gerard with Johnson, Goraeus and Fuchs, and had no objection against 'my Authour Dioscorides' (p. A4r). Their authoritative experience or learning gave validity to the remedies. Of course, more learned writers might give the qualitative degree of heat, cold, moisture or dryness of an illness and provide for it a remedy of an appropriate degree of a contrary quality (the cure by contrary quality). But even here a writer could always disagree with tradition and use his personal, subjective judgement to define anew the quality of a remedy – something which in any case he would have to do with newly discovered medicines, for instance, from the New World. In practice, only simples or remedies with very few ingredients could be allotted a specific qualitative degree (on a scale of one to four). In the case of polypharmacy or compound drugs the system broke down and the total mix of ingredients was usually presented simply as a cure for a condition without any analysis or rationalization of why it worked. What was important was the recipe itself. In this sense, it was a piece of aphoristic knowledge, and there were very many pieces of such knowledge as the lists of compound remedies appear endless.

It seems to me that in learned medicine in the early modern period we have a situation in which the desire to remain orthodox and to stay within the bounds of Galenic doctrine is very strong. The Renaissance saw a concerted move to get a 'purer' Galen into medicine, purged of Arabic and medieval Latin barbarisms. And if the period of 'Galen worship'[15] waned after the 1530s, by and large what innovations there

---

[15]   Marie Boas, *The Scientific Renaissance 1450–1630* (London: Collins, 1962), p. 135; for the philological results see R.J. Durling, 'A Chronological Census of the Renaissance Editions and Translations of Galen', *Journal of the Warburg and Courtauld Institutes*, 24 (1961), 230–305.

were within learned medicine were produced using Galen's theories and concepts. The shared admiration for classical medicine and the pressures of competition in the medical market place produced cohesion and conformity within learned medicine (though there were some exceptions).[16]

Now, what I have noted above about the existence of people creating personal knowledge in terms of the qualitative–humoral nature of things and their use of an aphoristic style of knowledge means that there was space within learned medicine for independent ways of gaining and expressing knowledge. On the whole, it was second-order knowledge dependent on a pre-existing Galenic framework, but it allowed the physician (and lay people, for they also made qualitative judgements) to feel that by using their senses they could assess for themselves the nature of illnesses, foods and the world around them. The aphoristic type of knowledge, whether derived from folk wisdom, personal experience or tradition and authority, did not threaten Galenic medicine. It was too brief and usually contained no theoretical statements, though theory might be implied. By the manner in which it was presented it could equally be new or ancient knowledge, and this may have given early modern writers, again, the feeling that they could contribute in a substantial way to learned medicine.

In other words, learned medicine in this period was not a rigid orthodoxy; there was flexibility, for instance, in creating narratives of what was going on inside the body, and in giving people the feeling that they could personally contribute to medical knowledge through their senses, and by adding pieces of information in an aphoristic, unargued way. Of course, the reason why this could happen without conflicting greatly with learned medicine lay in Galen's development of a qualitative medicine based on the senses and his openness to folk wisdom especially in the case of remedies. Another reason, and this may be worth comparative consideration, is that the personal–sensory basis of medical knowledge reflects the material conditions of life from the Greeks to the early modern period. Technology was simple, and in everyday life the senses were the main means of assessing the environment, food and people's ill or healthy conditions. But I have perhaps stressed the creative side to learned medicine too much. Orthodoxy and claims to know more than the opposition are characteristic of early modern medicine in England. The emphasis lay on pre-existing knowledge

---

[16] Exceptions relate to plague where a contagionist rather than a miasmatic theory began to be accepted by learned physicians and to the use of concepts of occult qualities and of the power of the 'total substance' of a remedy which, although discussed by Galen, were frowned upon by the majority of Renaissance learned physicians.

taught over a long period of time at university, and only if a practitioner
was initiated into this knowledge could he become a learned physician.

Epistemology and learned medicine

Most diseases and conditions had names. They were known. In the
heyday of a learned medical tradition it would have been surprising if it
had been otherwise. (Though as I write this I sense a tautology!) Lay
people were also confident that they could diagnose and name diseases.
In London, old women, often pensioners of the parishes, acted as
'searchers of the dead' and diagnosed the causes of death amongst
London's citizens for the bills of mortality. The published books of
remedies and the private manuscript collections were aimed at or
produced by lay people, especially women, and referred to the whole
range of illnesses. The medical culture of the time, both lay and learned,
did not lack confidence in diagnosing or naming an illness. (And where
doubts might exist there were sophisticated fail-safe procedures – a
patient might be labelled hypochondriac – in the modern sense – as the
seventeenth-century Nonconformist minister Richard Baxter found to
his cost.)[17] Or the case might be seen as being caused by witchcraft, a
practice which Richard Ady in 1655 castigated as 'a cloak for Physicians
ignorance . . . when he cannot find the nature of the Disease, he saith the
Party is bewitched').[18]

Of course, the learned physicians sought to differentiate their skill
from that of empirics and lay people. Learned medicine was presented
as the best possible type of medical knowledge, but as also complex and
full of difficulty. Galenic physicians like John Cotta and his North-
ampton colleague James Hart[19] stressed that the learning to be gained
from study in the universities alone provided the required degree of
knowledge and discernment to properly 'work the system', that is to
make use of the holistic potential of learned medicine.

The learned physicians stressed how they took into account many
more factors than did empirics. For instance, the differences between
diseases had to be considered along with the constitution, age and life-

---

[17]   See Andrew Wear, 'Puritan Perceptions of Illness', in R. Porter (ed.), *Patients and
        Practitioners: Lay Perceptions of Medicine in Pre-Industrial Society* (Cambridge: Cam-
        bridge University Press, 1985), p. 95.
[18]   Thomas Ady, *A Candle in the Dark: Or, A Treatise Concerning the Nature of Witches and
        Witchcraft* (London, 1655), p. 115.
[19]   John Cotta, *A Short Discoverie of the Unobserved Dangers of Severall Sorts of Ignorant and
        Unconsiderate Practisers of Physike in England* (London, 1612); James Hart, *Kliniki, or
        Diet of the Diseased* (1633); see also John Securis, *A Detection and Querimonie of the
        Daily Enormities and Abuses Committed in Physick* (London, 1566).

style of the individual patient. I am going to refer extensively to the work of an obscure but learned physician, Eleazar Dunk, as it gives a typical but detailed account of knowledge and medicine. In a letter published in 1606 he set out how the learned physician should think about a case when he defended the physicians against the empirics:

First the learned Physician is to search out the proper signes of this disease, and by them to distinguish it from others that hath some affinity with it: then he looketh into the cause of it ... he examineth the naturall constitution of the patient, his present state of body, his former course of life, his age, his strength, the time of the disease, the season of the yeare etc he considereth the qualities and quantity of the humours; from whence the matter of the disease floweth ... by what passages it moveth, whether swiftly, or slowly ... Out of an advised consideration of all these, first a diet is to be appointed: this cannot be the same in every one that laboureth of this sicknesse, but it requireth great variety and alteration agreeable to the foresaid circumstances. Then follow with the consultations of the meanes of the cure: what kind of evacuation is fittest whether opening a veine ...[20]

The learned physician's trademark was that he took into account the patient, and that it was the individual patient and not the disease that had to be treated, so that one remedy could not cure all who suffered from the same disease.

Such a view was also held by the highest in the land, James I, who in *A Counterblaste to Tobacco* (1604) wrote:

Yea, not onely will a skilfull and wary Physician be carefull to use no cure but that which is fit for that sort of disease, but will also consider all other circumstances, & make the remedies sutable therunto; as the temperature of the clime where the Patient is, the constitution of the Planets, the time of the Moone, the season of the yeere, the age and complexion of the Patient, and the present state of his body, in strength or weakness: For one cure must not euer be used for the selfsame disease, but according to the varying of any of the foresaid circumstances, that sort of remedy must bevsed which is fittest for the same.[21]

Dunk believed that empirics could be confused or mistaken about all the stages of diagnosis and treatment. His attack on empirics for their poor diagnosis allows us to learn what he saw as good diagnosis, especially the knowledge that was required in making it:

Diseases are knownen and distinguished by their signes ... because they [empirics] are ignorant, they must needs fall often into this fault [of wrongful diagnosis]. This is seldome discovered but when rationall Physicians have opportunity to look into their practise; then they see the disease taken to be in

[20]   Eleazar Dunk, *The Copy of a Letter Written by E.D. Doctour of Physicke to a Gentleman, by whom It was Published* (London, 1606), p. 24.
[21]   James I of England and VI of Scotland, *A Counterblast to Tobacco*, in *The Workes of the Most High and Mighty Prince, James* (London, 1616), p. 219.

the liver, when it is in the lungs or kidneis; to be in the heart, when it is in the head or mouth of the stomacke; to be in the brest, when it is winde in the stomache extending that region: and many such. What though they can judge of the gout, the palsie and the dropsie? So can simple women doe: but to judge rightly of the causes and the differences of these diseases, of the manifold differences of Agues, of simple and compound sicknesses and of sundry diseases of the head; that requireth Arte, which is not in any Empiricke. (pp. 25–6)

In therapy the empiric could also go wrong. As in the case of diagnosis some of the mistakes occur because of the greater complexity of learned medicine, with its many distinctions and differences. In a sense, learned medicine offered more possibilities in diagnosis, more courses of action in therapeutics and especially greater precision (at least in the eyes of learned physicians like Dunk):

Hence is a broad gate opened to a large field of medicines of sundry sorts, ointments, plaisters, syrups, potions etc. Some of these are very hot and much opening; some very cold and binding. In the use of these, and also of all the former things [Dunk had been describing bleeding, purging and fomentations], the Empirike is plunged into many doubts, and the patient into as many dangers: if he take away too little blood, he taketh not away the disease; if too much, he taketh away life: if he purgeth when he should open a veine, or doth this when that is required, he committeth a pernicious errour: if he iudgeth not rightly of the humour abounding, of the complexion etc. (of which only Arte is the competent iudge) he can attempt nothing in the cure safely, nor so much as appoint a fit diet. (p. 25)

Dunk continued in this vein, and the reader may well wonder if in reality the learned physician exercised such fine judgement as Dunk claimed. (See my 'Conclusion' for some comments on this.)

How did the learned physician avoid all these pitfalls? Where did he gain the necessary knowledge? Dunk answered, 'in the great variety of these doubts, difficulties and distinctions there is a necessary use of sound judgement, confirmed by long study and profound knowledge both in Philosophy and Physicke' (p. 25). Learning, reading and study was what constituted the 'Arte'. In relating to diseases and their differences Dunk wrote that 'the eye can not discerne colours but by the light, nor Physicians diseases but by learning'. The remedy of bleeding also led to 'doubts and difficulties as require much reading and deepe knowledge' (p. 27). Study made the physician. Dunk's little treatise *The Copy of a Letter Written by E.D. Doctour of Physicke to a Gentleman, by whom It was Published* pointed in its title page to the crucial role of study 'wherein is plainly prooved that the practise of all those which have not beene brought up in the Grammar and University, is always confused, commonly dangerous and often Deadly'.

Two questions need to be answered. Can we talk of epistemology in this context, and why did English learned physicians so emphasize their learning? If epistemology is the creation of new knowledge then I do not think that epistemology is involved in the learned physician's view of medical knowledge. However, that may be to rely too much on a modern view of epistemology which stresses new knowledge discovered especially through experience (though the use of reason or the mind obviously is not precluded, especially in relation to the classical period). Dunk's physician was taught; he learned from books. Empirics, on the other hand, 'learn by our perils, and they trie experiments by our death'. And he added:

Experience alone, with a little helpe of nature maketh men skilfull in mechanickall trades, in merchandise, and in other kinds of buying and selling; but the deepe knowledge conteined in the liberall sciences, and in other learning arising out of them, requireth much reading, long study, great meditation; and after the theorie or speculation of them is obteined, then practise and experience confirmeth and establisheth them: but without the former, the latter is weake, lame and maimed. (p. 32f.)

No nonsense here about the falsifying power of experience. In fact, experience is there to bolster learning – the expectation is that it will confirm it. Although Dunk recognized that Galen required both 'learning and Experience', and so could conclude 'therefore the best Empiricke is but a lame and left-legged Physician' (p. 33), he clearly gave priority to learning which alone taught the method of medicine, that is which taught the system of medical knowledge: 'It is a full consent of all learned in Physicke or Philosophy, That nothing can be happily done in the Art of Physicke without method and order: and it is as true that experience can not teach this method' (p. 33).

John Cotta's *A Short Discoverie of the Unobserved Dangers of Severall Sorts of Ignorant and Unconsiderate Practisers of Physicke in England* (1612) reflected the commonly held views of learned physicians and so followed many of the themes in Dunk's *Letter*. Cotta reiterated the point that personal experience (what was to be a key to knowledge for the new science of the seventeenth century) was inadequate for reaching a true and full knowledge of medicine. Only a true method and habit or disposition aided by books could do this:

The defect in the Empericke hence appeareth to be want of true methode and the habit of right operation and practise according to reason, (which is art) through which defect his actions must needs oft be reasonlesse, and by consequent as blind in their intention, so likely to be foolish in their issue and execution. For there must needs be in all actions want of much more neccessary knowledge then sense and experience can advance unto: and experience must needes witnesse against it selfe, that the longest age of experience doth nothing so fully furnish and instruct in many things, as much more speedily doth prudent invention; which though occasioned and helped by bookes and reading which are both keys unto all knowledge, and also rich storehouse of experiences ... yet do they [books] only glut the sense with stories of experiences past, but reason and judgement truly enrich the mind and give daily new increase and light before untried and unexperienced truths.[22]

So, maybe there was no epistemology of a serious sort in early modern learned medicine, apart from the odd disagreement over some qualitative, subjective, interpretation of the type noted earlier. Or, perhaps our use of the terms 'teaching' and 'epistemology' have to be altered. If the discovery of new knowledge by experience was precluded then it may be apposite to talk equally of the discovery, teaching or learning of medical knowledge through books. For if Paracelsus, Galileo and Harvey wanted to learn from the book of nature rather than from the books of the ancients they still retained from the latter the sense of personally learning. Such a sense of personal learning, which we now take for granted, forms a natural association with experience (that is, 'personal experience'). But if the distinction between discovery and teaching is blurred, as perhaps it has to be in any well-established medical learned tradition (are there comparative views on this?), then it may be easier to talk of epistemology in the context of how one learns, discovers or empathizes with a body of pre-established knowledge and acquires the Art and true 'reason and judgement'. Either that or we have to conclude that to talk of epistemology is not appropriate to learned medicine at this time, at least in relation to its basic theories and rules.

The second question as to why English Galenic physicians stressed learning so much does give rise to epistemological issues. As well as their general opposition to empirics, they were concerned with the rise of an ethnocentric medicine, that is an English medicine written in English books which sometimes claimed that there were specifically English remedies for English diseases. Classical medicine was Greek, but it was applied in the early modern period not only to other areas in the Mediterranean but also to countries north of the Alps. The question arose as to the universal applicability of this medicine. Clearly, Mediterranean and North European medicinal herbs were different.

But more fundamental differences were pointed out. As the Hippocratic text *Airs, Waters, Places* had indicated, the place in which someone was born and lived influences their constitution, their physical and psychological characteristics. The view then developed that the place where one was born was most natural to be in and the

22   John Cotta (note 19), p. 11.

healthiest. Christianity, from the early Church Fathers, also emphasized how God had put remedies on earth for man's use. This was repeated by writers such as Timothie Bright in his *A Treatise Wherein is Declared the Sufficiencie of English Medicines* (1580) and William Harrison in his *Description of England* (1586–7) to mean that God gave to each nation remedies specific for the diseases prevalent in it.

The claims of learned medicine to universality were thus curtailed and on this view some of the details of learned medicine if not its basic theories had to be modified. (Here the comparative dimension of, for instance, the applicability of Indian or Chinese medicine across large geographical areas would be interesting.) It tended to be opponents of learned medicine who argued for the ethnocentric approach, men such as Nicholas Culpeper (who repeated Bright's *Treatise* in his *School of Physick* (1659)) and who were concerned to prescribe to the poor cheap English herbal remedies that could be picked from English fields rather than expensive drugs from the Middle East, the Indies or America.

For Bright these latter remedies were 'things rather of superfluous pleasure than necessary reliefs and serving rather for a certain pomp than for maintenance of life'.[23] More specifically and pragmatically, Bright wrote that the English should not be dependent on supplies of drugs from 'heathen and barbarous nations' who, in any case, often corrupt or counterfeit them (pp. 8–9).

Bright also found theoretical reasons for dismissing foreign medicines. Not only did individuals have different temperaments or complexions (balance of humours) but so did nations. As the diet of Indians and Egyptians was different from that of the English, argued Bright, so would their humours and excrements also be different – which meant that the remedies to balance the humours in turn had to be different (pp. 19–20).

The universalism of classical medicine was also founded on its use of the universal scholarly language, Latin. Motivated by a Christian charitable desire to make their work available to all, to avoid obscurity and perhaps spurred on by a sense of nationalism and the example of the use of English in the Protestant religion, English medical writers began to write in their own tongue. Thomas Phayre in *The Book of Children* (1553) justified the practice, by stating that in the past 'Galen the Prince of this art being a Grecian wrote in Greek' and Avicenna, an Arab, in Arabic. Medicine in England, which was 'a thing that was made to be common to all', should not therefore be kept amongst a few.[24] A

---

[23] Timothie Bright, *A Treatise Wherein is Declared the Sufficiencie of English Medicines for Cure of all Diseases, Cured with Medicine* (London, 1580), p. 8.

[24] Thomas Phayre, *The Book of Children* (London, 1591), pp. a2r–a2v.

nationalistic local view of medicine could equally lead to the use of the vernacular and to locally produced remedies.

Language, of course, figured large in the claims of learned medicine to apply across all of Europe. If few students of learned medicine or their professors in the universities of North or South Europe knew Greek, the language of the *prisca medicina*, at least they were united by a shared knowledge of the next best, Latin. The use of Latin perhaps blurred geographical and national distinctions. It was a distinguishing mark of the learned physician as it helped to establish that he was learned.[25] It was also claimed that Latin gave a better type of medical knowledge, and also of philosophy, the basis of learned medicine. English books just were not good enough; with Latin one gained access to the best knowledge available.

The Salisbury physician John Securis, who had studied with the conservative Galenist Sylvius in Paris, defended learned medicine in his *A Detection and Querimonie of the Daily Enormities and Abuses Committed in Physick* (1566). To the objection that 'we have Englishe bokes enough to teach us divers medicins for diverse purposes',[26] Securis replied at length. Medicine could be understood only when placed in its philosophical context (which was expressed in Latin):

I answer that the englishe bookes teacheth nothinge of the trewe foundation of Phisike. For if there be any that doo it, howe can it be well understanded without logike and naturall philosophie. For Aristotle saith *Ubi desinit Physicus, ibi incipit medicus.* A man must first peruse naturall Philosophie, before he entre into phisycke. (pp. B1r–v)

Securis conceded that: 'to have some bokes of phisike in englyshe specially of the Simples, well and cunnyingly set foorthe for Surgeons, Apothicaries, yea and for sober and wyse men, that delyte to reade in suche thynges, and know not the Latine tongue, is not unmete nor hurtefull' (p. B1v). But Securis went to his main attack:

doo you thynke to have in youre Englyshe Bookes, all the perfecte knowledge that is required in Physicke? ... If Englyshe Bookes could make men cunnyng Physitions, then pouchemakers, threshers, ploughmen and cobblers mought be Physitions as well as the best yf they can reade.

Then wer it a great foly for us to bestow so much labour and study all our lyfe tyme in the scholes and universities to breake our braynes in readynge so many authours, to be at the lectures of so many learned menne, yea and the greatest follye of all were, to procede in any degree in the Universities with our great coste and charges, when a syr Johne Lacke Latin, a pedler, a weaver and

---

[25] A learned physician by definition had gone to university. There were no women at universities in England in this period.

[26] Securis (note 19), p. Aviii verso.

oftentymes a presumptous woman, shall take uppon them (yea and are permytted) to mynister Medicine to all menne, in every place, and at all tymes. *O tempora O mores, O Deum immortalem.* (pp. Biiv–r)

Latin (and its associations with the universities and learned culture) helped to mark out proper medicine. And in Latin there was to be had more medical knowledge than in English. Epistemologically, if I can use the word in a strained way, in Latin lay the key to finding the best and the most certain knowledge in medicine.

This was certainly the view of Dunk. In his *Letter* he wrote that a reason 'brought in defence of Empiriks is, That they reade English books sufficient to instruct them in their practise' (p. 35). His reply recognized that language could be a bar to the profession, but he emphasized that only if one knew Greek and Latin could medicine be grasped in a holistic sense. His reasons were pragmatic. Too little was written in English books, but also there is the sense that medicine is integrated into the whole corpus of learning, ignorance of which affects the proper understanding of medicine:

All the large volumes of Hipp[ocrates] Gal[en], Avicen[na], and all other famous Physicians both new and olde, were first written in the Greeke or Latine tongues, or afterward translated into one of them; the ignorance whereof hath in all ages beene accounted a strong barre to exclude all men from the profession of that Arte. That which is written in English is very littel and light in respect of the whole: neither can it be perfectly understood without the helpe of Grammer and Logicke, as every meane scholar will confesse. (p. 35)

Dunk was well aware of medicine as a learned profession and he compared it with the law and religion, both of which in his view required Latin at their highest levels. He noted that civil law (i.e., Roman law) depended on Latin (an obvious point!):

All nations Christian, wherein the civill is used, can not affoord one man of any meane account in that profession, that understands not the Latine tongue, wherein their large books are written. And I dare confidently affirme, that Physicke is as profound and intricate a study as the Civill law, and requireth as much reading and knowledge of tongues, as that doth. (p. 35)

Dunk also pointed to the example of religion as requiring a knowledge of Latin. Here, he was faced with a problem, for the Reformation had made the vernacular the norm. Dunk's answer is perhaps strained and shows how events were making his defence of Latin appear out of touch with the realities of early seventeenth-century England:

What though there be a profitable use of Ministers in our Church, that understand English books only, being yet able to execute their office in some commendable maner? yet this reason holdeth not in Empiriks: for first there is farre more Divinity than Physicke written in our vulgar idiome all the grounds and principles of religion are set forth at large in it; whereas no part of Hipp[ocrates], Gal[en] etc is translated into that tongue. Secondly, Ministers have farre greater help in hearing the learned of that profession, and in frequent conference with them: whereas Empirickes labour always to avoid the presence and company of learned Physicians ... As no Minister is able to confute a learned adversarie, that hath not skill at the least in the Latine tongue; so no Empirike is able to encounter with sicknesse, that great adversaire to nature, without weapons fetched from the Greek or Latine tongue. M. Latimer sayeth in one of his sermons, English Divinity will never be able to expell Popery out of this land and it may as truely be sayd; English Phyisicans can not cure English diseases. (pp. 35–6)

The learned professions in England were certainly changing and perhaps medicine too changed with them. Dunk forgot to mention that the civilians were being ousted from the English law, whilst Henry VIII had already abolished canon law. Moreover, English law in its attorneys provided practitioners akin to the empirics.[27] They used experience just as did the empirics (they were not allowed entry to the Inns of Court and their education), but this, argued Dunk, was no justification for the empirics or of experience. As one reads the learned physicians, whether Dunk, John Cotta or James Hart or even the great divine William Perkins who supported learned medicine, it is clear that the attack on experience is the counterpart to their support for learning. Their defence of learned medicine, although it echoed Galen's attack on empirics, also reflected the realities of the competitive medicine market place.

But by excluding experience, they confirmed that they were not interested in change. Or, at least this is how it appears in hindsight for change in medical knowledge was often to come from those who expressed a commitment to empiricism. On attorneys Dunk wrote:

This grand reason of experience is further urged of some by the example of Atturneys at the common law: most of these have nothing to direct them but experience and observation and yet sundry things passe thorow their hands as substantially and effectually performed, as by learned Councellers: therefore unlearned Physicians well instructed by experience, may do some cures as well as great scholars. The answer to this is easie: There are many things in law which belong merely to Atturneys, and require no learning: also they follow presidents and usuall formes, and many things which they doe, are plaine transcripts written out of books *verbatim*, wherein they cannot erre, if they folowe their paterne. But it is farre otherwise in Physicke: there is no usuall forme to follow in

[27] See C.W. Brooks, *Pettyfoggers and Vipers of the Commonwealth. The 'Lower Branch' of the Legal Profession in Early Modern England* (Cambridge: Cambridge University Press, 1986). Also Ronald A. Marchant, *The Church Under the Law* (Cambridge: Cambridge University Press, 1969); R.H. Helmholz, *Roman Canon Law in Reformation England* (Cambridge: Cambridge University Press, 1990).

iudging or curing of disease; things seldome fall out after the same maner; the Physician must alter and change his course, as the disease and accidents require, wherein experience can not guide him, but the rules of the Arte. (p. 34)

Attorneys were at this time often considered the dregs of the legal profession, and many barristers and judges would have concurred with Dunk's view that as the attorneys in doubtful cases 'ask the opinion of learned Councillers' so they depend on learning. Learned civil law had been limited to the Admiralty and Church Courts and was under attack from the common law courts by means of prohibitions preventing particular cases being heard in the civil courts, and canon law did not run in England. Yet the common law, despite its lack of classical antiquity and its potential to be exposed to experience (changing precedents, and the experiential assessment of juries) could still be considered learned, even if it was a native form of learning. Sir Edward Coke, the great exponent of the common law, supported learned medicine when in Bonham's case (1608–9) he judged that the College of Physicians of London could not convict someone of malpractice if they were unlicensed.[28] Coke felt that in this case the learning of a university graduate was sufficient to guarantee good practice. (He also condemned 'Mountebanks and cheating Quacksalvers' in his exposition of the witchcraft statutes.)[29] There certainly was a learned culture beyond medicine which shared some of its values, but it was also a culture which was not as static as the defenders of learned medicine might have hoped.

In the end, learned medicine precluded real change – that was precisely why it was learned, for the past supplied it with its learning (and its attack on its competitors made the orthodoxy more rigid). John Cotta described the 'True Artist' (the true physician), and stressed the constant and unchanging nature of learned knowledge in a way which echoes later ideas of unchanging laws of nature. Cotta wrote that the more studious men were the more they would know nature,[30] and of the latter he stated:

The order of nature in all her works is constant, full of wonder and unchanged truth in the continuall cohesion, sequence and fatall necessitie of all things, their causes and effects: wherein therefore how the Almigthie Dietie hath commanded all things by an unchangeable law to be ordered, is both true and necessarie wisdom to understand, and the true patterne, rule, and square of everie discrete, sober and wise designe and consultation. Hence upon the principles of nature stand everlastingly founded all arts and sciences ... And all true arts thus

---

28 See Harold J. Cook, 'Against Common Right and Reason: the College of Physicians versus Dr Thomas Bonham', *American Journal of Legal History*, 29 (1985), 301–22.
29 Sir Edward Coke, *The Third Part of the Institutes of the Laws of England* (London, 1797), p. 46 (1st edition, 1644).
30 Cotta (note 19), p. 117.

founded upon the undeceiving grounds of nature, in themselves are ever certtain and infallible, whose rules although discretion according to circumstance may continually diversly vary, yet can no time nor circumstance ever or at any time abrogate. (p. 118)

Medicine, in Cotta's view, was such a 'true art'.

Conclusion

This has been a paper about how knowledge was perceived in a fully developed tradition of learned medicine in a country where it was faced with significant competition. It may be that in this case we cannot talk of epistemology, or that learning is its own epistemology.

It might have been useful to explore how in reports of their cases learned physicians put their learning into practice. Did they practise what they preached and take into account the age, constitution, life-style etc. of the individual patient? But this has not much to do with epistemology; it is merely a question of whether the rules of learned medicine were properly applied or not. The data are, in any case, inconclusive. The case notes, for instance, of John Hall, Shakespeare's son-in-law, vary widely from the brief recitation of a disease and its remedy (in almost empirical fashion) to a consideration of a patient's constitution and diet.

As it turns out there is very little that is or can be new about the epistemology of the mature learned medicine of sixteenth- and early seventeenth-century England. Some of the pressures leading to change have been mentioned in the paper, and perhaps the very orthodoxy of learned medicine was a pressure in its own right.

Other reasons for changes in the epistemology of medicine in the seventeenth century are well known – Paracelsianism, the calls for medical reform during the Civil War and Interregnum, the mechanical and chemical approach of the new science, the associated emphasis on observation. But learned medicine itself did not change fundamentally, though it did accept chemical remedies, and by the end of the seventeenth century much of it had died out. Some structures remained, for instance, the six non-naturals (air, diet, exercise and rest, sleep and waking, the evacuations including sexual activity, and the passions of the soul or mind) which helped to pattern advice on regimen and the prevention of disease. Much of therapeutics (bleeding, purging, emetics, some drugs) also remained the same. But what was no longer held even amongst eighteenth-century 'regular' physicians was the view that theirs was an unchanging learned profession – there were too many systems and schools of medicine quickly succeeding each other for that to have happened, and, in any case, the moderns with their view of progress had won.

Yet the very survival of much of traditional learned therapeutics raises an epistemological question. In a sense, there was an epistemological void in therapeutics. It was impossible to know with certainty if a treatment was effective or not in a particular case. This was something which was not resolved until the nineteenth century and the use of statistical trials. This uncertainty allowed the fight between the learned physicians and empirics to be undecided and it also allowed old and new therapies to co-exist in the eighteenth century. As Henry Edmundson put it in his *Comes Facundus in Via, The Fellow Traveller* (1658):

It is a great Question what does the cure, the Vulgar will tell you the last thing they took did the cure, as the last thing they did caused the disease; Some physicians will ascribe it to the rarity and dearnesse, others to the variety and composition, others to the fitnesse and order etc. others think it is not the Physick or Physicians but Nature being disburthened returns to her functions by degrees, and men from weakness to a more cheerful condition, from a long hunger to a more greedy appetite etc. And some adde, that it is not Nature but the God of Nature which heals us, and as the Proverb is, God heals, and the Physician hath the thanks. It is Gods compassion on the poor man who contemneth no means but is without any. It is the reward of his patience. It is God's seeing his teares, or hearing his or the Churches prayers for him . . .[31]

In the eighteenth century the providential God was less conspicuous, but the uncertainty remained. So, at least, did one clear epistemological issue.

[31]   Henry Edmundson, *Comes Facundus in Via, The Fellow Traveller* (1658), pp. 111–12, cited in A. Wear, 'Interfaces: Perceptions of Health and Illness in Early Modern England', in R. Porter and A. Wear, *Problems and Methods in the History of Medicine* (London: Croom Helm, 1987), pp. 240–1.

Part 2

Chinese traditional medicine

9 Text and experience in classical Chinese medicine[1]

Nathan Sivin

Qualifications and lineages

What were the qualifications of physicians in ancient China? Who judged them? Were they unique to medicine? Few records survive from the centuries in which medicine emerged from the domain of the hereditary artisan to become a cumulative tradition, with its doctrines, not merely its techniques, transmitted in books. This process hardly began earlier than the unification of China in 221 BC, and was not fully accomplished before the first century. I will begin with two sources, one from the second century BC and one from perhaps a century later, that throw light on what made a doctor.[2]

The first is a long memorial in the biography of Ch'un-yü I in the first of the Standard Histories, Memoirs of the Grand Historian (*c.* 100 BC).[3] Ch'un-yü was descended from a noble family of present-day Shan-tung province that claimed to have held its fief for a millennium. He was Director of Granaries for the state of Ch'i. This position, if typical, was not a career but a sinecure passed down in his family. Fond of medicine in his youth, in 180 he began three years of study that made him the successor of an eminent doctor of his own village. He wandered from one court to another doctoring aristocrats and their women 'rather than treating his home as a home' as people of good family were expected to do. The historian makes the point that 'in some cases he did not treat people's medical disorders, which aroused resentment in many sick people'. In other words, he took his

[1] Copyright N. Sivin 1994. I use the modern form of the Wade–Giles transcription to romanize Chinese, and translate dates directly into the Gregorian system. I acknowledge with gratitude suggestions by Marta Hanson. For bibliographic abbreviations, please see the list at the end of this chapter.

[2] The important unpublished Ph. D. dissertation of David Keegan, ' "The Huang-ti nei-ching": The Structure of the Compilation; The Significance of the Structure', University of California at Berkeley (1988), has drawn attention to these sources and their connections.

[3] SC, *chüan* (hereafter ch.) 105, pp. 19–59.

prognoses seriously. Apparently practitioners did not have the luxury of refusing to care for those they could not help, at least not when summoned by the mighty. Ch'un-yü, in fact, excuses his peripatetic habits later in the memorial by arguing that his fear of being forced into the service of various monarchs made him in effect a refugee. He implies that rulers were often so dissolute that their ills were beyond curing.[4]

Resentment of his independence, the biography implies, led someone who had access to the palace *c.* 176 to charge Ch'un-yü with a serious offence. He was pardoned, not because he proved that he was innocent of this unspecified crime, but because his daughter wrote a moving plea on his behalf. His ordeal over, Ch'un-yü had already settled down in the capital when an imperial edict ordered a count of 'those who could determine correctly whether medical treatment [would result in] life or death. Which are the principal names among them?'

Ch'un-yü submitted a memorial claiming he belonged to this august group. His summary of the return edict's questions shows that the criteria went far beyond prognostic competence:[5]

What are my strongest skills? What illnesses can I cure?[6] Do I have books on [medicine] or not? Whence did I receive teachings on each [of them], and for how many years? Have these [teachings] been verified (*yen*)? Of what districts and villages [are my former patients]? What were the disorders? What was the state of [each] disorder after therapy?

He goes on to provide the first replies in the historical record to the questions with which this inquiry began. The qualifications itemized in the edict were partly artisanal, but they differ sharply from Western counterparts in their stress on the formal transmission of knowledge from master to disciple, especially in the form of written texts. The very existence of the memorial points to another significant difference. Evaluating formal credentials in early China is not the responsibility of other physicians, but of the emperor, or of the bureaucracy that acts in his name.

Written transmission is not merely the emphasis of the imperial edict, but also of Ch'un-yü's reply:

[4]   Ibid., p. 54.
[5]   The passages translated below are from ibid., pp. 21–3 and 56–9; see Keegan (note 2), pp. 226–7, 230–1. Keegan refers to the physician as Ts'ang. That was, however, not his surname but part of his title.
[6]   The verb *chih* does not correspond exactly to either 'cure' or 'heal', but means 'to order' medical – or social – disorder. On these concepts see Sivin, *Traditional Medicine in Contemporary China*, Science, Medicine and Technology in East Asia, vol. 2 (Ann Arbor, 1987), pp. 95–100.

When I was young I took delight in medicine. But the therapeutic formulas I tried were mostly ineffective.[7] In 180 I was fortunate enough to meet my teacher, Kung-sheng Yang-ch'ing of Yuan village in Lin-tzu district [modern Shan-tung province]. At the time he was over seventy, but I was able to meet and serve him. He said to me 'Get rid of all your formula books. They are all wrong. I have the Pulse Books of the Yellow Lord and Pien Ch'ueh (*Huang-ti Pien Ch'ueh mo shu*), and Diagnosis by the Five Colours (*Wu-se chen ping* or *Wu-se chen*, SC), transmitted from ancient predecessors. [Using these books it is possible to] know whether people will live or die. One can resolve doubtful cases and determine which are treatable. In addition [I have] books on the doctrine of drug therapy, most excellent ones. My family is well provided for. I love you, and intend to teach you all of my secret formularies.'

I replied with alacrity 'How fortunate I am! I had not dared hope for this.' I immediately left my mat[8] and made repeated obeisances.

He formally transmitted to me his Pulse Books (*Mo shu*, SC), Upper and Lower Canons (*Shang hsia ching*, SC, SW), Diagnosis by the Five Colours, Irregular and Regular [Disorders] (*Ch'i k'o shu*, SC), Gauging and Measuring (*K'uei-to*, SC, SW), External Transformations of Yin and Yang (*Yin–yang wai pien*, SC), The Doctrine of Drugs (*Yao lun*, SC), The God of Stone [Probes] (*Shih shen*, SC), and the Forbidden Book on Joining Yin and Yang (*Chieh yin–yang chin shu*, SC).[9] Receiving them, reading them, and getting a feel for them must have taken a year or so. The year after that I tried them out with some success. Still I had not yet mastered them. But by the time I had served him for three years or so, I was applying them to treat people's illnesses. In diagnosis and deciding whether the patient would live or die, their efficacy was most excellent.

Now Kung-sheng has been dead for more than a decade. I spent three years [with him]; at the time I was thirty-eight years old.[10]

---

[7] *Fang* may refer to drug formulas and procedures for acupuncture, moxibustion, diet, etc., in particular, or to techniques in general. I consistently translate it 'formulas' or 'formularies', but 'techniques' would be an equally defensible choice.

[8] A gesture of respect analogous to rising from one's seat today. At the time Chinese sat on mats rather than on chairs.

[9] '*Ch'i k'o shu*' occurs twice in the biography as *Ch'i k'o*, which might be translated 'Extraordinary Coughs', but is given as *Ch'i heng* in very similar lists of texts in SW, *p'ien* 46, sec. 8 and *p'ien* 77, sec. 3. As written in the late Chou or early Han, the two could easily be confused. The explanation at *p'ien* 46, sec. 8 (p. 130) supports the latter title but not the SC version. I provisionally follow Fuji Koretora, quoted by Takigawa, in emending to *Ch'i heng*. *Shang hsia ching* would normally refer to a book in two chapters. In translating *K'uei to* as two words rather than as a compound I follow Keegan (note 2), pp. 227, 359, n. 14; see also pp. 211–12. The meaning of *Shih shen* is highly problematic; *shih* may also refer to minerals. I tentatively follow Tamba no Motoyasu, cited in Takigawa.

For tables of books cited in the Inner Canon see Ma Chi-hsing, *Chung-i wen-hsien-hsueh* (The Study of Chinese Medical Literature) (Shanghai, 1990), pp. 63–5. Keegan, pp. 209–17, makes a good case that SW, *p'ien* 15 and 19 are descended from this tractate and the next, and reconstructs their complex lineage.

[10] Thirty-nine *sui*. Assuming 'at the time' refers to the year of Kung-sheng's death, Ch'un-yü was born *c.* 214, and the memorial was submitted not long after 167.

In reply to further interrogation, Ch'un-yü provides more details about his relations with Kung-sheng and describes his relations to another teacher.

I have been asked in what circumstances my teacher Kung-sheng received [his teachings], and whether he was renowned among the feudal lords of Ch'i. I reply that I do not know who Kung-sheng's [line of] teachers were.[11] His family was wealthy. Although he was skilled in medicine, he was unwilling to treat the illnesses of others [i.e., besides family and friends]. It must be due to this that he was not renowned. He also told me 'Take care that you do not let my sons and grandsons know you have studied my formulas.'

I have been asked how my teacher Kung-sheng met me and came to love me, so that he was willing to teach me all his formulas. I reply that I had not heard that my [future] teacher Kung-sheng was expert in the use of [medicinal] formulas. This is how I came to know about him.

When I was young I was fond of everything pertaining to [medicinal] formulas. When I tried them out, the results (yen) were for the most part excellent. I heard that in T'ang village, Tzu-ch'uan, there was one Kung-sun Kuang, who was skilled in the use of formulas transmitted from ancient times. I thereupon went to pay a formal call on him, and was fortunate enough to meet him and to serve him. He taught me his own formulas, Transforming Yin and Yang (Hua yin–yang, SC), and Methods to be Transmitted Orally (Ch'uan yü fa, §SC).[12] I received them and wrote them out. I wanted to receive all his other essential formulas, but Kung-sun said 'I have given you all the formularies I have; it is not that I begrudge you anything. My body is already worn out. I have no further use for them. These are the wonderful formularies that I received when I was young. I have given everything to you. Do not teach them to anyone!' I said 'It has been my great good fortune to meet you and serve in your presence, and to obtain all [your] secret formulas. I would die sooner than wrongly transmit them to anyone.'

I stayed on for some time with Kung-sun Kuang while he was living at leisure. I deeply discussed his formulas [with him]; I heard him say that they would be considered excellent for a hundred generations.[13] Kung-sun said with delight 'You are certain to become a national treasure. There are some [scholars of

---

11   *Ch'ing so shih shou* is ambiguous. It might also be understood as 'what [texts] Kung-sheng learned from his teacher'.

12   This sentence is problematic. Takigawa takes *Fang hua yin–yang* as a book title, but it makes no sense. I put the stop after *fang*, which makes the book title more comprehensibly *Hua yin–yang*. This remains a guess, since neither form of the title occurs in *Huang-ti nei ching* or in early bibliographies. The transmission of a text entitled *Yin–yang* is noted in SW, *p'ien* 77, sections 3/4 (p. 248). The final phrase, rather than being a book title, may mean 'and he transmitted to me some oral methods', that is, methods that had not been set down in writing. Books that purport to contain secret explanations meant only for oral transmission are not rare, but this one is exceptionally early. The commentators differ about whether the phrase is corrupt. See SC, ch. 105, p. 57. For an explanation of the symbol '§', see the Abbreviations, at the end of this chapter.

13   Since the object of the verb is not stated, this may also be understood as 'I would be considered. . .'. The attribution of the next assertion makes this reading less likely.

medicine] with whom I have been on good terms, but I am out of touch with them. A colleague living in Lin-tzu is skilled in [medical] formulas; I do not compare with him. His formulas are exceptional, not the sort that the uninitiated know about. Once, when I was in my prime, I made an effort to receive his formularies. But Yang Chung-ch'ien was unwilling, and said that I did not seem to be the right person. I should go with you to see him. He is bound to notice the delight you take in formulas. He too is elderly, and his family is well off.'

But at that time we did not go. It happened that Nan-yin, the son of Kung-sheng Yang-ch'ing, came to present a horse [to Kung-sun]. Because Kung-sun Kuang [in turn] sent the horse to the temporary royal residence, I had an opportunity to make friends with Nan-yin. Kung-sun also commended me to Nan-yin, saying '[Ch'un-yü] I is devoted to studies of regularities.[14] By all means treat him judiciously. He is a consummate scholar.' He thereupon wrote a letter introducing me to Kung-sheng Yang-ch'ing. That is how I came to know Kung-sheng. I was assiduous in serving him. That is how he came to love me.

I have been asked whether there are officials or commoners who have served me and studied my formulas, whether [anyone] has obtained all of them, and [if so] to what district and village [these disciples] belong. I reply: Sung I of Lin-tzu; he studied with me. I taught him the Five Diagnoses (*Wu chen*, §SC) for more than a year.[15] The King of Chi-pei sent his Palace Physicians Kao Ch'i and Wang Yü; they studied with me. I taught them Circulation Vessels (*Ching mo*, §SC), Vertical Orientations (*Kao hsia*, §SC), and Congelations in the Extraordinary Reticular Tracts (*Ch'i lo chieh*, §SC).[16] I discussed the locations of the [acupuncture] loci and how the *ch'i* should travel up and down,

14 Although *shu* literally means 'number', it was applied in the Han and earlier to any discipline that involved mastery of regular patterns, including methods of prognostication and other arts that were entirely qualitative. See, for instance, the passage in the Mencius: *Meng-tzu* (The Writings of Mencius), after 320 BC, HY, *p'ien* 6A.9, translated in D. C. Lau, *Mencius*, The Penguin Classics (Harmondsworth, 1970), p. 165, where it is applied to chess. On *shu* in science see Peng Yoke Ho, 'Chinese Science: the Traditional Chinese View', *Bulletin of the School of Oriental and African Studies*, 54 (1991), 506–19.

15 *Wu chen* is possibly an abbreviated title for *Wu se chen*. *Shang hsia ching*, like a number of other phrases in these passages marked with '§', may be either book titles or references to doctrines. Some occur as book titles elsewhere; for instance, SW, *p'ien* 77, sec. 3/4 (p. 248, a list of books) and *p'ien* 79, sec. 1/2 (p. 250) mention the Upper and Lower Canons. SW, *p'ien* 46, sec. 8 (p. 130), explains the meaning of this and other titles. 'Normal and Abnormal' is the title of *p'ien* 55 of LS. It is concerned with the use of acupuncture in accord with the state of the *ch'i* circulation. 'Circulation Vessels' is the general title of chs. 8–10 of *Huang-ti nei ching t'ai su* (Inner Canon of the Yellow Lord: Grand basis), 666/683?, cited from Kosoto Hiroshi (editor-in-chief), *Tōyō igaku zempon sōsho*, 8 vols. (Osaka, 1981), vols. 1–2. Other phrases in this passage are in a form that suggests a book title; thus Correspondences of the Four Seasons to Yin and Yang resembles the title of SW, *p'ien* 5. It is a reasonable hypothesis that, if one or more of the phrases in a list are book titles, all are titles.

16 It is impossible to be certain about the meaning of this last phrase. I take it in the sense of SW, *p'ien* 20, sec. 4/2 (p. 66): 'When the disorder is in the extraordinary reticular tracts (*ch'i hsieh*) . . . find the reticular tract in which there is a congelation and needle it to extract blood.' The sense of *Kao hsia* suggests that this text has to do with the relative positions of the body contents.

exit and enter, and its proper and pathological,[17] abnormal and normal
behaviour, in connection with indications for the use of the stone needle and
for determining the location for its use and for moxibustion. This took more
than a year.

At that time the King of Lin-tzu sent his Director of Granaries, Feng Hsin,
[who was assigned] to set his formulas in order(?).[18] I taught him the Method
of Deliberation (*An fa*, §SC), the Discourse on Abnormal and Normal
[Circulation] (*Ni shun lun*, §SC), the Method for Drugs (*Yao fa*, §SC),
Determining the Five Sapors (*Ting wu wei*, §SC), and Mixing Medicines (*Ho
chi t'ang fa*, §SC).[19] Tu Hsin, Household Aide to the Marquess of Kao-yung,
was an amateur of pulse diagnosis, and came to study it. I taught him the
Upper and Lower [Canons], the Circulation Vessels, and the Five Diagnoses
for more than two years.

T'ang An, of Chao village in Lin-tzu, came to study. I taught him the Five
Diagnoses, the Upper and Lower [Canons], the Circulation Vessels, Irregular
and Regular [Disorders], and the Correspondences of the Four Seasons to Yin
and Yang (*Ssu shih ying yin yang*, §SC).[20] Before he was finished he was
appointed Attending Physician to the King of Ch'i.

If read attentively, this document raises a number of interesting
questions. For instance, what does Ch'un-yü mean when he writes of
receiving texts, reading them, 'getting a feel for them', and practising
them?

Receiving, we are clearly told, is a formal process, which begins only
after one has been 'serving' the master as a disciple for some time. When a
text is 'received' (*shou*) it is not simply handed over, but ritually
transmitted and taught. At a certain point the disciple is allowed to copy it
out and read it, not necessarily in that order. *Tu*, 'reading', does not imply
reading quickly and silently. In ancient China, as in ancient Greece, prose
and poetry normally were chanted aloud. Early writings use the word in a
way that implies not just intoning, but studying and memorizing.[21]

Only after the words of a text are firmly lodged in one's mind does
'getting a feel for them' become an issue. This is the first stage that the

---

[17] I follow Wang Nien-sun, cited by Takigawa, p. 59, in adding *cheng* after *hsieh*.
[18] The meaning of *cheng fang* is unclear. I follow Tamba no Motoyasu (ibid.), in
considering the graph *ma* an accidental intrusion. The meaning 'case record' for *an*,
although common later, is not attested for the Han. I therefore accept the Takigawa
variant. Feng's title is also not a standard one.
[19] *Yao fa* may be a variant title or text of *Yao lun*. The Five Sapors are Five Phases
correlations of drugs. See Sivin (note 6), pp. 181–4.
[20] The last character, *ch'ung*, does not fit the context. Takigawa cites a laboured
explanation, but I suspect that the graph was erroneously introduced by a copyist. *Mo
shu shang hsia ching* [Pulse Book Composed of Upper and Lower Canons] may be a
single title, but *Shang hsia ching* appears as a separate title above (note 9).
[21] For reading in depth see the famous passage in the Mencius (note 14), ch. 5B.8 (Lau,
p. 158). *Tu* can also mean 'to punctuate' a text as one reads it, but this sense (usually
pronounced '*tou*') is not attested so early.

master does not directly mediate. The Chinese word for this step is composed of *chieh*, 'comprehend', and *yen*, which means, among other things, 'verify'. The discussion of the final stage uses the same yen in three slightly different senses, 'try out', 'success *or* succeed', and 'efficacy'. Here the context is no longer study but application in medical practice. Verification does not necessarily involve first-hand experience, but in this final instance it apparently does.

A second issue is motivations for transmission. Kung-sheng answers a question too obvious for the source to raise: why does he intend to pass on his texts outside his own family? His answer suggests that like his disciple he is not a hereditary physician. A hereditary doctor, whose texts were the foundation of his family's livelihood for generations to come, could have answered this question in only one way, namely that he had no son (and was too conventional to transmit them to his daughter). But Ch'un-yü's teacher says instead that his own family does not need them as a source of income. He is free to make a favourite disciple his medical heir.

The theme of guarding the text arises more than once here, as in other early medical writings.[22] Kung-sun Kuang warns Ch'un-yü about passing on the books that he has taught him. The latter's answer and his subsequent activity as a teacher indicate that the issue was not whether to pass them on – they could not in any case be allowed to die out – but to make sure they are not 'wrongly' transmitted, that they go to 'the right people'. Kung-sun himself had been refused access to certain texts because he 'did not seem to be the right person'. The master physician was expected to choose intellectually and morally fit disciples and prepare them to receive the canons. Virtue, as always in traditional societies, reflects social standing, but that is not all it implies.

The purpose of this highly ritualized teaching was not to pass on texts for their own sakes. The Confucian canon had to be kept intact because its teachings made it possible to be a responsible member of society and to realize one's aspirations and those of one's family. Similarly, the medical teachings were not abstract bodies of theory, but keys to diagnosis, prognosis, and therapy (see p. 195). Mastering them was a necessary step on the way to becoming a good doctor.

At another point in his memorial Ch'un-yü replies to a query about why the same disease may have different diagnoses (more often analyses of whole-body dysfunctions than identifications of diseases) and

---

[22] See, among other examples, the Ms. of the first century AD excavated at Wuwei, Gansu, in 1972, in *Wu-wei Han tai i chien* (Han Medical Documents on Wooden Slips from Wuwei, Gansu, Beijing, 1975), pp. 3b, 9a, 11b, 13b, 15a. The last of these citations says 'Interdicted; do not transmit even for a thousand in gold.' On similar warnings in SW see note 33 below.

different outcomes. He explains that the ancient sages provided distinctions in terms of pulses, yin–yang, and other cosmic patterns so that physicians could discriminate more finely than the names of diseases permit. Books are essential because they embody such distinctions.

Now my diagnoses are all [derived] from diagnostic books. This is the basis for the distinctions I draw. Just when the process of receiving my teacher's formulas was completed, he died. I therefore set out[23] the diagnoses and prognoses in the books, contemplated which were successful and which erroneous, and combined their pulse techniques. That is how I know about such things by now.[24]

If I understand Ch'un-yü correctly, he is saying that books preserve the experience of one's predecessors in a line that goes back to the archaic sages, and that with the proper initiation one can find in them by what amounts to induction the patterns of judgement that make skilled practice possible.

The second source that throws light on the making of physicians is the Inner Canon of the Yellow Lord (*Huang-ti nei ching*), probably of the first century BC. A number of passages describe rituals of transmission in a way that is idealized but readily recognizable to early readers. David Keegan has found in the Divine Pivot (*Ling shu*) details of an initiation that cast substantial light on Pien Ch'ueh's account.[25]

The Thunder Duke inquired of the Yellow Lord: 'Insignificant though I am, since you permitted me to receive your patrimony I have gone through the sixty bundles of wooden slips [on which] the Nine Needles [is written], ardently applying myself to them from daybreak to dusk. The bindings of the older ones are broken, and the slips of the newer ones are grimy,[26] but still I chant and memorize, never setting [the book] aside. [Nevertheless its meaning] is not yet quite clear in my mind. Where External Evaluation speaks of "binding together into one", I do not understand what it is saying. "[Seen as] large there can be nothing beyond it; [seen as] small there can be nothing inside it; there is no limit to it, large or small; there is no dimension for it, high or low" – how can one bind all that together? The talent and vigour of scholars varies, and their wisdom and power of reasoning may be superficial and narrow. They may be incapable of breadth and depth, or of driving themselves to study like my insignificant self. I fear that [the teachings] will be scattered and become extinct in later generations, inaccessible to our descendants. I venture to ask if there is any way

23 *Piao* may imply making a table or chart.
24 SC, ch. 105, p. 53.
25 LS, *p'ien* 48, sec. 1 (p. 396) = T'ai su, ch. 14, sec. 5, pp. 51–4 (vol. 2, pp. 107–10). The ritual content is omitted from the abridgement in *Huang-ti chia i ching* ('A–B' Canon of the Yellow Lord), between AD 256 and 282, in ITCM, ch. 4, sec. 1A, p. 1a. See Keegan (note 2), pp. 233–8, for this and a passage from LS, *p'ien* 28, sec. 1, that mentions oral transmission.
26 In both SW and T'ai su 'older' and 'newer' are interchanged, so that the text does not make sense, but Yang Shang-shan's commentary to the latter makes the correct order clear.

to epitomize them?'

The Yellow Lord replied: 'A most excellent question! There [is a synopsis that] my predecessors forbade to be wrongly and selfishly transmitted. An oath [must be sealed by] cutting the arm and smearing blood. If you really wish it, why not carry out the ritual purification?'

The Thunder Duke bowed repeatedly and then arose, saying 'Please command me with respect to this.' He purified himself for three days and then sought permission. 'I venture to make a request. Insignificant though I am, I hope to take the oath today at high noon.'[27]

The Yellow Lord accompanied him into the room where he had done the purifications, and carried out the cutting of the arm and the smearing of the blood. The Yellow Lord himself recited this formula:

> Today at the epochal time of yang
> We smear the blood, transmit the formulas
> He who dares defy these words
> Will surely suffer.

The Thunder Duke bowed repeatedly and spoke: 'Insignificant though I am, I receive it.' The Yellow Lord grasped his hand with his left hand, and with his right conferred the book on him, saying 'Take care! Take care! I will now explain it to you.'[28]

This document reveals the structure of the transmission. After being granted access to the manuscript, the disciple has gradually read, memorized, and reflected on it. He sets the ritual in motion by professing concern for the survival of the teachings. At that point he undertakes demanding physical and mental preparations. Such preparations conventionally include bathing, changing clothing, and meditation, as well as abstaining from meat, pungent vegetables such as onions, and sexual intercourse. They are not specific to textual transmission, but precede almost all solemn ceremonies.

The blood oath in a purified precinct is a most solemn affirmation, used for centuries before that time to give weight to agreements. Here it is called 'an oath [sealed by] cutting the arm and smearing blood'. The archaic form generally involved sacrificing animals and either sipping a bit of their blood or smearing it on one's mouth.[29] Here instead of a sacrifice the disciple presumably lets a little of his own blood (actually

---

[27] Literally, at 'the epochal time of yang'.

[28] The remainder of the chapter is, as promised, a summary of the External Evaluation text (*Wai ch'uai*, LS) from the Nine Needles (*Chiu chen*, SW) book, outlining pulsology and its applications. The title *Chiu chen* was often applied to the precursor of the extant LS.

[29] The oldest record known to me is for 547 BC, in *Tso chuan* (The Tso Tradition of Interpretation of the Spring and Autumn Annals), compiled between the third and first centuries BC, HY, Duke Hsiang, year 25/2, translated in James Legge, *The Ch'un Ts'ew with the Tso Chuen*, The Chinese Classics, vol. 5 (Hong Kong, 1872), p. 514b. It does not give details of the ritual.

the document does not specify whether one or both participants does this). This is less probably a peculiarity of the author's lineage than a local usage.[30] The significance of the oath is obvious. Blood as the agent of the ritual binds the teacher and his pupil as father and son, and establishes their relationship as one link in a lineage.

What is the disciple being prepared for? To possess the book, of course, in the sense that the master's copy (which he has already memorized) is entrusted to him so that he may make his own copy.[31] But beyond that, he has been designated a legitimate successor in the line of scholars who will keep the text in use, protecting it and teaching it to the next suitable person. The ritual does not complete his incorporation, for he has not yet fully internalized the revelation. That can happen only through the verbal guidance of his teacher.

Once the oath has been sworn, the teacher hands over the physical text and begins the oral teachings that allow the disciple to master the arcana. Another chapter in the Divine Pivot, in which the Yellow Lord asks Ch'i-po for an oral explanation of the Nine Needles canon, makes it clear that his teaching is not at all informal: 'It is what the former masters [of the lineage] have orally transmitted.'[32] Eventually many of these oral teachings were set down and themselves transmitted in writing, often accompanied by dire warnings against letting them fall into the hands of the unworthy.

The fundamental point of this is the continuity of the lineage, as the passage of the Basic Questions (*Huang-ti nei ching su wen*) that reveals the numerological basis of pulse lore affirms: 'I wish to learn the essential Way [of reading the pulse] in order to instruct my sons and grandsons and transmit it to later generations. I will inscribe it in my bones and marrow, store it in my lungs and liver. What I receive after the smearing of blood I will not dare to betray.'[33]

---

[30] In the second century the *Huai-nan-tzu* notes that 'the Hu [people of the north] drink wine from a skull cup, the Yueh [people of the south] cut their arms, and the people of the Central States smear blood [of an animal]. Although the means differ, the fidelity they imply is the same': Book of the King of Huai-nan, presented to the throne 139 BC, *Huai-nan hung-lieh chi-chieh* edn, ch. 11, p. 8b. There is no reason to connect the Inner Canon text directly with Yueh traditions, but in the century or so between the two books the Yueh usage may have spread.

[31] Keegan (note 2), pp. 245–6, argues plausibly that the two medical scrolls excavated at Ma-wang-tui in 1973 were copies made in connection with initiations, and that two slightly different versions of the same text, one on each scroll, were buried in the same tomb because they were transmitted, presumably to the same recipient, by different masters.

[32] LS, *p'ien* 28, sec. 1. For the whole passage see Keegan (note 2), p. 236.

[33] SW, *p'ien* 20, sec. 1. A few fragments of the corresponding *T'ai su* (note 15) passage survive in ch. 14. For a solemn warning against teaching the doctrine to 'the wrong person' and teaching inauthentic doctrines to anyone see SW, *p'ien* 4, sec. 3.

The opening sentences of the 'A–B' Canon of the Yellow Lord (*Huang-ti chia i ching*, late third century) make the same point by referring to the account in the Divine Pivot:

What medicine has accomplished is due to a long evolution. In high antiquity the Divine Husbandman first tasted plants to attain a knowledge of materia medica. The Yellow Lord consulted with Ch'i-po, Po-kao, Shao-shih, and their like ... and from this the Way of Needling was born. Their discourses were most remarkable. The Thunder Duke received his patrimony and transmitted it to his successors

whom the text goes on to enumerate. Medicine begins, in other words, with revelations by two legendary monarchs, the Divine Husbandman's canon of materia medica, and the medical doctrines of the Yellow Lord and his interlocutors in the various treatises gathered in the Inner Canon.[34] Medicine can continue its essential work only if these teachings are transmitted to practitioners in every generation.

Nothing in this account is peculiar to medicine. To take a single example, in the Mathematical Canon of the Chou Gnomon, also attributed to high antiquity, we find a similar account, in which one Jung Fang inquires after the secrets of mathematics that allow the cosmos to be measured.[35] His master refuses twice to teach him, ordering him each time to go home and let his thoughts on the subject mature. He returns after some days, admitting that, although he has exhausted his inner resources, his spiritual vitality and wisdom are insufficient to let him master the art without help. Only at this point, when the disciple confronts the limits of individual intellectual striving, does the teacher begin his explanations.

The pattern of transmission I have just described pervaded Chinese book learning. Confucius began philosophy by representing the few surviving texts of the early Chou dynasty (eleventh century BC) as relics of the archaic sages, containing all the wisdom needed for a good life in a good society. The truths were too deeply embedded in these texts; in the degenerate present only those initiated by a master could hope to comprehend them. As the sciences began separating out of philosophy, from the late third century BC on, they adopted a similar pattern, each claiming descent by direct transmission of a similarly revealed canon. Practitioners placed the founding revelators of some traditions, such as medicine, in the misty period before chronology began. This reach

34 Author's preface, p. 1a. This pattern does not begin with the Inner Canon, but is already visible in the Ma-wang-tui Mss.
35 *Chou pi suan ching* (Mathematical Canon of the Chou Gnomon), first century BC or first century AD, reproduction of 1213 Fukien edition in *Sung k'o suan ching liu chung*, 6 vols. (Beijing, 1981), vol. 1, ch. 1, pp. 11a–13a.

188   Nathan Sivin

toward a legendary past in part reflected Confucius' success in encouraging veneration for antiquity, and in part aligned these technical traditions with the very popular Huang-Lao intellectual movement of the Han.[36] At the same time, Han scientists and physicians asserted that they were linked with their semi-divine founders by an unbroken chain of transmission.

Sovereigns as innovators

The curious idea of sovereigns as technical innovators was not ancient. Traditional datings of classics assigned such ideas to the early Chou dynasty or earlier. Critical research has re-evaluated such dates almost across the board in the past decade or so. It now appears that accounts of legendary sages as culture-givers seldom predate the Han.[37] They reflect, in fact, a crucial transition in Chinese political, social, and intellectual life.

An effectively unified and centralized political order arose for the first time in the last three centuries BC. This first empire gradually ended the old system of patronage that distributed intellectuals, strategists, and other experts through the courts of ambitious rulers, competing for places but free to argue for very diverse points of view. By a hundred years into the Han, thinkers were officials. Those who spoke for the state were expected to portray cosmic order and state power as mirror images. The state, like the body, became a microcosm, resonating with the rhythms of the cosmos. This ideology portrayed the good society, the good life, and the arts of civilization as imperial grants.

Its foundations were being laid before the Ch'in state finished wiping out its rivals. In the Springs and Autumns of Lü Pu-wei (*Lü shih ch'un-ch'iu*, c. 239 BC), yin–yang has already become the order that drives the universe. This epochal book and its early Han successors provide a model for political order, which depends on creating hierarchical distinctions of authority – of those above and those below – and maintaining the unity of the state. Lü's book has transformed the soon-to-be emperor from a conqueror to a life-giver, to the maintainer of the only order that can survive. It can survive because it is not arbitrary but based on Heaven, the eternal standard. Dissidence or refusal to obey imperial regulations is thus unnatural.

---

[36] See the discussion of the Huang-Lao movement in Benjamin I. Schwartz, *The World of Thought in Ancient China* (Cambridge, Mass., 1985), pp. 237–54.

[37] For an excellent digest see Michael Loewe (ed.), *Early Chinese Texts. A Bibliographical Guide*, Early China Special Monograph Series, 2 (Berkeley, 1993 [publ. 1994]). A.C. Graham, *Disputers of the Tao, Philosophical Argument in Ancient China* (La Salle, Ill., 1989), gives other current datings and sources. See also note 2.

The idea that cognitive and technical innovation came from sovereigns, although the product of a special time and specific political circumstances, became deeply ingrained in medicine. It was repeated through the ages, especially but not only by medical authors who were the recipients of state support. Here, for instance, is the preface of Sun Ssu-mo to his Formulas Worth a Thousand, the most important medical handbook of the seventh century:[38]

Pure and impure parted; above and below separated;[39] [the division of] heaven, earth, and man was founded; that of the Five Phases fell out; the myriad things [were formed, all] pristine: [this process of cosmic formation is] indescribable.

The Firemaker Lord (Sui-jen) came forth, contemplating the Dipper and the North Star and thence naming the directions, initiating the metamorphoses of fire. Lord Fu-hsi arose and followed [the Firemaker Lord's precedent] by drawing the Eight Trigrams and instituting [the work of] the kitchen. Once the culinary arts [lit., 'the flavours'] were practised, illness burgeoned. The Divine Husbandman, that great sage, pitying the black-haired people [i.e., the masses of his subjects] on account of their many illnesses, tasted the hundreds of herbs so that he could cure them, but [medicine] was still not perfected. When the Yellow Lord received the Mandate [of Heaven to rule], he invented the nine needles [used in acupuncture] and discussed the circulation system with Ch'i-po, the Thunder Duke, and other masters of techniques. Becoming conversant with [the nuances of medicine through] the questions and challenges he put to them, mastering the patterns of meaning, he put [all that he had learned] into the canonical discussions [i.e., of the Inner Canon]. Thus later generations [of physicians] could follow it and thrive.

In the Spring and Autumn era there were the excellent physicians Ho and Huan;[40] in the time of the Six States, Pien Ch'ueh; in the Han, the Director of Granaries [i.e., Ch'un-yü I] and Chang Chi; and in the Wei, Hua T'o. All of them investigated the arcana and penetrated the subtleties [of medicine]. They used only two or three herbs, and not more than six or seven charges of moxa, but there was no disease they failed to cure. From the Chin and Liu Sung dynasties on, although eminent physicians have continued to appear from time to time, they have been unable to cure five or six [patients] out of ten. This is because the passions of people today are overwhelming, their resolution inconstant. Their behaviour is abandoned; they lack self-cultivation.

This is a thoroughly mythical account of the origins of medicine, beginning with a cosmogony packed into the first sentence (possible because all the themes that appear in this excerpt were familiar to every

---

38 Sun Ssu-mo, *Pei chi ch'ien chin yao fang* (Essential Formulas Worth a Thousand in Gold, for Urgent Need), completed 650/659, reprint of Edo igaku edn of 1849 (Taipei, 1965), prefaces, p. 6. For his biography see Sivin, *Chinese Alchemy: Preliminary Studies*, Harvard Monographs in the History of Science, vol. 1 (Cambridge, Mass., 1968), ch. 3.
39 This phrase implies social as well as cosmic distinctions.
40 Cited in *Tso chuan* (note 29), Duke Chao, year 1/appendix 8 and Duke Ch'eng, year 10/5.

reader by Sun's time). Once the universe has attained its final shape, legendary emperors invent the arts of civilization. As civilization – especially gastronomy – spawns illness, they perfect medicine and grant it to their subjects. Only after the Yellow Lord reveals the Inner Canon do physicians come into their own. When the golden age is over, China, bereft of sages, is abandoned to history.[41]

Lineages of eminent physicians gradually illuminate the truths that without them could barely be glimpsed in the murky depths of the Inner Canon. Theirs is an effort not of innovation but of recovery. But physicians can never literally reinstate the medicine of high antiquity. Living in a debased order, their patients lack the effortless self-discipline that, as the opening chapter of the Basic Questions emphasizes, made health and longevity the norm when society was young. Perfect bodies, in other words, require perfect politics. And that doctors do not control.

The persistence of revelations

The theorists of the new state in the Ch'in and Han periods – Lü Pu-wei (d. 235), Liu An (?180–122), Tung Chung-shu (c. 179 – c. 104), and others – were highly catholic in their use of sources. Between the mid-third and late second century they drew on all of the influential intellectual currents of their time, from Huang-Lao thought to Confucianism, despite the antipathy of the Ch'in First Emperor and the initial disdain of the Han's founder for the literati ritualists. Tung succeeded c. 136 in restricting imperial support to five Confucian classics. But he and his predecessors, in the process, had transformed Confucianism from the humanism of Confucius, Mencius, and Hsun-tzu into a synthesis that kept one eye on the family and the state and the other on the cosmos.[42] They drew on what they found useful in all the intellectual trends of the transitional period, even on the statist doctrines that had encouraged the Ch'in regime's contempt for Confucius' values. Despite that catholicity, this first neo-Confucianism was not in practice tolerant of its rivals. The orthodoxy that Tung and his successors demanded left no room for alternative teachings.

---

[41] It was customary in orthodox writing to call the present emperor, no matter how wretched his rule, a sage, but this courtesy was not necessarily extended to the ruling houses of previous dynasties.

[42] Michael Nylan and Nathan Sivin, 'The First Neo-Confucianism, An Introduction to the "Canon of Supreme Mystery" (T'ai hsuan ching, ca. 4 BC)', in Charles le Blanc and Susan Blader (eds.), *Chinese Ideas about Nature and Society, Studies in Honour of Derk Bodde* (Hong Kong, 1987), pp. 41–99.

Despite its yearning for a single orthodoxy, the new Confucianism of the Western Han was not a single, consistent doctrine. The synthesizers mentioned above took very different tacks.[43] Their constituencies varied.

Many orthodox scholars ignored the trend, more concerned with the preservation of the classic texts than with their sociopolitical significance. The First Emperor's attempt to confiscate the Confucian classics in private hands, and the general destruction at the Ch'in-Han transition, had led to the loss of several canons, prompting an abiding fear that more would be lost. Most of these texts lost before the Han were eventually recovered in more than one version, but the upshot was continuing arguments, and recurrent polarization of the scholarly world, over which version was authentic. Attempts 'to re-establish the lost unity (or effect the unification) of the Confucian classics, to reintegrate the fragmented canon', and to impose 'visions of completeness and perfection' on ancient works both narrow in scope and markedly imperfect, were in large part responsible for the flood of commentaries from the Han to the last days of imperial China.[44]

That deep urge to build a seamless canon out of tattered remnants of an imagined Golden Age was equally formative in medicine. We know little about the origins of the Inner Canon, and practically nothing about its relation to the lost Outer Canon that accompanied it, or to the several other paired inner and outer canons of medicine that circulated in the Han.[45] It has been widely understood for about a decade that the Inner Canon is not a book with a single point of view but an unintegrated compilation of short writings. Some sections duplicate or rearrange parts of others; some provide conflicting explanations of the same concept or phenomenon; some explicate or take issue with others.[46]

Through the history of medicine there has been a tension between the

---

[43] For instance, Charles Le Blanc, *Huai-nan tzu. Philosophical Synthesis in Early Han Thought. The Idea of Resonance (Kan-Ying). With a Translation and Analysis of Chapter Six* (Hong Kong, 1985), shows that the juxtaposed doctrines in the *Huai-nan-tzu* were meant to demonstrate the superiority of Taoist (or, as we would say today, Huang-Lao) teachings as a pattern for the emperor's self-cultivation.

[44] John B. Henderson, *Scripture, Canon, and Commentary. A Comparison of Confucian and Western Exegesis* (Princeton, 1991), pp. 45, 105.

[45] The best starting point on this vexed topic is Li Po-ts'ung, *Pien Ch'üeh ho Pien Ch'üeh hsüeh-p'ai yen-chiu* (A Study of Pien Ch'üeh and the 'School of Pien Ch'üeh') (Xi'an, 1990).

[46] Keiji Yamada, 'The Formation of the Huang-ti nei-ching', *Acta Asiatica*, 36 (1979), 67–89, and Keegan (note 2). For comprehensive lists of inconsistencies see Maruyama Masao, *Shinkyū igaku to koten no kenkyū*, *Maruyama Masao tōyō igaku ronshū* (Studies in Medical Acupuncture and Moxibustion and their Classics. Collected Essays of Maruyama Masao on Oriental Medicine), 2nd edn (Osaka, 1977, 1979), pp. 268–74 *et passim*, and Ma Chi-hsing (note 9), pp. 65–6.

'visions of completeness and perfection' that gave force to its classicism, and the need to resolve obtrusive contradictions in the canons. This tension was reinforced by the conviction that with the passing of time the true significance of this legacy was slipping away. The outcome, over about three hundred years, was a succession of new writings meant to reassert the integrity of the ancient ones, while explaining how to understand what seems contradictory as actually consistent. For the Inner Canon there were several such syntheses in the second and third centuries AD. Three of these survive, the Canon of Eighty-one Problems [in the Canons] of the Yellow Lord, the 'A–B' Canon of the Yellow Lord, and the Canon of the Pulse.[47]

That the word *ching* occurs in even the earliest citations of the three titles implies that these too are canons; the original titles put them in the Yellow Lord tradition.[48] But their forms differ considerably. The Canon of Eighty-one Problems takes a new dialogue form, apparently the sequel of an initiation: a teacher imparts oral explanations in response to a disciple's questions about difficult points and disparities in the Inner and possibly the Outer Canon. In resolving these questions it is innovative in a number of ways – most of them clinical, as Maruyama has pointed out.[49] The 'A–B' Canon continues the form of the Inner Canon, as a series of dialogues between the Yellow Lord and his courtier Ch'i-po reconciling the content of the Basic Questions and two other books in the same tradition that have not survived. The Canon of the Pulse sets out in the form of a systematic handbook an account of the ch'i circulation system and the diagnosis of its malfunctions, drawing on sources from the Yellow Lord and other textual traditions.[50] We can readily see that these ching are canons not by virtue of mere age or form, but because they claim to belong to – to preserve, restore, and reveal – archaic traditions.

Later medical handbooks, even those similar in form, gave up this emphasis on revelation to identify themselves with what began to evolve as a genre. Nevertheless the production of ching did not end in the third

[47]   *Huang-ti pa-shih-i nan ching* (Canon of Eighty-one Problems [in the Inner Canon] of the Yellow Lord), probably second century AD, in *Nan-ching pen i; Huang-ti chia i ching* (note 25); and *Wang Shu-ho, Mo ching* (Canon of the Pulse), c. 280, ITCM.

[48]   Henderson (note 44), p. 50, reminds us that the word '*ching*' was used very loosely in the Chou and Han dynasties. In Ch'in and Han texts it usually implied scriptural authority connected with a lineage of transmission.

[49]   Maruyama Masao (note 46), pp. 281–9. As Ma Chi-hsing has pointed out, of quotations from 'the canon' in the *Nan ching*, nine are found in the extant SW, thirty-eight in the extant LS, and seventeen in neither: note 9, p. 102.

[50]   The Canon is explicitly a pastiche. See the detailed study in Kosoto (note 15), vol. 8, pp. 333–402. According to their count, 56 per cent of the text is quotations from extant precursors, and the remainder is probably taken from lost books. What was added by eleventh-century editors remains uncertain.

century. 'Canons' that situate themselves in the Yellow Lord tradition appear as late as the T'ang. The last medical scripture in the grand style could claim imperial origin with complete confidence. The brief Canon of Sagely Benefaction (*Sheng chi ching*) was compiled by command of the Emperor Hui-tsung (which made it in effect his composition), and was promulgated for use in the medical schools in 1118. It is, like the Inner Canon, a work of fundamental doctrine underlying practice. It begins, in fact, with a definition of health that resembles Aristotle's definition of virtue:

One yin and one yang [i.e., their constant alternation] are called the Way; bias toward yin or bias toward yang is called disease. Those who fail clearly to understand the Way have never been able to cure man's diseases. Yin and yang illuminate each other, overlap each other, order each other; the four seasons succeed each other, give rise to each other, kill each other; the Five Phases in turn become sovereign, are set aside, serve as minister.[51]

Human beings, born and living in their midst, conform to yin and yang, are attentive to the four seasons, and regulate [themselves?] by the Five Phases. With the median comes felicity; with excess comes calamity; with licence comes disease.

The emperor's surrogates digested the clinical details of medicine in a companion work, the General Record of Sagely Benefaction (*Sheng chi tsung lu*), twenty times as long. Its preface recapitulates the theme of imperial innovation, with some interesting thoughts on the relation between political and medical reform:[52]

In archaic times the Divine Husbandman and the Yellow Lord ... tasted the diverse plants in order to distinguish [the medicinal uses of] each, and studied the diverse ailments in order to preserve life. In determining names [for the former?], in choosing classifications [for the latter?], in establishing correct relations between monarch and minister and instituting the functions of assistants and emissaries [in drug formulas], in making these apparent in the writings in the Grand Basis and the Jade Tablets, and in the inquiries of the Thunder Duke and Ch'i-po, it would seem that they have revealed the hidden treasures of the gods. Fathoming the transformations of yin and yang, they have traced to their origins the patterns of inborn nature and destiny. Thus [the legacy of these sages] partakes in the powers of heaven and earth that spread over and bear up [humanity] ... In the Sage [emperor]'s reforming of the world, the root is above and the ramifications below. If [the reforming impulse] is not manifested above, the Way of Therapy will not be

---

[51]   *Sheng chi ching* (Canon of Sagely Benefaction), compiled by imperial order and issued 1118, in *Chen pen i shu chi ch'eng*, vol. 9, preface. The point is that each phase predominates during part of a cycle, then giving way to its successor, and carries out ancillary functions when it is not predominant.

[52]   *Cheng-ho sheng chi tsung lu* (General Record of Sagely Benefaction of the Regnant Harmony Era), compiled by imperial order 1111–17, issued 1122, 2 vols. (Beijing, 1952) (reprint, 1982), preface, p. 1.

established. If it is not manifested below, the tools of therapy will not be put to use. What the Canon [of Sagely Benefaction] discusses is the Way. When the physician masters it, he can fully manifest his divine powers. What this General Record contains is the tools. When the physician uses them he stops illness.

In the language of this document, to an even greater extent than in those already quoted, familiar elements of political and medical discourse intersect. Monarch and minister, assistant and emissary are classifications of drugs that organize their use in prescriptions.[53] In this hierarchy of functions, all are equally necessary and each has its place, but order and health emanate from the top. 'Root and ramifications' in medicine implies therapeutic priority; the physician treats the fundamental imbalance, not peripheral symptoms. In politics the root is the unique place of the sagely emperor – sagely by definition. Most striking, the compilation of medical books, from the viewpoint of a flesh-and-blood emperor, is not a mere technical act, but an essential aspect of social reform. The state is concerned with every aspect of order. *Chih*, as I have already remarked, is the verb for imposing order on both the chaos of human impulse and on the innumerable disorders of physiological function.[54]

I have argued so far that formal medical qualifications mainly had to do with ritual induction into fictive lineages that existed to transmit from one generation to the next charismatic revelations in writing, accompanied by explanations that might be either written or oral. Founding revelations were generally ascribed to royal figures of high antiquity. The writings of those who founded segmented lineages might eventually be given practically equal status. This happened because the claims of their successors, sometimes several generations later, prevailed. The most famous instance of this segmentation, which spawned four important traditions between the late twelfth and mid-fourteenth centuries, was typical in that the founders drew on Han and pre-Han classics to temper the novelty of their own therapeutic emphases rather than seeking to supersede the classical doctrines.[55]

53   The *locus classicus* is SW, *p'ien* 74, sec. 5.5. *P'ien* 74 is widely regarded as a T'ang addition to the Inner Canon. On the use of these rubrics in the formulary literature see Watanabe Kōzō, 'Tso wei p'ei fang yuan-tse te "chün ch'en tso shih"' ('Monarch, Minister, Assistant and Emissary' as Principles of Prescription), *Chung-hua i shih tsa-chih*, vol. 3 (1954), pp. 187–90.
54   See note 6.
55   See Jutta Rall, *Die vier grossen Medizinschulen der Mongolzeit*, Münchener ostasiatische Studien, vol. 7 (Wiesbaden, 1970), Li Ts'ung-fu and Liu Ping-fan, *Chin Yuan ssu ta i-chia hsueh-shu ssu-hsiang chih yen-chiu* (Studies of the Academic Thought of the Four Great Physicians of the Chin and Yuan Periods) (Beijing, 1983), or, better, [Jen Ying-ch'iu], *Chung-i ko-chia hsueh-shuo* (Doctrines of the Schools of Classical Chinese Medicine) (Shanghai, 1980). See also Yiyi Wu, 'A Medical Line of Many Masters: A Prosopographical Study of Liu Wansu and his Disciples from the Jin to the Early Ming', *Chinese Science*, 11 (1994), 36–65.

All of my examples have come from élite medical teachings. As one would expect, they reflect the world view and values of China's educated few, a largely hereditary office-holding group before the present millennium, but one based increasingly on wealth and achievement from the eleventh century on. It was doctors and literati from the upper social strata who could leave records, so most physicians about whom we know anything at all belong to them rather than to the ranks of the hereditary doctors. There is every reason to believe that the latter remained the great majority of physicians. We know practically nothing about the practitioners who could not be called physicians – the priests and other popular healers – who actually were the peasant majority's only source of therapy.

In the early imperial period we rarely find traditions of medical practice spanning more than one generation in scholar-official families. Their orientation toward civil service tended to discourage other careers. Medicine became considerably more popular among the privileged, however, from the thirteenth century on, as they became more numerous and their access to official appointments more uncertain.[56]

Variegated though this picture of health care is, it does not limn a profession. Medical authors do not speak for even a coherent occupation, for therapy was diffused through every level of society. The common universe of discourse that they defined was not shared by all those who healed the ill. It drew, rather, on the cosmology that physicians shared with other members of the élite. Concepts changed not just as health care changed, but as the élite changed. When physicians said, as they frequently did in late imperial China, that someone who cannot serve as a good minister of state can at least be a good doctor, they made a connection central to their system of values.

Theory and practice

Finally I will argue that if we wish to understand how Chinese physicians before modern times understood what they were doing, the notion of 'theory' may be more distracting than helpful. It becomes problematic when it is considered without reference to practice, as frequently happens in modern writing on the history of science and medicine. Theory was not unrelated to practice even in the era of the Scientific Revolution in Europe.[57] It is not valid in any ancient civilization. In

---

[56] Documented for one region of China in Robert P. Hymes, 'Not Quite Gentlemen? Doctors in the Sung and Yuan', *Chinese Science*, 8 (1987), 9–76.

[57] Lesley B. Cormack, '"Good Fences Make Good Neighbors": Geography as Self-Definition in Early Modern England', *Isis*, 82 (1991), 639–61.

Greece, for instance, what mainly determines the level of abstraction and the concern with therapy in a given document is audience; a Hippocratic book that originated as a popular oration will be slanted differently from one arguing a point for colleagues. Galen does not divide theory and practice. They were first separated, as Andrew Cunningham has shown, in the institutionalized teaching of Galen during a period of social collapse 'round about the sixth century'.[58]

No closely analogous break occurred in China. The consistency with which medical authors were practitioners is remarkable by Occidental standards. In many years of searching I have found only a handful of exceptions, almost entirely in the last three hundred years.

Authors by and large agree on what the literature is for. All medical writings, including canons, were meant to be applied as we saw Ch'un-yü I applying them (p. 179). Physicians at first distinguish two kinds of writing. The first is canonical works. They convey the fundamental doctrines, including spiritual and moral doctrines, that make good practice possible. The second is books that supplement these classics with detailed explanations, therapeutic methods, and so on. The General Record of Sagely Benefaction, for example, called these two categories 'the Way' and 'the tools' (p. 194 above). They correspond to the scripture that the teacher transmits in a line that begins with the archaic sages, and his explanations to the initiate (p. 186). Early writings specify that the explanations be oral, but many extant formularies and handbooks undoubtedly record such explanations. They become increasingly monographic, their topics narrowing from the ch'i vessels used for moxibustion (second century BC) to broad classes of medical disorders (c. AD 200) and finally to diseases of the throat (late eighteenth century), etc.[59]

In late imperial China, largely from the sixteenth century on, text-books that provide a systematic curriculum, incorporating the gist of canons and explanations alike, become an important medical genre. The reasons for this transition are not at all clear. Rising population meant

---

[58] Andrew Cunningham, 'The Theory/Practice of Medicine: Two Late-Alexandrian Legacies', in Ogawa Teizo (ed.), *History of Traditional Medicine, Proceedings of the 1st and 2nd International Symposia on the Comparative History of Medicine – East and West* (Osaka, 1986), pp. 303–24.

[59] Examples of the three types are *Tsu pi shih-i-mo chiu ching* (Moxibustion Canon for the Eleven Foot and Arm Circulation Vessels), before 168 BC, in *Ma-wang-tui Han mu po shu* (Documents on Silk from the Han Tombs at Ma-wang-tui), vol. 4 (Beijing, 1985); Chang Chi(?), *Shang han tsa ping lun* (Treatise on Cold Damage and Miscellaneous Disorders), 196/220, critical edn of *Shang han lun* in Ōtsuka Keisetsu, *Rinshō ōyō Shōkanron kaisetsu* (Osaka, 1966); and Cheng Hung-kang, *Ch'ung lou yü yueh* (Jade Key to the Storeyed Tower, a Monograph on Throat Disorders), before 1787, printed 1839 (Beijing, 1956).

fewer official appointments for examination graduates, and blurred the career boundaries between élite and *hoi polloi*. It is certainly due in part to the ready availability of printed books, which make study without a teacher feasible, and which are attractive to teachers with many pupils. Textbooks in the Ch'ing are not peculiar to medical education, but can be seen in every field of instruction.

Keeping in mind that the various genres of early medical writing were complementary, we can see that the canons were not meant to be, nor were they, used as bodies of theory to be studied apart from therapeutic work. A better word for them is 'doctrine'. They were not learned as preparation and set aside. To the contrary, we can see from the beginnings to the present day that clinical work gradually reveals to the physician the meaning of canons memorized before his career begins. But this is a reciprocal process. Understanding of the canons, as it deepens, organizes and gives meaning to diagnostic and therapeutic acts.

It is interesting that this ideal survives in the educational system of 'Traditional Chinese Medicine' since the 1950s. This major component of China's contemporary health care system superimposes Western institutionalization on classical medicine, moving it in decidedly non-classical directions. In 'colleges of TCM' career instructors – who may or may not be seasoned practitioners – now teach standardized curricula of five years or longer, which include substantial anatomy, biochemistry, etc. These courses generally include only excerpts from the classics, or translations of two or three canons into modern vernacular. Most students encounter the ancient language for the first time in such schools, and cannot learn much of it. Many young graduates freely admit (at least to a foreigner) that they do not comprehend yin–yang, Five Phases, Six Warps, and so on, deeply enough to base diagnosis on them. Many, after they begin practice, rely instead on modern nosology and diagnostics.[60]

Despite these portentous changes, which prompt the question of whether traditional medicine can survive, the basic doctrines that medical students are taught remain tightly bound into practice. Judith Farquhar, an anthropologist whose field work made her a student at a college of Traditional Chinese Medicine, puts it thus, 'medical discourse is consequential discourse. It is not idle speculations or descriptive rhapsodies emitting from philosophers in mountain retreats, rather it is concrete action with the simple goal of relieving specific forms of

---

[60] See Sivin (note 6), p. 176, and Sivin, 'Reflections on the Situation in the People's Republic of China, 1987', *American Journal of Acupuncture*, 18 (1990), 325–43.

suffering.' In other words, concepts cannot be applied in textbook fashion, even though they have come to be taught in textbooks.

Doctors seek *guidance* from the experience recorded in the archive [i.e., in writing] and accumulated in the clinic rather than as an authoritative or cut-and-dried solution ... Once medical action is seen as a complex operation of evaluation, intervention, observation, and re-evaluation ... experience can present itself as the only stable reality of medicine and as hierarchically encompassing both 'knowledge' and 'method'.

What doctors taught in a given tradition are expected to agree on is not knowledge of such matters as diagnosis, which develops only through individual experience, but patterns of planning therapy once the imbalance of vital functions is identified. 'Knowledge is individual but therapy is social.'[61]

The values underlying the modern curriculum thus assume that the reciprocal relation of doctrine and practice will somehow allow further generations, despite the demise of traditional world views in the society at large, to continue making the living connection between canon and clinic – if not when newly graduated, then as experience accumulates over the course of a career. Whether that is wishful thinking only time will tell.

Conclusion

Elsewhere in this volume G.E.R. Lloyd has summed up what our joint research suggests are significant differences between Greek and Chinese answers to these questions. Can medicine be called an art or a branch of knowledge, and if so, why? What distinguishes the true practitioner from the layman or the quack? What justifies the doctor's claim to truly know? Let me make the basis of these comparisons clearer by adding to Lloyd's conjectures about the Greek answers my working hypotheses about early China.

First, in China medicine's status as an art was not in question. It did not depend on parallels with philosophy or conscious epistemology, which remained occasional but marginal indulgences. This status was warranted by long traditions of practice. That of hereditary servitors served a social purpose too useful for their aristocratic clients to question; later the unified Ch'in and Han states acknowledged it by incorporating Imperial Physicians in their bureaucracies.

Medicine was often called 'the way of benevolence', which character-

---

[61]   Judith Farquhar, 'Knowledge and Practice in Chinese Medicine', unpublished Ph.D. dissertation, Univ. of Chicago (1986), pp. 201–7.

istically emphasizes not the cognitive but the moral character of its foundation. This usage was not medical in origin. It was borrowed from political thought; the philosopher Mencius first uses it to describe the ruler's natural concern for a living animal.[62] It and many equally complimentary descriptions – comparisons of the physician to a minister of state, analogies with the redemptive mercy of *bodhisattvas* – are potent clues. They insist that clinical practice is an altruistic calling, and never admit that it can be a mere livelihood. They indicate a self-consciousness very different from that of the hereditary servants of noble houses who first shaped medicine as an occupation.

These claims of elevated ethical status suggest a reply to the second question: the basic Chinese distinction was between the relatively few literate, well-born physicians who left the enormous written record, and the plebeian practitioners of every stripe, generally illiterate for most of Chinese history, who cared for the overwhelming majority of the population. The early social transformation of medicine that produced scholar-physicians has often been overlooked on the ground that medicine did not become a respectable career for members of the élite until the second millennium AD. But the fact remains that most of the physicians who left written records before AD 500 were, like Ch'un-yü I, learned aristocrats, and that their emphasis on textual transmission indicates some fledgling solidarity. Physicians certainly never formed a discrete occupational group, but the Greek model of public battles between individuals and schools never took hold either.

That solidarity survived the larger metamorphoses of the Chinese élite away from an aristocracy of birth that turned it in the eleventh century AD into an increasingly mobile class based on literacy, wealth, and office-holding. This is not to say that the scholarly lineages I have described agreed with each other on questions of doctrine and practice, but that they stood together against the majority, the illiterate and marginally literate practitioners, empirics, religious healers, and others, especially those who dared appropriate the dignity of the physician. As time passed there were few disputes between peers on technical or epistemologic issues, but many accusations that others, definitely not peers, were quacks.[63]

The criterion of the true practitioner is thus inseparable from that of true knowledge. As I have suggested, both are settled by membership in

---

[62] *Meng-tzu* (note 14), *p'ien* 1A.7; tr. Lau, p. 55.

[63] Paul Ulrich Unschuld, *Medical Ethics in Imperial China. A Study in Historical Anthropology*, trans. M. Sullivan (Berkeley, 1979), judiciously selects but unreliably translates documents rife with such accusations. He interprets them oddly as attempts by 'Confucian thinkers' to deny 'scarce resources' to physicians 'outside Confucianism'.

a lineage of properly initiated masters who transmit authentic, written medical revelations.

This social form, by no means confined to medicine, is founded on the pattern of the family. It made possible the move from a society where birth largely determined livelihood to a diverse and flexible system of occupations. We may see it in medicine as an adaptation of the hereditary family's transmission of a patrimony. This was not a monolithic pattern, for the privilege of serving went not only from father to son but occasionally to son-in-law or disciple. Its transformation was responsible for a new medicine, a free-for-all between every conceivable variety of practitioner, but with medical prestige newly concentrated at the top of the social scale, and the ranks of the doctors at the apex increasingly closed against incursions by the lower orders. The signs that such conflict increased even though the scholar-physicians retained all the advantages are an index of social mobility.

From the point of view of the élite physicians – the only point of view about which we are well informed for the Han – epistemology was not necessary to true knowledge. That was settled once and for all by initiation. As a familiar saying puts it, 'those who study it are as the hairs on an ox; those who succeed are as the horn of a unicorn. This is purely a matter of whether one has received the transmission'.

[64]   Ts'ui Hsi-fan(?), *Ts'ui Kung ju yao ching chu chieh* (Master Ts'ui's Canon, the Mirror of Emplacing the Elixir, with Annotations), tenth century, TT 60, S135, preface, p. 1a; see also *Huang-ti chiu ting shen tan ching chueh* (Canon of the Nine-vessel Divine Elixir of the Yellow Lord, with 'Oral' Explanation), TT 584–5, S885, ch. 3 (c. AD 1000), pp. 2b–3a. The first sentence entered the Standard Histories, applied to *belles lettres*, in Li Yen-shou et al. (eds.), *Pei shih* (Standard History of the Northern Dynasties), 659, in Chung-hua Book Co. edn of standard histories, ch. 83, p. 2779.

GLOSSARY

an 案

An fa 案法

Chang Chi 張機

Chang Yü-ch'u 張宇初

Chen pen i shu chi ch'eng 珍本醫書集成

cheng fang 正方

Cheng-ho sheng chi tsung lu 政和聖濟總錄

Cheng Hung-kang 鄭宏綱

Cheng-t'ung tao tsang 正統道藏

Ch'i heng 奇恆

ch'i hsieh 奇邪

Ch'i k'o 奇咳

Ch'i k'o shu 奇咳書

Ch'i lo chieh 奇絡結

chieh 解

chieh-yen 解驗

Chieh yin-yang chin shu 接陰陽禁書

chih 治

Chin Yuan ssu ta i-chia hsueh-shu ssu-hsiang chih yen-chiu 金元四大醫
家學術思想之研究

ching 經

Ching mo 經脈

Ch'ing so shih shou 慶所師受

Chiu chen 九鍼

Chou pi suan ching 周髀算經

chüan 卷

Ch'uan yü fa 傳語法

Ch'un-yü I 淳于意

ch'ung 重

Chung-hua i shih tsa-chih 中華醫史雜誌

Chung-i ko-chia hsueh-shuo 中醫各家學說

Chung-i wen-hsieh-hsueh 中醫文獻學

Ch'ung lou yü yueh 重樓玉鑰

fang 方

Fang hua yin-yang 方化陰陽

Ho chi t'ang fa 和齊湯法

hsieh cheng 邪正

Hua yin-yang 化陰陽

Huai-nan hung-lieh chi-chieh 淮南鴻烈集解

Huai-nan-tzu 淮南子

Huang-ti chia i ching 黃帝甲乙經

Huang-ti chiu ting shen tan ching chueh 黃帝九鼎神丹經訣

Huang-ti nei ching chang-chü so-yin 黃帝內經章智索引

Huang-ti nei ching ling shu 黃帝內經靈樞

Huang-ti nei ching su wen 黃帝內經素問
Huang-ti nei ching t'ai su 黃帝內經太素
Huang-ti pa-shih-i nan ching 黃帝八十一難經
Huang-ti Pien Ch'ueh mo shu 黃帝扁鵲脈書
I t'ung cheng mo ch'üan shu 醫統正脈全書
Jen Ying-ch'iu 任應秋
Kao hsia 高下
Kosoto Hiroshi 小曽戸洋
K'uei-to 揆度
Kung-sheng Yang-ch'ing 公乘陽慶
Kung-sun Kuang 公孫光
Li Po-ts'ung 李伯聰
Li Ts'ung-fu 李聰甫
Li Yen-shou 李延壽
Liu An 劉安
Liu Ping-fan 劉炳凡
Lü Pu-wei 呂不韋
ma 馬
Ma Chi-hsing 馬繼興
Ma-wang-tui Han mu po shu 馬王堆漢墓帛書
Maruyama Masao 丸山昌朗
Meng-tzu 孟子
Mo ching 脈經
Mo shu 脈書
Nan-ching pen i 難經本義
Nan-yin 男殷
Ni shun lun 逆順論
Ōtsuka Keisetsu 大塚敬節
Pei chi ch'ien chin yao fang 備急千金要方
Pei shih 北史
piao 表
p'ien 篇
Pien Ch'ueh ho Pien Ch'ueh hsueh-p'ai yen-chiu 扁鵲和扁鵲學派研究
Rinhō ōyō Shokanron kaisetsu 臨床應用傷寒論解説

Shang han tsa ping lun 傷寒雜病論

Shang hsia ching 上下經

Sheng chi ching 聖濟經

Shih chi 史記

Shih shen 石神

Shiki kaichū kōshō 史記會注考證

Shinkyū igaku to koten no kenkyū, Maruyama Masao tōyō igaku ronshū 鍼灸医学と古典の研究、丸山昌朗東洋医学論集

shou 受

shu 數

Ssu shih ying yin yang 四時應陰陽

Sun Ssu-mo 孫思邈

Sung k'o suan ching liu chung 宋刻算經六種

Takigawa Kametarō 瀧川龜太郎

Tamba no Motoyasu 丹波元簡

Ting wu wei 定五味

Tōyō igaku zempon sōsho 東洋醫學善本叢書

Tso chuan 左傳

Tso wei p'ei fang yuan-tse te chün ch'en tso shih 作為配方原則的君臣佐使

Tsu pi shih-i-mo chiu ching 足臂十一脈灸經

Ts'ui Hsi-fan 崔希範

Ts'ui Kung ju yao ching chu chieh 崔公入藥鏡註解

tu 讀

Tung Chung-shu 董仲舒

Wai ch'uai 外揣

Wang K'en-t'ang 王肯堂

Wang Nien-sun 王念孫

Wang Shu-ho 王叔和

Watanabe Kōzō 渡邊幸三

Wu chen 五珍

Wu-se chen 五色診

Wu-se chen ping 五色診病

Wu-wei Han tai i chien 武威漢代醫簡

Yang Chung-ch'ien 楊中倩
Yao fa 藥法
Yao lun 藥論
yen 驗
Yin-yang wai pien 陰陽外變

BIBLIOGRAPHIC ABBREVIATIONS AND CONVENTIONS

HY   Harvard-Yenching Sinological Index Series

ITCM   Wang K'en-t'ang (ed.), *I t'ung cheng mo ch'üan shu* (Main
       Artery of the Orthodox Medical Tradition, a Complete
       Collection), 1601, reprint of Beijing 1907 edn (Taipei,
       1975)

LS   *Huang-ti nei ching ling shu* (Inner Canon of the Yellow Lord:
       Divine Pivot), probably first century BC, in Jen Ying-ch'iu
       (editor-in-chief), *Huang-ti nei ching chang-chü so-yin*
       (Beijing, 1986)

S   Item number in K.M. Schipper, *Concordance du Tao-tsang.
       Titres des ouvrages*, Publications de l'Ecole Franççaise
       d'Extrême-Orient, vol. 102 (Paris, 1975)

SC   *Shih chi* (Memoirs of the Grand Astrologer), completed *c.*
       100 BC, in Takigawa Kametarō, *Shiki kaichū kōsho*, 10 vols.
       (Tokyo, 1932–4)

SW   *Huang-ti nei ching su wen* (Inner Canon of the Yellow Lord:
       Basic Questions), probably first century BC, in Jen (see
       above, explanation of LS)

TT   Chang Yü-ch'u et al. (eds.), *Cheng-t'ung tao tsang* (Taoist
       Patrology of the Regnant Concordance Era), promulgated
       1444, Commercial Press edn

   Authors of books in Chinese or Japanese are given in the notes with
surname first.
   In references to lost books, phrases in the translation that may be the
names of doctrines rather than book titles are preceded by '§'. Other
sources in which the same titles occur are noted.

10 Visual knowledge in classical Chinese medicine

Shigehisa Kuriyama

The main fact, then, about a flower is that it is the part of the plant's form developed at the moment of its intensest life; and this inner rapture is usually marked externally for us by the flush of one or more of the primary colours.   John Ruskin, *Queen of the Air*

How should we understand the strange disparities between the human body described in classical Greek medicine, and the body envisaged by physicians in ancient China? How is it that this basic and most intimate of human realities came to be conceived by two sophisticated civilizations in radically diverging ways?

We glimpse the legacy of this divergence in illustrations from two works of later Chinese and European medicine – the *Shisi jing fahui* by the Yuan dynasty physician Hua Shou (Plate 1), and Andreas Vesalius' *Fabrica* (Plate 2). Viewed side by side, the illustrations each betray 'lacunae'. In Hua Shou's figure, we miss the precisely articulated muscles of the Vesalian man; and indeed, traditional Chinese medicine had no true equivalent for the notion of muscle. Fascination with musculature was a peculiarly Western phenomenon. Conversely, the points mapping out the acupuncture man eluded Vesalius' vision of the body – necessarily, since they were, even to Chinese eyes, invisible. Thus, when Europeans in the seventeenth and eighteenth centuries began to peruse Chinese medical literature, the descriptions of the body they encountered appeared to them like accounts of an imaginary land – 'fantastical', one English physician would deem them, 'absurd', would judge another. Chinese 'anatomy' was unlike anything Galen or Vesalius had ever seen.

These were not timeless differences. The canonical understanding of acupuncture networks emerged only in the Han dynasty (206 BC to 220 AD); systematic dissection was a Hellenistic innovation. Still, by the end of the Han dynasty in China, and by the time, in the Greek world, of Galen (129–200), the characteristic contrasts between the traditional European and Chinese conceptions of the body had already crystallized.

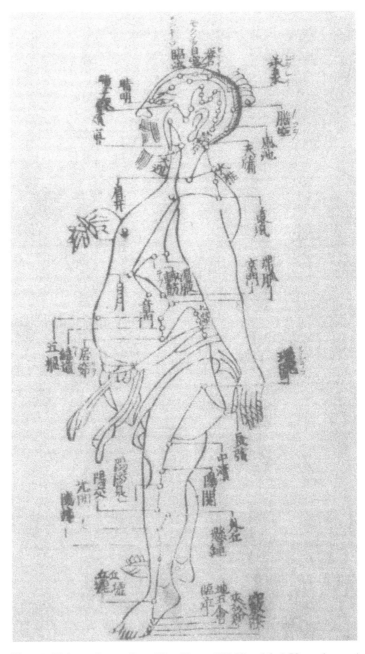

Plate 1: Chinese figure, from Hua Shou, *Shisi jing fahui* (Yuan dynasty)

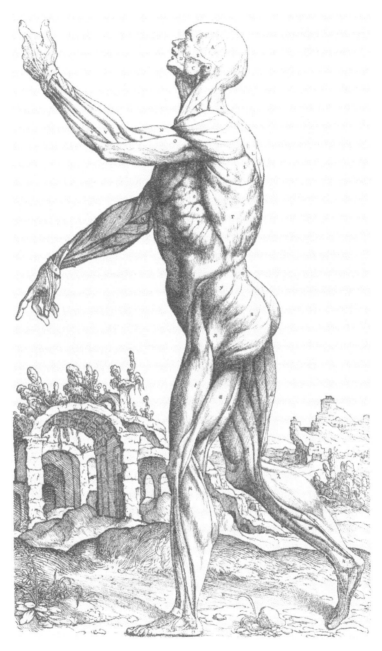

Plate 2: Vesalian figure, from Andreas Vesalius, *De humani corporis fabrica libri septem* (1543)

The disparities depicted in Vesalius and Hua Shou go back to Greek and Chinese antiquity.

I propose, in this essay, to explore one contrast in particular: the difference in ways of seeing. Specifically, I want to try to shed some light on the nature of visual knowledge in Chinese medicine, and its relationship to the Chinese understanding of the body.

Superficially, there may appear to be no relationship. One might think, that is, that the disparities between Plates 2 and 1 mirror the contrast between looking and not looking, and that the distinctiveness of the Chinese conception of the body lay precisely in the fact that Chinese physicians ignored the evidence of the eyes. One could think this without dismissing Chinese notions as fantasy. It could be that, instead of relying on sight, Chinese physicians drew on alternative, non-visual approaches to the body. This much is certain: Chinese physicians never recognized most of the detail observed by Greek dissectors, and they incorporated invisible structures that dissections could never justify. Much of the baffling otherness of the Chinese conception of the body lay in its resistance to the claims of anatomy.

We would be wrong, however, to attribute all or even most of the strangeness of the Chinese body to an exotic visual indifference. The contrast between looking and not looking confuses not seeing *anatomically* with not seeing at all; and it is historically false. The neglect of dissection in ancient China went hand in hand with an extraordinary faith in what sight could reveal. Chinese physicians, like Greek anatomists, looked, and looked intently. Only they somehow saw differently.

The legend of Bian Que testifies to the special affinity between medicine and the gaze. The most renowned physician of antiquity originally had no connection to medicine. He was managing a boarding house, when a guest named Changsang Jun drew him aside. 'I possess secret skills', Changsang revealed to him, 'but I am old, and want to pass them on'. Changsang pulled out an elixir, and explained, 'Drink this with fresh dew for thirty days, and you will know things.' Bian Que did as he was instructed, and soon was able to see through walls, and inside bodies.[1]

Bian Que's transformation into 'the Hippocrates of China' thus turned on the acquisition of penetrating insight. If his name became synonymous with medical acumen it was in part because he could see, literally, what others could not. His celebrated diagnosis of Duke Huan

[1] *Shiji*, vol. 6, ch. 105, p. 2785. For bibliographic abbreviations, please see the list at the end of this chapter. For a thorough and acute analysis of the available sources on Bian Que see Yamada Keiji, 'Henjaku densetsu', *Tōhō gakuhō*, 60 (1988), 73–158.

is a case in point: Bian Que tracked the course of Duke Huan's illness not by questioning him, for the Duke himself had no consciousness of being sick, or by smelling or touching him, but just by peering at him from a distance.[2]

The mystique of insight was not confined to hagiographic legend. We find it echoed as well in the basic texts of classical medicine. To gaze and know the illness, the *Nanjing* teaches, is called 'divine' (*shen*); to listen[3] and know is 'sagely' (*sheng*); to question and know is 'crafty' (*gong*); to touch and know is 'skilful' (*qiao*). Divine insight crowned a hierarchy of ways of knowing. The *Lingshu* ranks and characterizes perceptual skills slightly differently, but it too gives priority to the 'enlightened' (*ming*) gaze.[4] The *Shanghan lun* puts it plainly: the physician who gazes and knows belongs to the top class (*shanggong*); the physician who questions and knows is average (*zhonggong*); the physician who touches and knows is inferior (*xiagong*).[5] Medical mastery required an exceptional eye.

Sight, of course, has long lain at the heart of Western epistemology. On the one hand, the experience invoked to found knowledge has been primarily visual experience, so that discourse on science has regularly conflated sight and perception, observation and experience, *autopsia* and *empeiria*. On the other hand, a venerable tradition has also treated theoretical reflection upon this experience – the very acts of thinking and knowing – as forms of seeing.[6]

This has led some scholars to identify the hegemony of the visual as a distinctively Western trait, rooted perhaps in the nature of Indo-European languages.[7] But Chinese philosophers too speak of the obscurity (*xuan*) and the fine-grained subtlety (*wei*) of the Way, and of the brightness (ming) of intelligence, and of the contemplation (*guan*) of

---

[2] Ibid., p. 2793. A variant of the same episode is recounted in the *Hanfeizi*, ch. 21, *juan*, 7, pp. 2b–3a.

[3] *Wen*. This actually encompasses both listening to the timbre of voices, and smelling body odours.

[4] *Lingshu*, ch. 4, p. 275.

[5] *Shanghan lun, juan*, 1, p. 19a.

[6] Bruno Snell, reflecting on the Homeric concept of *noos*, or 'mind', reminds us that the verbal form *noein* means to 'acquire a clear mental image of something. Hence the significance of noos. It is the mind as the recipient of clear images, or more briefly, the organ of clear images ... Noos is, as it were, the mental eye which exercises an unclouded vision': Snell, *The Discovery of the Mind in Greek Philosophy and Literature*, trans. T.G. Rosenmeyer (New York: Dover, 1982), p. 13. Along these lines, one might add that *idea*, Plato's term for the objects of true knowledge, is a participle of the verb *horaō* ('I see'). Plato was apparently the first to speak of the 'eye of the soul' (*to tēs psychēs omma*). See *Republic*, 533d, and Paul Friedlander, *Plato I: An Introduction*, trans. Hans Meyerhoff (Princeton: Princeton University Press, 1969), p. 13.

[7] See, for instance, Stephen A. Tyler, 'The Vision Quest in the West, or What the Mind's Eye Sees', *Journal of Anthropological Research*, 40 (1984), 23–40.

cosmic principles. And in Chinese medicine, both what was known and what it meant to know were inseparable from the act of seeing.

It is not enough, therefore, in studying Chinese notions of the body, to pursue alternatives to visual knowledge. We must also investigate an alternative visual style.[8] Though Chinese physicians, like Greek anatomists, invested sight with immense significance, they saw in a manner that, from the anatomical perspective, can seem like a failure to look. My essay explores this different way of seeing, its nature and mystique, and its implications for how and what Chinese physicians knew.

The object of the gaze

What is it, exactly, that the eyes can know? What things seen justify the prestige of sight? The Chinese medical classics give a surprising answer: to see is to see *se* – as in *wuse*, 'the five colours'. If the eyes of the Hellenistic dissector were trained on structures, the Han dynasty physician fixed on hues.

We come straight to the heart of the matter. Fingers feel the texture of the skin, the warmth and consistency of the flesh, the movements of the pulse; the nose smells the patient's body and excretions; the ears take in voice pitch, groans, and the reports of the patient's experiences. The eyes observe many things – physiques, gaits, postures in sleeping, oedemas, skin eruptions; but above all, they gaze at colour (*wangse*). Practically, colours command the most consistent and sustained visual attention. Theoretically, colours define the function and rationale of sight. In traditional Chinese medicine, the equation of seeing with seeing se is a basic and unquestioned given.

This is puzzling. Were we ourselves asked what a doctor should see, the word 'colour' probably wouldn't spring immediately to mind. We might well include the patient's facial hues among things to observe; yet while it seems enough to reply 'Smell' to the query 'What should the nose discern?', it seems odd to distil ocular evidence to colour. What motivated this focus? How did attention to se relate to the mystique of insight? And most fundamentally, what did seeing se really mean? These are the key questions.

A face tinged with yellow or red, the *Neijing* teaches, signals fever;

---

8   Particularly suggestive for the relationship between sight and science is Svetlana Alpers, *The Art of Describing. Dutch Art in the Seventeenth Century* (Chicago: University of Chicago Press, 1983). I have also addressed the theme of visual styles in 'Between Eye and Mind: Japanese Anatomy in the Eighteenth Century', in Charles Leslie and Allan Young (eds.), *Paths of Asian Medical Knowledge* (Berkeley: University of California Press, 1992), pp. 21–43. My approach to the theme there, however, is quite different from the one I pursue in this paper.

white means cold; and green and black, pain.[9] In fevers of the liver, redness first appears on the left cheek; in fevers of the lung, on the right cheek; in cardiac fevers, on the forehead.[10] This was one form of seeing se: noting changes in facial hue and relating them to changes in the body. While we may be sceptical of certain diagnoses, the spirit of this kind of observation is familiar enough. We too make inferences from pallor, or feverish flush, or jaundice, about the health of those in whose faces these appear. In itself, there is nothing perplexing about Chinese physicians attending to facial colours.

What puzzles is that colours should be judged paramount – that Chinese physicians should equate seeing with seeing se, and that seeing se should reign supreme over other ways of knowing. For the value of colours as indicators of pain, fever, and cold doesn't seem to justify the judgement. Not only are pain, fever, and cold just some of many conditions that a physician must recognize, but they are broad symptoms with countless nuances and possible causes. Were such vague states all that it revealed, it would be hard to understand the insistence on se.

There was, in fact, another, more influential interpretation, which endowed colour with cosmic as well as somatic significance. Each of the five basic colours of green, red, yellow, white, and black corresponded to one of the five phases (*wuxing* = wood, fire, earth, metal and water) of cosmic change. By observing the hues tingeing a patient's face, the physician could determine the phase governing the patient's condition. A florid countenance, for instance, bespoke the dominance of fire; a visage with yellowish tints, the waxing of earth.[11] Nuances of shade, differences in when and where various hues appeared, and the indications of other senses could add practical complexities; but the principle was simple: to see was to see colour, because the five colours linked the eye to the five-fold transformations pacing the cosmos.

This approach to colour already figures prominently in the canonical classics of the Han dynasty, and defines the theoretical framework for all post-classical commentary on diagnostic sight. It remains, today, the rationale for studying se commonly given by modern textbooks of traditional medicine.

Its appeal isn't hard to understand. By equating the scrutiny of colour with scrutiny of the five-phase rhythms of biocosmic change, this

[9] *Suwen*, ch. 39, p. 113; see also *Lingshu*, ch. 49, p. 401. Sometimes, black is deemed to mean something different from green. See *Suwen*, ch. 56, p. 151, and *Lingshu*, ch. 74, p. 455.
[10] Ibid., ch. 32, p. 94.
[11] The colour–phase correspondences ran as follows:

colour	green	red	yellow	white	black
phase	wood	fire	earth	metal	water

interpretation embedded visual knowledge firmly in the yin-yang/five-phase framework of classical medical theory. Moreover, physicians weren't alone in investing colour with great meaning. For political theorists, the five colours evoked the rise and fall of dynasties. White was the colour of the Shang dynasty; red, the hue of the succeeding Zhou. The latter's conquest of the former was presaged, legend had it, by the capture of a white fish and the appearance of a beam of light that transformed itself into a bright red crow.[12] The first Qin emperor linked the fortunes of his own dynasty with the water that conquers red (Zhou) fire, and ordered black (water's chromatic correlate) for official banners and ceremonial dress.[13]

Nor were the implications of hue confined to succession in time. Colour also articulated the partition of space, and was associated with the dynamics of the four quarters. Sima Qian describes a ritual whereby the emperor erected a mound of earth of the five colours as altar to the spirits of the land. The mound was made of green soil on the east, red soil on the south, white soil on the west, black soil on the north, and covered with yellow soil on top. When a prince was enfeoffed with land to the east, he received some of the green soil; a prince whose fief lay in the south received red soil; a prince whose fief lay in the west received white soil; and a prince whose fief lay in the north received black soil. Each then would take this soil to his fief, and build an altar around it, covering it with some yellow earth that he would also receive.[14]

To imagine colour was thus to imagine power. Chromatic conscious-ness suffused Han culture, finding expression in court banners and ritual utensils, in clothing and architectural design. All this makes the scrutiny of hues in Han medicine appear eminently natural. The cosmic resonance of the five colours seems to provide ample reason to fix on se.

In what follows, however, I will argue that there is more to the matter – that the focus on se also engaged concerns beyond those framed by the five-phase correspondences. Though sanctioned by tradition, the asso-ciation of colour with cosmic rhythms illuminates only one aspect of the Chinese gaze. It leaves some important issues obscure.

Some unexplained puzzles

One obscurity concerns the mystique of the gaze. Nothing in five-phase analysis suggested that the eyes were more discerning than the ears or

---

[12]   Shiji, vol. 1, ch. 4, p. 120.
[13]   Ibid., ch. 6, pp. 237–8.
[14]   Ibid., vol. 4, ch. 60, p. 2115. See also the commentary to the Shujing, 'Yu gong', juan, 6, p. 6b.

the nose, or that the five colours gave better access to cosmic change than, say, the five sounds or five smells. The theory of five-phase correspondences didn't make visual knowledge special. Yet, somehow, it *was* special.

Now someone might protest that the hierarchy that privileged sight was only an ideal, and didn't mirror actual practice. There is much to this – the most detailed diagnostic lessons of the *Neijing* and *Nanjing* elaborate not visual inspection, but the semeiotics of the pulse. The biographies of the famed Han dynasty physicians Chunyu Yi, Guo Yu, and Hua Tuo, in contrast to Zhou legends of Bian Que's clairvoyance, all highlight sphygmological skill. In Guo Yu's most famous feat, for instance, he was not allowed to see his patient at all, but had, instead, to make his diagnosis just by feeling two wrists thrust through curtain openings.[15] This eventually became the standard image of medical expertise: the notion of medical consultation became inseparably fused to the examination of the pulse.

Still, the mystique of insight can't be so casually dismissed. Even if the primacy of the gaze were only an ideal, it would still require explanation as an ideal. Moreover, the real issue may lie less in the dichotomy of real and ideal, than in historical change. Pulse examination emerged relatively late in the development of ancient Chinese medicine, probably emerging as a major technique only in late Warring States and early Han times.[16] This suggests that the contrast between the biographies of Bian Que and Guo Yu mirrors, at least in part, the contrast between Zhou and Han dynasty medicine.

Even after pulse-taking became the prime method of diagnosis, inspection of se remained its necessary complement. A special binary logic made them inseparable: reliable assessment of the pulse required weighing ocular evidence, and vice versa. If the indications of colour and the pulse matched each other, if, for example, both pointed to a wood ailment, then the patient would live; if they diverged, if one signalled wood and the other metal, the patient would die.[17] The ear, nose, and tongue might add supplemental hints, but the crux of judgement lay in the dialectic of hand and eye. Knowing se remained vital to knowing the body. Why? The correspondence between the five colours and the five phases doesn't give the answer.

A second puzzle concerns the generality of the fixation on se. For the

---

[15] For a translation of the account in the *History of the Later Han*, see Kenneth J. DeWoskin, trans., *Doctors, Diviners, and Magicians of Ancient China. Biographies of Fang-shih* (New York: Columbia University Press, 1983), p. 75.
[16] See Yamada (note 1), p. 120.
[17] *Nanjing*, 13.

fixation was not, it turns out, confined to physicians. 'The way the mouth is disposed toward tastes, the eye toward colours (se), the ear toward sounds, the nose toward smells, and the four limbs toward ease is human nature ...'[18] The philosopher Mencius echoes here the standard partition of the senses in ancient China: colour is to the eye what taste is to the mouth, and sound to the ear.[19] Colour is not one object of sight, any more than smell is one object of the flair – it is *the* object of sight, the perception of which defines the eye's proper function. In this sense, it isn't surprising that Chinese physicians should scrutinize colours. Just as Greek study of anatomical structures was rooted in a broader philosophical discourse on forms, so the fixation on se engaged commitments that reached well beyond medicine. But what commitments? What bound the human eye, not just the diagnostic gaze, to se?

Besides broadening the puzzle's scope, Mencius' remarks hint again at the incompleteness of any account that interprets se in terms of the five colours alone. Mencius (371–289? BC) was born more than a century before the compilation of the *Lüshi chunqiu* (240 BC), which offered the first systematic application of five-phase analysis to a theory of cosmic correspondences. Although the *Mencius* contains some two dozen references to se, the phrase wuse doesn't appear even once. More to the point, neither in Mencius' comments on colour nor in these early references to the five colours is there any suggestion that the eye fixes on colours *because* there are five colours, or *because* of a connection between colour and cosmic change. Almost certainly, the marriage of sight and se cannot be explained by five-phase analysis alone.

The meanings of se

Perhaps the commitment to colour is actually not so odd. Aristotle too, in his treatise on psychology, asserts that the object of sight is 'the visible' (*to horaton*), and then elaborates, 'The visible is colour.'[20] And if we count white and black as colours, as the Chinese certainly did, we too must recognize colour as essential to sight: without distinctions of light and dark we would be unable even to distinguish shapes. We would see nothing at all.

Colours often reverberate, moreover, with mystical associations. In their burial rituals, the *Liji* tells us, the people of Shang times 'treasured [the colour] white'.[21] The most important of Shang rituals, the *liao*

18   *Mencius*, 7B.24.
19   See for instance *Zhuangzi*, ch. 12, *juan*, 5, p. 11a.
20   *De anima*, 2.7.
21   *Liji, juan*, 6, 'Tangong', p. 113.

sacrifice, called specifically for the burning of a white dog; and inscriptional references, in other contexts, to white cows, white horses, white pigs, and white deer seem to confirm the symbolic resonance of white in Shang culture.[22] Long before the interpretation of colours was systematized and rationalized by five-phase theorists, in other words, the Chinese attached deep significance to colours – and in this they were like many other cultures.

Yet such considerations take us only so far. For one, they are never explicitly acknowledged. When Mencius and others connect the eye to se, they appeal neither to the symbolic significance of hues, nor to the perceptual priority of shades over forms. But there is an even more decisive limitation: these and other reasons for fixing on colour cannot fully account for the equation of seeing with seeing se, because seeing se was not just a matter of seeing colours. Although se was a common term in pre-Han writings, in the majority of cases it did not signify colour – at least not simply and directly. It meant other things.

The related compound yanse offers instructive hints. In modern Mandarin, yanse is the standard word for colour. To learn the hue of a friend's new Toyota, one asks about its yanse. The term is ancient, however, and is invoked already by Confucius – but with a different meaning. 'Confucius said, "When in attendance at a gentleman one is liable to three errors. To speak before being spoken to by the gentleman is rash; not to speak when spoken to by him is to be evasive; to speak without observing the expression on his face (yanse) is to be blind." '[23] For Confucius (551–479 BC), yanse meant not colour but facial expression. And this typifies classical usage: nowhere in early Chinese writings does the term indicate an abstract notion of hue. In its origins, yanse referred exclusively to the look on a person's face.

Now the character yan designates the face, or more precisely, the forehead; and from this one might infer that se by itself meant something like look, or appearance. Later, indeed, in post-classical Buddhist usage, se signifies the realm of phenomenal appearance, as opposed to noumenal emptiness (kong). Were this its sense in antiquity, the equation of seeing with seeing se would be trivial, for se would encompass all sensory perceptions. But in pre-Buddhist writings the term is not metaphysical. Most often, it evokes not appearance in general, but specifically the appearance of the face. Whenever Confucius went past the station of his lord, 'his face suddenly changed expression (se), his step became brisk, and his words more laconic ... When he had

[22] Nakajima Yosuke, *Goshiki to gogyō. Kodai chūgoku tenbyō* (Tokyo: Bon Books, 1986), p. 89.
[23] *Analects*, 16.6.

come out and descended the first step, he relaxed his expression (yanse) and no longer seemed tense.'[24] In this passage, the *Analects* speak of facial expression first as se, then as yanse; but the two terms are clearly synonymous. In late Zhou and Warring States usage, mien, not hue, was se's most common sense.

Mencius thus observes the hungry look (*jise*) of the people under a tyrant, and the joyful expression (*xise*) of a people blessed with a generous king, and Zhuangzi spots the woeful mien (*youse*) of those who have yet to awaken to the Way.[25] Eventually, with the rise of five-colour/ five-phase analysis, the association of se and colour becomes fairly common. Even so, the Han dynasty *Shuowen*, the earliest Chinese dictionary, defines se as 'the spirit (*qi*) [that appears in] the forehead', and much later, the Qing commentator Duan Yucai could still explain, 'Yan refers to the space between the eyebrows. The mind appears in the spirit, and the spirit appears in the forehead. This is what is called se.' The modern *Cihai*, in fact, still gives 'spirit of the face' (*yanqi*) as se's first meaning, citing Duan's comments for support. Colour is listed as the second sense.

This suggests one explanation (I shall later advance another) for why the Chinese spoke of *gazing* upon se. Modern summaries of traditional diagnostic inspection often convey the impression of a straightforward task: one looks at the hue on the patient's face and determines which of the five phases is ascendant. Yet the standard verb for examining se, *wang*, 'to gaze', intimates a subtler challenge. The earliest inscriptions represent wang by a graph for the eye combined with the depiction of person stretching forward (朢). In its mature version (望), the character shows a person straining to catch a glimpse of the distant moon. Both forms of the character reflect the etymology of the term: wang, 'to gaze', was cognate with wang, 'to be absent', and *mang*, 'to be obscure'.[26] In other words, wang (to gaze) expressed the effort to see what can be perceived only darkly, or from far away. Seeing se somehow involved a straining of the eyes, the reach toward something absent or obscure.

The interpretation of se as countenance gives one source of this sense of straining. For what do we see, when we see a look? Raised eyebrows, a glimmer in the eyes, quivering lips, the lack or flush of colour – all these are doubtless part of what we take in. But mostly, we don't attend to

24   Ibid., 10.3.
25   *Mencius*, 1A.4, 3B.9, 1B.1; *Zhuangzi*, ch. 18, *juan*, 6, p. 18b; ibid., ch. 20, *juan*, 7, p. 9a.
26   See Tōdō Akiyasu (ed.), *Kanwa daijiten* (Tokyo: Gakushū kenkyūsha, 1978), p. 619. Tōdō also points out etymological connections to terms such as *mu* (慕), 'longing (for what is not there)', and *mu* (募), 'to recruit (to fill a vacancy)'.

them separately and consciously, any more than we read a book letter by letter. Rather, what we see – or think we see, for it is often difficult to be sure – are hesitation or impatience, despair or longing, shiftiness or candour. We gaze, that is, upon attitudes and inclinations, which are distinctly visible, yet hard to see distinctly. This is what gazing upon se originally entailed. The medical study of facial hues, I suggest, arose out of a tradition long fascinated by facial expressions. The puzzle of the Chinese gaze is thus only partially about colour. It is also about reading faces.

Se as expression

The obvious reason to study facial expressions is that they express. From them we learn much about those around us. To speak without observing the countenance of one's interlocutor, as Confucius says, is to be blind.

Of course, reading faces requires finesse; expressions are at best translucent, and people dissimulate. Already the *Shujing* cautions against selecting officers on the basis of cunning words and an ingratiating face (*qiaoyan lingse*);[27] and Confucius, for his part, evinces a constant wariness of the chasm between façades of benevolence, friendliness, and bravery, and a person's actual disposition.[28] But such warnings don't so much deny the face's truth as signal the need for perspicacity.

Skilful observers can see through pretence. They can even discern silent thoughts and hidden plans. Wang Chong recounts how Duke Huan of Qi once plotted with his minister Guan Zhong to attack Lu. Mysteriously, even before they had announced their plans, word of the impending expedition had spread. 'There must be a remarkable sage in the land', Guan Zhong remarked. How else to explain the exposure of unspoken designs? Suspecting a certain Dongguo Ya, he summoned him and asked,

'Were you the one who announced the attack on Lu?'
'Indeed.'
'I said nothing about attacking Lu. How did you know?'

It was a matter of apprehending intentions, Dongguo Ya explains. He had simply read Guan Zhong's face (se). He had learned to see when Guan Zhong was joyful, when pensive, when riled for battle. By observing the minister's expression and connecting it with the current political situation, he had divined what was in store.[29]

[27] *Shujing*, Zhoushu: 'Jiong ming', *juan*, 19, p. 8b.
[28] *Analects*, 12.20; 17.10.
[29] *Lunheng*, vol. 2, ch. 79, pp. 1089–91.

Another tale relates how the observant Chunyu Kun once astonished King Hui of Liang by his insight into the king's wandering thoughts. Wang Chong comments, 'The intention was inside the breast, hidden and invisible, but Kun was able to know it.' How? 'He scrutinized the face to peer into the mind' (guanse yi kuixin).[30]

In the amazement aroused by such access to secrets we find the chief source of sight's mystique. Even in Wang Chong's rational account, the acuity of observation is impressive. But Wang's rationalism, as is well known, was exceptional, and his explanation explicitly sought to refute widespread belief in supernatural prophecy. He was arguing, that is, against a popular tradition that saw Dongguo Ya and Chunyu Kun not just as astute observers, but as diviners – seers who, like Bian Que, saw what was hidden inside bodies, in minds, in time.

This is another, and perhaps the direct, reason for speaking of 'gazing' (wang) upon colour: the link between seeing and divining. Physicians gazed at a patient's look (wangse) and predicted the course of illness, much as another class of diviners gazed at the air (wangqi) and prophesied the fate of armies and states. Wangqi was a mantic technique that became especially popular in the Qin and Western Han dynasties – at the same time, that is, that medicine was beginning to crystallize into its classical form.[31] Its premiss was that shifts in climate, in political fortunes, and above all in the momentum of battles appeared first in subtle atmospheric changes.[32] When clouds floating above an army assume the form of a beast, wangqi experts taught, then the army will triumph. Wispy, clear white clouds signal a ruthless leader with fearful troops. Greenish-white clouds which dip low presage victory; clouds reddish in the front and rising warn that the battle cannot be won. In some regions the atmosphere is white, in others red, in yet others the lower sky is black and the upper air is blue. 'One divines by matching the clouds and the five colours.'[33] To gaze at qi was at once to scrutinize far-away clouds and qualities of air, and to peer into the obscurity of things to come.

Medical inspection of se shared much with this atmospheric

---

[30] Ibid., pp. 1091–2.
[31] Onozawa Seiji, Fukunaga Mitsuji and Yamanoi Yū (eds.), Ki no shisō (Tokyo: Tokyo Daigaku Shuppankai, 1978), pp. 154–6; 183–4; 230.
[32] The intimate ties between wangqi and military concerns are detailed in chs. 4 and 5 of Sakade Yoshinobu, Chūgoku kodai no sempō (Tokyo: Kembun shuppan, 1991), pp. 128–83.
[33] Shiji, vol. 3, ch. 27, pp. 1336–7. In his biography of Xiang Yu, Sima Qian relates that before his meeting with Liu Bang, Xiang Yu consulted a wangqi expert who warned him against attacking Liu Bang's troops because the clouds above them had assumed the shape of the dragon and tiger tinged with the five colours – a sure sign of heavenly backing (Shiji, ch. 7, 'Xiang Yu benji').

prognostication. In both wangse and wangqi the seer strained to detect the first and most ethereal manifestations of change. When a particularly powerful pathogen attacks the body, the *Lingshu* explains, 'the patient shivers and trembles and moves the body'. The illness appears in violent shaking that no one can miss. But when the pathogen is of a less virulent sort, the symptoms are initially much subtler. 'The illness can first be seen in the face (se), even though it may not appear in the body. It seems to be there, but not there; it seems to exist, yet not exist; it seems to be visible, and yet invisible. No one can describe it.'[34] To gaze and know things – the pinnacle of medical acumen – is to know things before they have taken form, to grasp 'what is there and yet not there'. As an illness becomes more serious, its corresponding colour intensifies, but if the colour fades 'like clouds completely dispersing (*yun chesan*)', the illness will soon pass. One observes whether the colour is superficial or sunken to know the depth of the illness, whether the colour is dispersed or concentrated to know the proximity of crises. 'By concentrating the mind in this way, one can know the past and present.'[35] Before an illness crystallizes in the body, it announces itself in the face, in an altered air.

Western commentaries on Chinese medicine and philosophy regularly stress the holistic unity of the Chinese body/self. Viewed against the dualisms that so decisively shaped the Western understanding of the human condition – the radical oppositions of divine soul and corrupt flesh, of immaterial mind and material body – the absence of such polarities leaps out as the critical difference. But the attention to dichotomies alien to Chinese thought has often led to neglect of distinctions that the Chinese did make. The form–face distinction is one of them.

The distinction, to be precise, is between *xing* (form) and se. Form and se (*xingse*), Mencius explains, are our natural endowment.[36] The phrase xingse echoes several others: *xingshen* (form and spirit), *xingsheng* (form and vitality), *xingqi* (form and breath). We get the general drift: human beings consist of form and something more. In a sense, we seem not far from the division of body and soul. There is a difference, though. For what separates this something more from mere form, se from xing, is not an ontological chasm, but degrees of perspicuity. As the *Lingshu* passage suggests, there are aspects and phenomena – gross morphology, the shaking of the limbs and trunk – that are as plain as day. Then there are those aspects, still visible, but fleeting and dim, that 'seem to be

---

[34] *Lingshu*, ch. 4, p. 275.
[35] Ibid., ch. 49, p. 401.
[36] *Mencius*, 7A.38.

there, but not there, seem to exist and yet not exist'. Se corresponds to the latter.

The difference in perspicuity corresponds simultaneously to the distinction between those aspects of the person which change slowly, or only under the impact of great force, i.e. xing, and that aspect which responds with exquisite sensitivity. Physicians treasured se because of its responsiveness to the most filigree changes. Physique and physiognomy evolve over months and years; by the time an illness reshapes these, it has usually been long at work. Yet well before an illness emaciates and disfigures, it appears in fugitive and ineffable changes in look. The physician who gazes and knows, who truly sees se, recognizes realities that remain invisible to others until much later.

There is a more general, moral dimension as well. According to Confucius, the person who has 'got through' (*da*) and grasped the Way is 'straight by nature and fond of what is right, *sensitive to other people's words and observant of the expression on their faces* [my emphasis], and always mindful of being modest.'[37] 'The expression on their faces' here translates the single term se. By ranking it alongside such cardinal virtues as rectitude, righteousness, and modesty, Confucius endows the observation of faces with a stature that we ourselves don't normally accord it. We have no difficulty, however, in imagining why Confucius thinks this way: the reason surely lies in his vision of moral development, which intertwines self-cultivation with interpersonal relations. To respond appropriately to others we must understand them; to understand them we must attend carefully to their words and faces.

Yet what is it that we must understand in others? What do faces and words express? Let us first consider words. A familiar way of conceiving them is to think of them as symbolic substitutes for intentions and ideas. To understand a word, in this view, is to grasp the idea that the word represents. Such a conception traditionally underlies the request for definitions, and questions like, 'What do you mean by that term?' But this is not the model of language motivating the Confucian insistence on verbal sensitivity. 'Knowing words' (*zhi yan*) is one of the two special skills that Mencius believes set him apart. He explains, 'When words are extravagant, I know how the mind is fallen and sunk. When words are depraved, I know how the mind has departed from principle. When words are evasive, I know how the mind is at its wit's end.'[38] 'Knowing words' thus has little to do with clear definitions, or grasp of particular terms. Rather, to know words is to hear the attitudes and states of mind

---

[37] *Analects*, 12.20.
[38] *Mencius*, 2A.2.

from which words spring. Sensitive listening is listening to the uninten-
tional overtones of intentional speech.

The same holds true for faces. To the observant eye se expresses even
those inclinations that a person wants to conceal, even velleities foreign
to a person's own awareness. When people 'change expression' (bianse),
or 'make a face' (zuose), they often do so suddenly, spontaneously –
boran bianse, boran zuose, fenran zuose, furan zuose[39] – without premedita-
tion, seized by surprise or anger. Such phrases remind us of the easy
transition from expression to hue. We could translate as well, 'suddenly
change colour', or 'suddenly colour' – or more expansively, 'blenched in
shock', 'flushed with rage', 'blushed in shame'. In se, people manifest
their true colours, as it were. When Confucius emerged from an official
audience, he manifested his yanse – translators say, 'he relaxed his
expression' – letting down his guard, allowing his feelings to show
through. In seeing se, we see the self.

Stunned and humiliated by the biting criticism of a mysterious
gardener-sage, Zi Gong 'lost his se':

Dazed and rattled, he couldn't seem to pull himself together (bu zi de, lit.,
couldn't regain self-possession) and it was only after he had walked on for some
thirty li that he began to recover. One of his disciples said, 'Who was that man
just now? Why did you change your expression and lose your colour (shi se) like
that Master, so that it took you all day to get back to normal (zhongri bu zi fan,
lit., recover yourself)?'[40]

To lose se was thus at once to lose colour and to lose the self.

Earlier, I contrasted the long-term character of changes in form (xing)
to the ethereal volatility of se. But of course facial expressions don't
change randomly, nor do they just reflect the provocations of the
moment. They express as well long years of unconscious habits and
deliberate disciplines. Chinese thinkers knew this well: se made claims
upon their attention not just as something seen, as an object, but also as
something to be subjectively cultivated. While denouncing meretricious
demeanours, Confucius himself made mastery of expression central to
self-cultivation. 'There are three things which the gentleman values most
in the Way: to stay clear of violence by putting on a serious countenance,
to come close to being trusted by setting a proper expression on his face,
and to avoid being boorish and unreasonable by speaking in proper
tones.'[41]

Two of the three most valued things thus called for management of

---

[39] See Mencius, 5B.9, 1B.1; Zhuangzi, ch. 12, juan, 5, pp. 7a, 10a; Analects, 10.3.
[40] Zhuangzi, ch. 3, juan, 5, p. 7b. The translation is from Burton Watson, trans., The
Complete Works of Chuang Tzu (New York: Columbia University Press, 1968), p. 135.
[41] Analects, 8.4.

the face; the third concerned speech. Note again the linkage of se and words, and note also that what mattered in speech was not so much the ideas explicitly opined, as the implicit spirit of discourse (ciqi). The expressiveness of the face was like the expressiveness of one's tone of speech. 'Zi Xia asked about being filial. The Master said, "What is difficult to manage is the expression on one's face (senan). As for the young taking on the burden when there is work to be done or letting the old enjoy the wine and the food when these are available, that hardly deserves to be called filial." '[42]

Taking on the onerous chores, providing for elderly parents – these are things that filial children must do, but they don't suffice to make one filial. The performance of filial duties must be accompanied by an appropriate expression on the face. This is what is hard. It is as in the performance of rites: 'Unless a man has the spirit of the rites, in being respectful he will wear himself out, in being careful he will become timid.'[43] Anyone can pronounce certain words, walk, clasp their hands, bow. They are easy: one decides to do them, and does them. But tone of voice, bearing, facial expression, the precise spirit of the rites – these are a different matter. Like walking and bowing, they are subject to the will, but one's control over them is more tenuous, indirect, less consistent. They require patient cultivation over time, repeated practice.

Se thus expressed the years of lived life – and this sometimes in the most concrete sense. Zhuangzi speaks, for instance, of a seventy-year-old sage whose complexion (se) was that of a young babe.[44] The biography of Hua Tuo marvels at how the arts of rejuvenation gave him the countenance (se) of youth even in old age.[45] In both cases, se translates either as complexion or face, and probably encompasses both. In judging age we observe, in part, facial expression – whether someone looks experienced or untested, life-weary or callow. But we also weigh the colour, softness, and sheen of the skin. As an indicator of age or health, se was thus synonymous with seli, where li referred to the pores of the skin, and seze, where ze evoked the skin's lustre. Seli and seze thus evoked skin hue and texture, the life manifest at the body surface. The sage and Hua Tuo were men who were old in years but who looked young. This is another aspect of people's looks, whether they appear youthful or decrepit.

We find an interesting parallel to Chinese ideas of se in the Homeric notion of chrōs. For chrōs too pointed toward the expressively tinged

---

[42]   Ibid., 2.8.
[43]   Ibid., 8.2.
[44]   Zhuangzi, ch. 19, juan, 7, p. 3b; see also ch. 6, juan, 3, p. 7a.
[45]   Sanguo zhi, 'Hua Tuo zhuan'. See DeWoskin (note 15), pp. 140, 150.

face. The divide between the cowardly and the brave, the captain of the
Cretans observes, is clear: 'The colour [of a coward] is ever-changing'
(*trepetai chrōs alludis allē*; Fitzgerald translates, 'This one's face goes
greener by the minute'), whereas 'The colour [of the brave one] never
changes.'[46] But chrōs was also the vital body. It refers, for example, to
the body of Patrocles, preserved by nectar and ambrosia,[47] or the body
of Achilles, which must (or so Agenor thinks), like that of all mortals, be
susceptible to attack by bronze spears.[48] Hector's body/flesh (chrōs),
despite being subject to desecrations, remains strangely preserved.[49]
The subsequent rise of humoral analysis in Greek medicine doubtless
owed something to this vision of body as flesh tinged with life.

The predominance of yellow or black bile, phlegm or blood readily
appears in facial hues of yellow or black, or white or red. Thus Greek
physicians too took account of colour in their diagnoses, and Galen
could even identify sight with the apprehension of chromatic change.[50]
But two differences bear notice: (1) se in Chinese medicine engaged an
intensity of interest and had a range of significance unmatched by
colours in Greek medicine; and (2) Chinese colours were not humoral.
The *Lingshu* explains that poor blood circulation leads to loss of lustre in
the face and hair,[51] and that is as close as the Chinese classics come to a
humoral account. But this raises an important question: if not as a
mixture of coloured fluids, how *did* Chinese physicians imagine the hue
that tinged the face? Why *does* the face have colour? Before we can
answer this question, we first must look more closely at the alternative
against which I am contrasting the scrutiny of se. We must examine
anatomical seeing.

The anatomical perspective

If by anatomy one means cutting open the body and looking, then it is
inexact to say that the ancient Chinese showed no interest in it. The
Lingshu speaks explicitly of the possibility of 'dissecting and in-
specting',[52] and the *Hanshu* biography of Wang Mang records that in 16
AD a dissection was actually performed.[53] Both passages, however, are
brief, and neither records specific observations. Moreover, they are the

[46] *Iliad*, 13.278–84.
[47] Ibid., 19.38–9.
[48] Ibid., 21.567–8.
[49] Ibid., 24.413–14.
[50] Galen, *De symptomatum differentiis*, 1.1., K 7, p. 44.
[51] *Lingshu*, ch. 10, p. 305.
[52] Ibid., ch. 12, p. 311.
[53] *Hanshu*, vol. 5, ch. 69B, pp. 4145–6.

only explicit references to medical dissection up through the Han dynasty.[54] They are isolated exceptions.

Still, the two share an intriguing peculiarity. They both evince a concern with measurement. The body of Wangsun Qing was dissected, the Mang biography reports, and the measurements of the five viscera recorded. The *Lingshu* is more expansive. 'The height of the heavens, breadth of the earth, these lie beyond the human capacity for measurement', it explains. But the human body is immediately accessible and of modest proportions. One can make measurements along the body surface, and after death one can dissect. By dissection one determines the consistency of the solid organs, the size of the hollow organs, the amount of food in the system, the length of the vessels, the clarity or turbidity of the blood and its amount, which vessels have more blood and less qi, and which vessels the reverse. All these have their norm, their measure (*dashu*).

The *Neijing* and *Nanjing* offer, in fact, some remarkably detailed numbers. The mouth, the *Lingshu* reckons, is 2.5 *cun* wide; from the teeth to the back of the throat is 3.5 cun; the capacity of the oral cavity is 5 *he*. The tongue weighs 10 *liang*; it is 5 cun long and 2.5 cun wide. The stomach weighs 2 *jin* 2 liang; it is 2 *chi* 6 cun long, and measures 1 chi 5 cun in its circumference; its capacity is 3 *dou* 5 *sheng*. The bladder weighs 9 liang 2 *zhu*; it is 9 cun wide and its capacity is 9 liang 9 he. The list goes on for each of the organs.[55] On the body surface, of course, an abundance of precise distances map the many sites of acupuncture.

My point is this: there is more than one way to cut open the body and look. On the rare occasion(s?) when the Chinese dissected, they focused mostly on features other than those that interested Hellenistic dissectors. But this example of an alternative mode of dissection suggests that we cannot be satisfied with interpretations of Greek anatomy that see it simply as the expression of some vague 'empirical spirit'. Greek anatomy represented *one way* of looking at the body. It reflected the will to observe in a *particular manner*.

Full elucidation of this manner would obviously require a separate

---

[54]   The passage in the Wang Mang biography is the *sole* mention of dissection to be found in any of the official histories (*zhengshi*) that so voluminously document Chinese history. Medical sources, however, make clear that dissections did occur in later periods. For a survey of dissections in traditional China, see Watanabe Kōzō, 'Genzon suru Chūgoku kinsei made no gozō roppu zu no gaisetsu', in his *Honzō no kenkyū* (Osaka: Takeda Kagaku Shinkōkai, 1987), pp. 341–452.

[55]   *Lingshu*, chs. 31 and 32, pp. 359–62; *Nanjing*, 42 and 43. For a more detailed review of classical Chinese 'anatometrics', and translations of many of the relevant passages, see Yamada Keiji, 'Anatometrics in Ancient China', *Chinese Science*, 10 (1991), 39–52.

essay. Here I can only briefly and dogmatically state two themes that I think especially pertinent to the contrast with the Chinese gaze.

The first is intentional design. Aristotle concedes, in *Parts of Animals*, that 'it is not possible without considerable disgust to look upon the blood, flesh, bones, blood-vessels and similar parts of which the human body is constructed'. But these, he stresses, are not what anatomy is about. The aim of dissection is not to see the immediately sensible materials *per se*, which are repulsive, but rather to contemplate (*theorein*) the purposive design of Nature. As long as one trains one's eyes to somehow see beyond the matter of which animals are composed and to apprehend the whole configuration (*he holē morphē*), the Form as it reflects Nature's ends, then this gruesome enterprise of anatomy can even be characterized as beautiful.[56]

What makes anatomical sight possible, then, and defines its aims, is a psychology of purposive intent. In Plato's teleology, the creator of the universe is a sort of craftsman. But craftsmen, as Socrates reminds us, 'do not choose and apply their material to their work at random, but with the view that each of their productions should have a certain form (*eidos*)'.[57] In making a table or couch, the craftsman 'fixes his eyes on the idea or form'.[58] Creation is thus an act of copying, a translation of a visual image into material form. And so it goes also with the Demiurge. When he fashions and shapes the world he too must keep in view 'the pattern of the unchangeable'.[59]

It is this original intention that dissectors like Galen would try to apprehend. 'Rid your mind of the differences in material, and look at the pure art itself', he urges.[60] While the common man never gets beyond the matter which makes up things, the scientist (*technitēs*) marvels at how Nature, the great craftsman, 'does nothing in vain'. To see and know the body is to see and know the motivating intentions behind it. Seen anatomically, the body expresses forethought.

The second theme to which I want to draw attention is that of volition. The Vesalian figure with which I began the essay elegantly exemplifies the prominence of muscles in the anatomical view of the body. Galen, in his *Anatomical Procedures*, devotes no fewer than four of the first nine books to their dissection. Interestingly, however, the term 'muscle' does not appear in the Homeric epics. Plato refers frequently in his *Timaeus* to the body's flesh and sinews, but also makes no mention of muscles.

---

[56] *Parts of Animals*, 645a.
[57] *Gorgias*, 503e.
[58] *Republic*, 10.596b.
[59] *Timaeus*, 29a.
[60] *De usu partium*, book 3, 3.

Muscles do appear in the Hippocratic treatises, but surprisingly rarely. Even in those Hippocratic works where one might expect the most detailed attention to musculature, such as the treatises on *Surgery* and on *Fractures*, the preferred term is not muscles, but flesh (*sarx*). In a pattern paralleling that found in China, the Greek author of *Fractures* thus speaks of 'bones, tendons, and flesh', rather than bones, tendons, and muscles.[61] It is only after Hippocrates that muscles become a central feature of the Greek understanding of the body.

Now one might suppose that post-Hippocratic fascination with muscles sprang from the rise of Hellenistic anatomy. Hellenistic physicians, one might think, spoke specifically of muscles rather than generically of flesh, because they, in contrast to their Hippocratic predecessors, probed below the surface of the skin, and distinguished individual muscles from each other.

However, by approaching muscles simply as objects of visual apprehension, the appeal to anatomical experience alone neglects the chief characteristic of the new discourse on muscularity: whereas flesh referred primarily to the visual and tactile perception of somatic bulk, Greek physicians in late antiquity invoked muscles to analyse the body's movements. Muscles were not just flesh perceived with enhanced perspicuity; they were organs invested with a specific and unique function.

We see this most immediately in organs like the stomach, the uterus, the bladder, and above all, the heart. For the modern anatomist, these are all muscular structures; for Galen they were not. Galen cites a variety of distinctions between such organs and true muscles – the course of the fibres, colour, taste – but the decisive difference is this: the latter obey the bidding of the will, the former do not. Although the heart, with its densely compressed flesh, may look muscular, it can't really be a muscle because it moves of its own accord.[62] We can't control it as we command the muscles of the arms and legs; we cannot start or stop it as we wish.

Galen's treatise *On the Motion of Muscles* thus concentrates as much on exploring the conundrums of action and intention as on detailing muscular function.[63] It testifies to the inseparability, in late Greek medicine, of interest in muscularity and the analysis of agency. Some somatic processes, Galen notes, go on without our attending to them, and we cannot directly influence them even if we wished. Such is the

---

[61]   *Fractures*, 2. See also Aristotle, *Parts of Animals*, 2.8.
[62]   Galen, *On the Motion of Muscles*, 1.3, *K* 4, p. 377; *On the Usefulness of the Parts of the Body*, 6.8, *K* 1, pp. 319–20; *On Anatomical Procedures*, 7, *K* 2, pp. 610–15.
[63]   *On the Motion of Muscles*, *K* 4, pp. 367–464.

case with digestion and pulsation. But there is also an important class of activities, such as walking and talking, which depend directly upon our will. We can choose to walk faster, or slow down, or stand still. We can alter the cadence of our speech. We can do all this because we have, in addition to the stomach, and intestines, and arteries, these special organs called muscles.[64] Muscles, as Galen defines them, 'are the organs of voluntary motion'.[65] Their activities express the impulses of the soul. They allow us to choose the pace and character of our actions, and this choice, by distinguishing voluntary actions from involuntary processes, confirms us as genuine agents.

In two different ways, then – in the study of somatic structures as the manifestation of intentional design, and in the fixation on muscles as the organs of the will – Greek anatomical vision was shaped by the assumptions and concerns of Greek psychology. And this is what we should expect. For it is commonly acknowledged that how we see something is influenced by what we imagine the thing to be. But in the case of the body, that imagined object is ourselves. This brings me to my main thesis. It is that the differences in how Greek and Chinese physicians looked at the body, as an external object, derived in large measure from differences in how they conceived and experienced themselves from within, as persons.

Someone could object that for the Greeks neither volition nor intentionality (though the argument in the latter case is murky) were uniquely human. Animals had them too. But this approximation of the human and the animal, which we know had important practical consequences for the development of Greek anatomy, itself offers an intriguing contrast to the Chinese understanding of the person.

The flowering spirit

I have talked loosely thus far of se's expressiveness – of faces mirroring feelings and inclinations, of hues reflecting a person's five-phase status. To conclude, I want to press for greater precision: exactly how was se related to what it expressed?

The relationship between a person and a person's look is surely not the same as that between the decision to start walking and the contraction of the relevant muscles. Showing a look involves more than just a decision; one can try to look filial, but effort alone hardly ensures success. Nor is the relationship between se and what it expresses like

[64] Galen, *On the Usefulness of the Parts of the Body*, 16.2, *K* 2, p. 380: 'For voluntary motion Nature has constructed in animals one kind of instrument called muscle.'
[65] Galen, *On the Motion of Muscles*, 1.1, *K* 4, p. 367. This definition opens the work.

that between the artefacts of Plato's craftsman and the ideas of which these artefacts are the material realization. It isn't a matter of foresightful design.

Of course, volition and intention have their part: people often strive for a certain look, and this effort influences how they do, indeed, look. The *Analects*, for instance, harken repeatedly to the expressions assumed by the Master. But looks that are truly commanding, or reverent, or benevolent – as opposed to mere façades of authority, or reverence, or benevolence – can't be summoned at any time, or by anyone who might will them. Something more is required. We've noted, moreover, that it is often precisely in one's unguarded moments that se expresses most – despite oneself. The limited role of will and purposive design holds all the more in the case of se as it expresses age or health: one's colour, the lustre and elasticity of the skin, and a look of youthfulness and vitality – or the absence thereof – only indirectly, if at all, express the will, as the sum of countless decisions and indecisions spanning months and years.

How, then, should one imagine se's expressiveness? More to the point, how did the ancient Chinese conceive it? I suggest that they conceived it botanically. 'Colour', the *Suwen* explains, 'is the flower (or flowering) of the spirit (*sezhe, qi zhi hua ye*)'.[66] 'The heart gathers together the essences of the five organs ... The flowering visage (*huase*) is the bloom [of this essence].'[67] And again, 'The heart gathers together the vessels. It flowers in the face (*qi rong se ye*)'.[68] Se expressed the person much as blossoms express the plant.

It is easy to overlook such remarks; botanical analogies in Chinese medicine are so common. The analogy to plants underlies, for example, the relationship between the various organs and the parts of the body that each governs: when the spleen ceases to nourish, the flesh becomes soft and the tongue wilts (*wei*); when the kidneys cease to nourish, the bones become desiccated (*ku*).[69] Similarly, the mutual correspondence between spirit on the one hand, and se and pulse on the other, is like that between trunk and branch, roots and leaves (*benmo genye*).[70] According to the *Nanjing*, the source of vital breath (*shengqi*) serves as the body's stem and roots; when the roots are severed, the branches and leaves wither.[71] Such examples could easily

---

[66]   *Suwen*, ch. 17, p. 50.
[67]   Ibid., ch. 81, p. 254.
[68]   Ibid., ch. 10, p. 34.
[69]   *Lingshu*, ch. 10, p. 305.
[70]   Ibid., ch. 4, p. 275.
[71]   *Nanjing*, 8. This explains how it can happen that a person with an ostensibly healthy pulse suddenly dies. It is as in the case of plants: when the roots are suddenly cut, the plant may, judged by the flowers and leaves, initially seem to be in good health.

be multiplied. While the classical texts of Chinese medicine use many metaphors to interpret the body, none is as pervasive as that of plant growth and development.

I think it important that we not treat the image of the flowering face as just another instance of this common trope. I urge, on the contrary, that we take this image as a clue to the deeper implications of the analogy to plants. For it suggests that the botanical vision of the body was a vision in the literal as well as figurative sense. Chinese physicians did not merely speak of se as flower; they saw it as such.

I mean two things by this. Most immediately, I mean that physicians studied the face in much the same way that a gardener judges the condition of plants. Obvious signs of a plant in faltering health include limpness, shrivelling, and desiccation, and Chinese physicians used the same terms to describe the sickly body. But it is perhaps the colour and lustre of the blossoms and leaves that offers the subtlest and most revealing index of vitality.

My neighbour happens to be an avid horticulturalist, whereas I myself tend to neglect my yard. Each spring, the difference becomes embarrassingly apparent: my neighbour's azaleas blaze with a rich brilliance of colour that bespeaks the care and fertilized soil on which they have been painstakingly nourished; my own azaleas (planted by a previous owner) have the recriminatingly pale hues of plants long left to scrounge for survival in Georgia clay. The leaves of my neighbour's plants literally shine with lustrous vitality; mine look distinctly dull and drab. And so it went too, in Chinese medicine, with the contemplation of facial hues. Even more fundamental than the distinctions between the five colours was the contrast between lustrous and lacklustre shades of the same colour – between, for example, the glistening white, red, and black of pig's fat, the cock's crown, and the feathers of the crow; and the lifeless white, red, and black of dried bones, coagulated blood, and soot. The former portended recovery; the latter signalled death.[72]

Greek physicians also acknowledged similarities between animals (including human animals) and plants. While voluntary motion separated the zoological from the botanical realm, both animals and plants nourished themselves and grew. This is why growth and nutrition were deemed functions of the so-called vegetative soul. But in China the botanical parallel didn't apply merely to select, lower aspects of the human economy; it characterized human nature itself.

[72] *Suwen*, ch. 10, p. 34. See also *Suwen*, ch. 17, p. 50.

In defence of what later become the cornerstone of Confucian orthodoxy, Mencius turned to plants to illuminate the essential goodness of human nature. All humans, he argued, are born naturally good. But the four qualities that make up this goodness – benevolence, rightness, rites, and wisdom – are like four shoots whose development requires careful cultivation. One must constantly attend to them; yet one cannot *force* them to grow. Witness the folly of the man from Song:

> There was a man from Song who pulled at his rice plants because he was worried about their failure to grow. Having done so, he went on his way home, not realizing what he had done. 'I am worn out today', said he to his family. 'I have been helping the rice plants to grow.' His son rushed out to take a look and there the plants were, all shrivelled up.[73]

Self-cultivation and the cultivation of plants require an effort that differs from the exertion involved in, say, moving a rock. It is not a matter of just deciding, and immediately pushing or pulling – of what one might call muscular will. This brings me to the second, deeper sense in which scrutiny of se matched the contemplation of a plant's bloom.

In an earlier paragraph, I proposed a connection between Greek anatomical study and two influential models of human expression – one centred on the articulation of intentions, the other emphasizing the manifestation of the will. Neither of these models played much part in Chinese self-definition. Rather, the crucial model in China was that of the growth and health of plants. Human beings were like plants not just in 'physiological' functions, such as growth and nutrition, but in their moral development and in their personal expressiveness – in the way they grew and revealed themselves as persons.

Whence the focus of the Chinese gaze on se. 'Benevolence, rightness, the rites, and wisdom', Mencius observes, 'are rooted (*gen*) in the heart, and give rise to an expression (se) that appears pure and luminous in the face (*mao*)'.[74] In a similar vein, the *Guoyu* identifies the face (mao) with the flowering of feeling.[75] Conversely, if se is the flower (*hua*) of the spirit, 'Flower', a common gloss has it, 'is se'.[76]

From the image of the expressive flower we could head in various directions. We could pursue, for instance, the socio-economic origins of

---

[73] *Mencius*, 2A.2.
[74] *Mencius*, 7A.21.
[75] *Guoyu, juan*, 11, 'Jinyu. Part 5', p. 109.
[76] See, for instance, *Hanshu, juan*, 27C, 'Wuxing zhi', vol. 3, p. 1442.

the Chinese predilection for botanical analogy. Or we might speculate about the analogy's consequences – about how it may have contributed to the relative indifference of Chinese physicians toward questions of structure and function. But these are matters for future study. What I hope to have shown in this essay is the importance of the problem of visual knowledge in Chinese medicine, and its affinity to the problem of imagining and being persons.

[77] In a recently published study, Derek Bodde observes that, 'Since very early times the Chinese were apparently much more interested in crops and plants than in animals.' He then goes on to cite Ho Ping-ti on the backwardness of Chinese animal husbandry:

> Throughout China's long historic periods the agricultural system ... has always been lopsided in favor of grain production, with animal husbandry playing a subsidiary role ... Among relevant [early cultural] traits, the most noticeable was the lack of sufficient knowledge to make and use dairy products ... The Chinese had yet another peculiar trait, namely, the unusually late beginning and persistent underutilization of draft animals for cultivation.

See Ho Ping-ti, *The Cradle of the East, An Inquiry into the Indigenous Origins of Techniques and Ideas of Neolithic and Early Historic China 5000–1000 B.C.* (Hong Kong, Chinese University of Hong Kong, and Chicago: Chicago University Press, 1975), pp. 113–14. The passage is cited in Bodde, *Chinese Thought, Society, and Science. The Intellectual and Social Background of Science and Technology in Pre-Modern China* (Honolulu: University of Hawaii Press, 1991), p. 311.

GLOSSARY

benmo genya 本末根葉

Bian Que 扁鵲

bianse 變色

boran bianse 勃然變色

boran zuose 勃然作色

bu zi de 不自得

chi 尺

Chunyu Kun 淳于髡

Chunyu Yi 淳于意

Cihai 辭海

ciqi 辭氣

cun 寸

da 達

dashu 大數

Dongguo Ya 東郭牙

dou 斗

Duan Yucai 段玉裁

fenran zuose 忿然作色

furan zuose 怫然作色

gen 根

gong 工

guan 觀

Guan Zhong 管仲

guanse yi kuixin 觀色以窺心

Guo Yu 郭玉

Guoyu 國語

Han 漢

Hanshu 漢書

he 合

hua 華

Hua Shou 滑壽

Hua Tuo 華陀

huase 華色

jin 斤

jise 飢色

ku 枯

li 理

liang 兩

liao 寮

Liji 禮記

Lingshu 靈樞

Lu 魯

Lüshi chunqiu 呂氏春秋

mang (to be obscure) 茫

mao 貌

ming 明

Nanjing 難經

Neijing 內經

qi 氣

qi rong se ye 氣榮色也

qiao 巧

qiaoyan lingse 巧顏伶色

Qin 秦

Qing 清

se 色

seli 色理

senan 色難

seze 色澤

sezhe, qi zhi hua ye
  色者、氣之華也

shanggong 上工

Shanghan lun 傷寒論

shen 神

sheng (sagely) 聖

sheng (measure of weight) 升

shengqi 生氣

shi se 失色

Shisi jing fahui 十四經發揮

Shujing 書經

Shuowen 說文

Song 宋

Suwen 素問

wang (to gaze) 望

wang (to be absent) 亡

Wang Chong 王充

Wang Mang 王莽

wangqi 望氣

wangse 望色

Wangsun Qing 王孫慶

wei (subtlety) 微

wei (wilts) 萎

wen (listen/smell) 聞

wuse 五色

wuxing 五行

xiagong 下工
xing 形
xingqi 形氣
xingse 形色
xingshen 形神
xise 喜色
xuan 玄
yan 顏
yanqi 顏氣
yanse 顏色
youse 憂色

yun chesan 雲撒散
ze 澤
zhi yan 知言
zhonggong 中工
zhongri bu zi fan 終日不自反
Zhou 周
zhu 銖
Zhuangzi 莊子
Zi Gong 子貢
Zi Xia 子夏

ABBREVIATIONS

Guoyu	*Guoyu. Zhanguo ce* (Changsha: Yuelu shushe, 1988)
Hanfeizi	*Hanfeizi* (Taipei: Zhonghua shuju, 1982)
Hanshu	*Hanshu*, 5 vols. (Taipei: Dingwen shuju, 1981)
K	C.G. Kühn (ed.), *Claudii Galeni opera omnia*, 20 vols. (Hildesheim: Georg Olms Verlagsbuchhandlung, 1964)
Liji	*Liji zhengyi* (Shanghai: Guji chubanshe, 1990)
Lingshu	*Huangdi neijing zhangju suoyin* (Taipei: Qiye shuju, 1987)
Lunheng	Juang hui (ed.), *Lunheng jiaoshi*, 2 vols. (Taipei: Shangwu inshuguan, 1983)
Nanjing	*Huangdi bashiyi nan jing*
Neijing	*Huangdi neijing*
Shanghan lun	*Shanghan lun* (Taipei: Zhonghua shuju, 1987)
Shiji	*Shiji*, 6 vols. (Hong Kong: Zhonghua shuju, 1969)
Shujing	*Shangshu zhengyi* (Taipei: Zhonghua shuju, 1979)
Suwen	*Huangdi neijing zhangju suoyin* (Taipei: Qiye shuju, 1987)
Zhuangzi	*Zhuangzi* (Taipei: Zhonghuan shuju, 1979)

11   A deathly disorder: understanding women's health in late imperial China

Francesca Bray

The subject of this paper is how physicians in late imperial China (*c.* 1500–1850) understood women's bodies and health problems. Two questions raised in this paper relate closely to issues explored by Lesley Dean-Jones. First, did orthodox Chinese physicians, all of whom were men, feel any uncertainty about their knowledge of the female body? And second, what value did they place on women's testimony about their bodily states and experiences? In the third part of the paper I look at patterns of medical reasoning and choices of diagnosis in the case of a single, sex-specific health problem, amenorrhoea, which physicians and lay people alike thought of as life-threatening. The late imperial gynaecological texts on amenorrhoea offer interesting insights into levels of medical causality, the relationship between professional and lay reasoning, and the power of words to influence therapeutic choice.

Knowing the other sex

Orthodox physicians in late imperial China included literati and hereditary physicians. The literati doctors were also well trained as scholars and more deeply versed in general philosophy than the hereditary physicians, but both groups had studied the medical canonical texts and shared a cosmological understanding of the nature of the human body and its disorders. These physicians were exclusively male. Did they, like certain Greek physicians, have any doubts as to their understanding of the female body?

Such uncertainty clearly relates to how the physical difference between the sexes was understood. In the Greek medical tradition, the explanation of sex differences centred mainly on a contrast in reproductive form and function from which other secondary differences derived. Women's health, constitution and behaviour was often explicitly linked to their wombs, a distinct anatomical organ which men do not have themselves; they could not experience its sensations, though they could examine it. The kind of understanding thus reached by a male medical

236   Francesca Bray

profession was objective, not subjective. The question arose in Greece whether such knowledge was adequate, or did male physicians need to consult women to reach a truly empathetic understanding of female experience and ailments?

In dealing with women's bodies Chinese physicians were not faced with this issue of understanding the other, because sex differences were conceived of as a question of degree rather than one of essential nature. The Chinese medical conception of the body was not anatomical, but functional and processual.[1] Differences between male and female were explained in terms of relative predominance of yin and yang. Chinese medical thought saw the male body as more dominated by male vital energy, yang qi, the female body by its female counterpart, yin qi; in late imperial texts it is usually said that the processes of the female body are dominated by yin qi in its material manifestation, blood, while the processes of the male body are dominated by non-material qi energy.

But of course men also have blood and women also have qi. The difference between male and female is conceived in terms not of two separate essentialized categories, but rather of a continuum of probability. Most women will have more yin characteristics than most men; at the same time individuals in the phase of growth and maturation will be more yang than those in a phase of ageing and decline, so that they will occupy different positions along the continuum according to their age and variations in their health.[2]

The process of sexual maturation is described in the canonical Huangdi neijing and thereafter as broadly the same in both sexes, though it occurs two years later in males. Puberty marks the ability to procreate, and in both sexes it results from the full development of the Kidney system:

When a girl [reaches the age of] twice seven, her Kidney qi is abundant and she acquires her reproductive capacities, tiangui. Her ren tract goes through, and the

[1] See the papers by Farquhar, Kuriyama and Sivin in this volume.
[2] In pre-Song texts there is no separate branch of medicine devoted exclusively to women's disorders, though there are manuals of obstetrics. But in the Song dynasty (960–1279) a general intellectual concern with classification and systematization led, in medicine, to a reformulation of medical 'disciplines' (ke) that included two new categories: gynaecology (fuke or nüke) and paediatrics (erke). In her work in progress on women and gender in late imperial China, Charlotte Furth points to a historical evolution of fuke: in the Song many physicians felt that women (and children) would experience a particular disorder differently from men because of differences in balance between yin and yang which affected the manifestation of the disorder. Song fuke works accordingly were not confined to the discussion of female reproduction and its attendant problems, but also included discussion of gender-specific manifestations and treatment of common complaints. But by late imperial China fuke works concentrated almost exclusively on reproductive function and problems.

greater *chong* tract flourishes,[3] her menses flow regularly and she can bear children ... When a boy [reaches] twice eight, his Kidney qi is abundant and he acquires his reproductive capacities. His seminal essence overflows and drains, he can unite yin and yang [have sex] and have children.[4]

The *Huangdi neijing* describes progressive sexual maturation and decline in terms of the Kidney system, the reproductive tracts, and hair and teeth, which are the external features of the Kidney system. Genitalia are not mentioned, nor certain features that we consider important secondary sexual characteristics such as breasts. The womb is not mentioned in discussions of reproductive characteristics; it comes up only in discussions of pregnancy and childbirth, as the organ in which the foetus develops and from which it is born. It is not a synecdoche for woman, nor a ruling feature of her constitution.

Since the differences between the male and female body are understood in terms of the relative predominance of shared characteristics, the general problem of mastering the nature of the 'other' does not arise. Chinese medical writers, all male, do not express any doubts about their grasp of the principles and processes of the female organism, nor do they mention reservations about their capacities to understand the generalized female experience of sickness. Mastering the characteristics of an individual case is, however, recognized as presenting particular problems if the patient is female.

Diagnosis and gender

Diagnostic procedures in late imperial China were quite different from those with which we are familiar today. The physician did not normally feel the brow for fever, palpate the limbs or torso, or auscultate, let alone poke around inside any orifices. By our standards, the approach was definitely hands off. The purpose was also different. The Chinese concept of disorder, *bing*, does not correspond to our modern notion of disease. A Chinese disorder, though it has similar origins in all patients, will *manifest* itself differently in individual patients, according to the

---

[3]   Qi circulates through the body along tracts. The ren and chong tracts are the tracts associated with the reproductive functions.

[4]   *Huangdi neijing* (The Canon of Interior Medicine of the Yellow Lord), from the *Suwen* chapter 'On Ancient Heavenly Truth': Nanjing School of Traditional Medicine (ed.), *Huangdi neijing suwen shiyi* (Annotated Modern Translation of the *Suwen* Chapter of the *Huangdi neijing*) (Shanghai: Kexue Jishu Press, 1983), pp. 4–5. The *Huangdi neijing*, the most authoritative source of traditional medical doctrine, was traditionally ascribed to the legendary Yellow Emperor, but recent scholarship suggests that it is the work of several authors compiled in the first century BC or early first century AD. However, the two books which form the core of the canon, the 'Basic Questions' (*Suwen*) and the 'Divine Pivot' (*Lingshu*), did not exist in their present form before the eighth century.

exact circumstances in which it was contracted and the particular constitution of the patient; it will also evolve over time in ways that vary between patients. Diagnosis must therefore identify a disorder category in its particular manifestation, *bian zheng*. For this, a complete description and case history was essential.

There were differences in the most favoured diagnostic technique according to school or period, but basically diagnosis comprised four essential methods involving all the senses. The Chinese doctor *looked* at the patient's complexion, *smelled* (and tasted) his breath and bodily odours, *listened* to his account of his disorder, and *touched* his wrist during the complex procedure of taking the pulse. In the late imperial period, not vision, but hearing and touch turned out to be the most important source of knowledge for the physician himself.[5]

Determining the manifestation type depended not only on the physician's powers of perception, but also on his ability to communicate with the patient and his or her family. The 'Ten Questions' formulated by the master diagnostician Zhang Jiebin in the seventeenth century[6] comprise (in order): feelings of cold and fever; sweating; how the head and body feel; elimination; appetite; how the chest feels; hearing; thirst; pulse and complexion; and finally qi and savour (matching the medical properties of the prescription to the patient's needs). The first eight categories were questions that the physician needed to ask the patient. They would inform him of the superficial phenomena: the exposure to cold, the overindulgence in wine, the aches, the restlessness, the periodicity of fevers, the incidence of diarrhoea, that defined the manifestation of the patient's disorder.

We have access to the Chinese physician's and his patient's experience only as they appear in the written narrative of the case-history, and we really have very little knowledge of how a physician was likely to select, arrange or re-phrase the information provided by the patient, or how his judgement might be affected by the patient's presentation. Both the texts on diagnosis and the case-histories, however, give the impression that

---

5   See Kuriyama, this volume, on the importance of vision in earlier texts. In the People's Republic today, 'traditional' physicians may well include such quantitative data as a patient's temperature, blood pressure, or the result of an X-ray in their evaluation. However, as far as I can tell, in the field of fuke no absolute measurements or descriptions resulting from a direct examination of the reproductive organs occur in any treatises until well into the twentieth century.

6   Zhang Jiebin's *Shiwen pian* (Treatise on the Ten Questions) was published in the seventeenth century; Lin Zhihan's *Sizhen juewei* (Selection of Subtleties in Diagnostic Technique) of 1723 includes Zhang's work in j.3 with a four-page commentary of his own. See Zhang Jiebin, *Jingqiu quanshu* (Complete Works of [Zhang] Jingqiu) (Beijing: Renmin Press, 1991), j.1/16–24; Lin Zhihan, *Sizhen juewei* (repr. Beijing: Zhongguo Shudian, 1987), j.3/26a–38b.

the physician accepted what the patient told him as reliable and relevant.[7] Zhang Jiebin's 'Ten Questions' seem designed to make sure that no information is omitted, rather than to eliminate categories of irrelevant information that the patient might volunteer.

Chinese mores required that women live in seclusion, meeting only the men they were related to by birth or by marriage. Diagnosing female patients was acknowledged to be more difficult, because social convention severely restricted the direct sensory contacts between physician and patient. The twelfth-century pharmacologist Kou Zongshi first wrote on the special problems involved in diagnosing female patients from good families. They would not let their faces be seen, obscured their pulses by draping their wrists, found questioning onerous, and failed to take medicine as prescribed.[8] In fact, Kou lamented, of the four normal methods of diagnosis two were more or less ruled out; looking was impossible and pulse-taking was made difficult, so only questioning and smelling remained. This complaint became a trope in the late imperial gynaecological literature. Indeed even questioning was considered difficult, since it might well have to proceed through an intermediary, husband, father or servant.

There was, however, no epistemological difference drawn between the information provided by male and female patients. Physicians in late imperial China do not say that female patients provide unreliable information because they are irrational, hysterical or otherwise worse witnesses than men, nor do they ever question women's knowledge of their own bodies.[9] Yet, we have seen, they do complain that

---

[7]   This may be connected to the fact that the majority of cases involved patients of élite or at least middle-class standing, who would often be conversant with medicine themselves. Being a physician did not confer social status or prestige, and except in the case of élite scholars who practised medicine in their spare time, to cure family members, or for charitable reasons, the patient's social rank was often higher than that of the physician.

[8]   Quoted in the slightly later work by Chen Ziming, *Furen daquan liangfang* (Good Prescriptions from the Compendia of Gynaecology) (1237) (repr. Beijing: Renmin Press, 1985), pp. 64–5.

[9]   In an interesting parallel with my arguments below about the power of words to affect medical understanding, there are indications that learned diagnosis in late imperial China was influenced by the lay understanding of yin as female, or socially weak. Disorder characteristics came in paired categories, such as repletion and depletion, and a physician might hesitate between yang depletion and yin repletion in his choice of diagnosis. Such choices do seem to have been influenced by the sex and social standing of the patient. Charlotte Furth has analysed over four hundred cases taken from late imperial works, and she finds that physicians were more likely to label an illness a yin disorder when it was grave, or when the patient had low social status, and/ or when the patient was a woman: Charlotte Furth, 'Gender, Class and Kinship in Ch'ing Dynasty Medical cases', unpublished paper presented at the Workshop on Family Process and Political Process, University of California, Davis, April 1991.

communication with female patients is difficult. Does this complaint arise because the patient must collaborate with the physician as an active creator of the case-history, or is it because the physician just has less access to a passive source of information? Is accurate diagnosis of women more difficult simply because the information gleaned through an intermediary is incomplete or imprecise? Or does direct conversation with the patient mean the physician can follow up on simple questions to build up a more detailed picture? Unfortunately I have not found any explicit discussion of these issues in the medical writings.

Naming causes

This section attempts to link medical understandings of causality and patterns of diagnostic interpretation to the power of words. I take as my case the various constructions of amenorrhoea by physicians and patients, all operating within the broad framework of Chinese classical medical knowledge.[10]

The key terms of medical explanation had rather precise technical meanings as used by physicians, but they were also common terms in everyday language. In vernacular use such terms might have had very powerful significance, related to but not identical with their technical medical meaning. I suggest this overlap could have affected the interpretation of lay person and medical specialist alike, in particular their attributions of causality. One important term that affected perception and explanation of menstrual disorder was *tong*, which in everyday parlance meant 'to circulate', 'to pass through', or 'to pervade'; it was closely connected in everyday usage with ideas of health and efficient function. The coinage of the realm, for example, was stamped with the words *tong bao*, 'circulating treasure'. Applied to the body tong had the connotation of 'vital circulation', as in the circulation of qi and blood. Any impairment of this circulation had, for the lay person, profound emotive dimensions that predisposed a patient to adopt immediate and heroic measures to restore health by removing

---

[10] I shall not take into account here the ritual, religious or 'folk' dimensions of healing discussed by Sivin in this volume, but shall confine myself to discussions and treatments of amenorrhoea within the framework of classical medical understanding. On the nexus of biomedical, Chinese medical, religious, and social beliefs attached to menstruation in Taiwan today, see Charlotte Furth and Ch'en Shu-yueh, 'Chinese Medicine and the Anthropology of Menstruation in Contemporary Taiwan', *Medical Anthropology Quarterly*, 6.1 (March 1992), 27–48.

the blockage.[11] Here I shall argue that even sophisticated physicians were not entirely immune to the powerful resonance of this word.

In diagnosing any disorder, physicians of different degrees of competence operated at different levels within the framework of Chinese medical explanation. A good physician would make his analysis in terms of root causes. Superficial symptoms elicited by questioning and observation of the patient were linked to the pulse results which provided an in-depth image of a specific form of imbalance in yin and yang, impaired circulation of qi and blood, and consequent malfunction of one or more organ systems. The aim was to establish the fundamental causes of the disorder, the course which it was running, and the stage which it had reached so far. In consequence the physician could work out a series of treatments to restore normality a step at a time.

A scholarly physician of little skill, or an uneducated doctor, was likely to stay at the surface of things, to identify one symptom as the central problem and therefore to treat the symptom itself rather than the root of the disorder.

Amenorrhoea: a deathly disorder

In Chinese medical treatises, menstrual regularity is singled out as the key to female health from the *Huangdi neijing* onwards. Amenorrhoea is not a disorder in itself, but signals some fundamental dysfunction that could well develop into a fatal sickness. It is therefore taken very seriously in the medical writings of all periods, including today.[12] The monthly circulation and renewal of female blood is one of the most fundamental of natural cycles, *jing*. Almost every late imperial work on women's medicine begins with an essay on the importance of menstrual regularity and the dangers of irregular cycles and of amenorrhoea. Whatever the training or status of the author, the message is the same: menstrual regularity or regulation is not simply crucial to fertility but also fundamental to female health. Chinese of all social and educational levels believed firmly that the failure to menstruate signified not just temporary infertility but complex and urgent health problems. The sixteenth-century scholarly physician Xu Chunfu writes:

[11] Another dimension, of course, is that amenorrhoea can signal early pregnancy, so that 'treating amenorrhoea' may in fact be a euphemism for administering an abortifacient. I refer to this question only incidentally here, since I deal with it at length in a forthcoming work, *Fabrics of Power: Technology and Culture in Late Imperial China*; the final chapters examine the nexus of social and medical techniques of reproduction.

[12] Charlotte Furth, 'Blood, Body and Gender: Medical Images of the Female Condition in China 1600–1850', *Chinese Science*, 7 (1986), 43–66; also Furth (note 10).

If the menses are not regulated then all kinds of disorders will succeed each other, becoming so severe that they cannot be cured. This includes infertility. The [*Huangdi nei*]*jing* says: the disorders of the two yangs always begin in the Spleen system but are sometimes hard to get at and manifested indirectly. If a girl has no menses, should it be transmitted as wind-wasting (*fengxiao*) or as breathing-anger (*xifen*),[13] then all her life the sufferer cannot be cured. This is even more true of the Heart system, which belongs to the category of yang and governs the blood. The Spleen system enfolds the blood and thereby activates qi. If the menses do not come through, it is invariably because there is an insufficiency of the activities of the Heart system. Worry damages the Spleen system, [this damage is then] a cause of exhaustion syndrome (*laojuan*), the grain qi [energy produced from food] is not transmitted, the Metal of the Lung system which nourishes the Water of the Kidney system is lost, and there is nothing to build up the menstrual blood. The bodily secretions dry up day by day. If by the fourth or fifth time [the menses] have not been regulated, they will gradually cease altogether. The depletion will cause damage as an internal Heat syndrome, the symptoms of bone-steaming (*guzheng*) and consumption (*laozhai*)[14] will develop, and [the disease] will suddenly become incurable. Therefore we should nourish the Heart system so that the blood will increase, and aid the Spleen system so that the qi is properly distributed. If these two procedures are co-ordinated, the qi will be luxuriant and the blood will be active, and the prerequisites for regulated menses will be achieved.[15]

Medical writers differ in the details of their categorizations of menstrual irregularity or amenorrhoea. Some, for instance, distinguish between women of different constitution or child-bearing history in whom the same symptom, amenorrhoea, may stem from different fundamental causes. For example, the eighteenth-century gynaecologist Wu Daoyuan writes in his introduction to his first chapter, on 'Menstrual Regularity', that amenorrhoea is likely to have different causes in multiparous women (in whom it is caused by damaged blood), in plump, pale-complexioned women (in whom it is caused by damp phlegm), and in thin, dark-complexioned women (in whom it is caused by exhaustion of blood and stagnation of qi).[16]

In one popular eighteenth-century work on women's health, written in easily memorized short verses, we find the following variations under amenorrhoea, collectively classified as 'blocked menses', *jingbi*: (i) stagnation of the blood, with retention of blood in the uterus caused by a Cold pathogen (the text says this condition resembles the amenorrhoea

---

[13] *Fengxiao* denotes emaciation due to emotional upsets; *xifen* is a Heart system disorder.
[14] Fatal wasting diseases equivalent to the Western syndrome of terminal consumption.
[15] Xu Chunfu, *Gujin yitong daquan* (Complete Ancient and Modern Medical Compendium) (1556) (repr. Taipei: Xinwenfeng Press, 1978), p. 5374.
[16] Wu Daoyuan, *Nüke qieyao* (Absolute Essentials of Gynaecology) (1773) (repr. Beijing: Zhongguo Shudian, 1987), j.1/1b–2a. This work was written when the author was seventy-five.

of early pregnancy); (ii) deficiency of blood, associated with repressed emotions and often resulting in fatal wasting diseases; (iii) drying up of the blood from excessive sex or too many pregnancies, likely to produce emaciation, coughing and 'bone-steaming'; (iv) amenorrhoea caused by chronic coughing or consumption; (v) intermittent amenorrhoea associated with menopause; (vi) intermittent amenorrhoea in young virgins, which was no cause for worry unless it resulted from some fundamental deficiency in blood or qi; (vii) amenorrhoea of nuns, unmarried women or widows, whose frustrated emotions damaged the Liver and Spleen systems.[17]

So amenorrhoea was a symptom of any one of a number of fundamental causes. First the possibility of pregnancy had to be considered. If this was ruled out (see below), then the amenorrhoea had to be considered in the framework of imbalances of yin and yang, or disorders or insufficiencies of blood or qi, which at a higher level were translated into a dysfunction of one or other of the organ systems. In medical theory, the disorders amenorrhoea accompanied fell into one of two general categories: yin depletion or blood stagnation. Each called for completely different forms of prescription. Educated physicians frequently criticized 'quacks' and women for uncritically attributing amenorrhoea to blood stagnation and treating it as a cause rather than a symptom. They often invoked ignorance or bad faith as the reasons for this tendency. But I suggest that part of the appeal of the stagnation diagnosis lay in its explanation of amenorrhoea as 'blockage', as a damming up of vital circulation, tong.

Levels of causality

The passage by Xu Chunfu, quoted above, is a discussion of the ways in which amenorrhoea 'is transmitted', zhuan. In the beginning of his analysis Xu quotes the Neijing, writing of menstrual irregularities as very basic 'disorders of the two yangs' with their primary manifestation in the Spleen system. He goes on to illustrate successively severe stages resulting from this original basic problem, suggesting that the course of the disorder can follow different paths, perhaps according to the constitution or emotional predisposition of the patient. Although Xu speaks of amenorrhoea 'being transmitted' in various forms, he does not

---

[17] Wu Qian, Fuke xinfa yaojue (Essential Esoterics of the New Gynaecology) (eighteenth century) (repr. Taipei: Xuanfang Press, 1981), pp. 20–3. Here it is clearly the lack of a normal married sex life which is seen as the root of the problem, whereas in the case of the drying up of the blood, sexual excess was the root of the damage. Moderation, physical and emotional, was the key to health.

actually go so far as to speak of the phenomenon as causal in its own right. An educated physician was obliged to situate causality at a more profound level even than this dysfunction in a fundamental natural cycle. He had to place any specific case of amenorrhoea as one of a network of symptoms, in order to identify the underlying problem and the appropriate treatment.

Xu writes of amenorrhoea as a *precursor* of debilitating and sometimes fatal disorders. But I think we can extend the significance of amenorrhoea beyond the level of correlation in Xu's mind to that of instrumentality: amenorrhoea not as a *primary* but at any rate as a *secondary cause*. Chinese medical theory shared with ordinary culture the belief that the interruption of a natural process was dangerous *per se*, as we can tell from medical discussions of miscarriage and abortion.[18]

In dealing with amenorrhoea, skilled physicians would leave aside the superficial effects to treat the disorder at its source,[19] and yet they were also obliged to deal more immediately with the dangers of impaired blood circulation which amenorrhoea signalled, in other words to treat the amenorrhoea as a secondary cause. A woman whose menses stopped would be likely to construe the lack of blood as a primary cause, and many unskilled or unscrupulous physicians would agree and treat her accordingly. But part of the reason for this therapeutic choice lay in the use of words, namely the conventional grouping of all cases of amenorrhoea under the general category of '*blocked* menses'.

Powerful words

A number of terms were used in medical writing to describe the category of amenorrhoea. Chief among them were: *yueshi* (the monthly event) or jing (cycle) *bu lai* (fails to come) or *bu tong* (does not come through); and jing bi (the cycle is *blocked*). All of these terms used common lay vocabulary, and writers do not attempt to justify their choice on technical grounds by providing distinctions or precise definitions. The last term, 'menstrual blockage', seems to have been the most common, and is a category in almost every Chinese medical work on female disorders. (It is far more common than the more neutral terms of bu lai or *wu jing*, absence of menses.)

Learned and experienced physicians clearly took this term as a

---

18 Francesca Bray, 'Abortion in Pre-Modern China: Ethics and Identity', unpublished paper presented at the Workshop on Gender and Sexuality in East and Southeast Asia, University of California, December 1990.
19 E.g. Xu Chunfu (note 15), p. 5380, writing on the widely used blood tonic *siwutang*, 'four-ingredient decoction'.

convenient label covering a far greater complexity of phenomena. 'Blockage' was in fact their least likely diagnosis. Amenorrhoea might reflect a range of deep-seated problems affecting the balance of yin and yang and the production of blood, and manifested through the dysfunction of one central organ system which then affected others. However this might be, we may say that the blood was affected in one of two basic ways: either it was depleted and/or dried up; or it was stagnant or blocked. Either of these conditions affected not only menstrual flow but the circulation of nutrition and energy in the body. The physician's first task, then, was to restore the circulation of a healthy flow of blood. Once that had been achieved, the deeper levels of the problem could be addressed and treated with a sequence of prescriptions until full health was restored.

But the way to restore a healthy flow of blood was different in each case. If the blood was diagnosed as depleted or dried up, supporting and replenishing drugs would be administered to build it up. This broad category of diagnosis seems to have been the most common among distinguished physicians, if the number of cases cited in the texts is any indication.[20] But the second category was deeply problematic. As Wu Qian mentioned, 'stagnation of the blood', i.e. real 'menstrual blockage', resembled the amenorrhoea of early pregnancy. Such stagnation was viewed as causal in its own right and required treatment with powerful blood-vivifying (*huo*), activating (tong) or dispersing (*san*) prescriptions to restore circulation.

One problem was that the principal drugs in such prescriptions were also well known to be abortifacients – if a woman was pregnant she would almost certainly lose the child. Even if she was not pregnant, such drugs could easily cause dangerous haemorrhages. To identify a case of amenorrhoea with 'blockage', then, was to enter a situation of risk.

And yet at the same time, the very notion of blockage was extremely threatening. Chinese popular notions of health give enormous importance to the concept of vital circulation, tong. A healthy person, or one affected by a mild but chronic disorder, will be inclined to think in terms of balance, nourishment and replenishment, and eat and take tonics or other prescriptions accordingly. But any interference with natural circulation would be considered an acute and serious symptom, requiring immediate treatment.

---

[20] In fact there were a number of standard prescriptions which could be obtained ready made up at any druggist's, containing tonic and replenishing plants, and which a woman would take if she felt any weakness or fatigue associated with female complaints. (Today they can be found on the shelves of a surprising number of Californian drugstores and grocers' stores.)

Therapeutic choices

Blocked circulation of the vital fluids is particularly dangerous. If qi is blocked, then death is imminent; if blood is blocked, then qi will soon follow; absence of sweating, constipation or retention of urine too are seen as serious symptoms by physicians as well as ordinary people. While today Westerners and Chinese alike often contrast the 'gentle, gradual' effects of Chinese prescriptions to the drastic and immediate action of biomedical drugs, such a characterization is a modern ideological construct, which has been possible only since Western drugs became available to the Chinese for the treatment of acute disease. 'Heroic medicine' was as much in demand in late imperial China as it was anywhere else; a physician who made his patient defecate, vomit and sweat could be *seen* to be producing results.

While drawing blood European-style was not part of the Chinese repertory, causing blood to flow through the prescription of drugs was a very common response to 'female disorders'. Elite physicians might rail against quackery, and the ignorance of unskilled doctors who treated a fundamental disorder at the level of its most superficial symptom. Nevertheless, categorizing amenorrhoea as a 'blockage' of vital circulation and treating it accordingly probably corresponded to most patients' understanding of the problem: for them, the blockage was the problem, not a symptom. This level of attributing causality was shared by many healers too. Not surprisingly, drugs to bring on the menses and restore this vital circulation, *tongjingyao*, were very commonly prescribed by physicians of all kinds.

A wise physician would hesitate before prescribing these drugs. If there was any chance at all of a pregnancy, he would first administer a pregnancy test:[21]

A woman of twenty-seven whose menses had already stopped for three months. Some [doctors] suspected that her menses were blocked. I was called in ...

[21] Pregnancy is the only medical condition for which standard tests, consisting of prescriptions that are not in themselves therapeutic, exist in late imperial Chinese medicine. However, a physician was in essence constantly testing the accuracy of his diagnosis by observing whether his prescription produced results consistent with that diagnosis. If not, both diagnosis and therapy would have to be reconsidered. Judith Farquhar, 'Time and Text: Approaching Chinese Medical Practice through Analysis of a Published Case', in Charles Leslie and Allan Young (eds.), *Paths to Asian Medical Knowledge* (Berkeley: University of California Press, 1992), pp. 62–73, gives a fine example of this empirical approach in China today.

[Describes pulse characteristic of pregnancy.]²² I said, 'this is no light illness – she is pregnant'. I prescribed *xiongguitang*²³ and there was a slight movement in her abdomen, indicating that she was pregnant. After several months she did indeed give birth to a child.²⁴

If a woman or her physician suspected that she was pregnant, usually taking missed periods as an indication, then she could take a mild medication such as *xiaoyaosan* or Buddha's hand powder, fushousan,²⁵ as a test. According to Chinese medical theory, the main ingredients of these formulae nourished and activated the blood. If she was not pregnant, it was believed, these drugs would produce a menstrual flow. If nothing happened, the chances were she was pregnant.²⁶

If the pregnancy test proved negative and the diagnosis of blockage was confirmed, then blood-vivifying or blood-moving drugs would be prescribed, but with great caution because they were extremely dangerous if misused. A skilled physician might include such drugs in a prescription, but usually only as a minor and relatively inactive ingredient. The knee-jerk response to the problem, however, was to prescribe the blood-vivifiers, activators or dispersers as the main ingredient or ingredients of the prescription, often with dramatic results.

The eighteenth-century physician Xu Dachun reports several cases of women worried about amenorrhoea being treated by less scrupulous or

---

22 There are numerous descriptions of the pulses characteristic of the successive stages of pregnancy. The eighteenth-century physician Xu Dachun diagnosed pregnancy in a woman who had missed her menses for three months when he found that her pulse was 'rapid, blending, the foot portion slippery': Xu Dachun, *Yilue liushu, nüke zhiyan* (Medical Compendium in Six Books, Experiences in Gynaecology), j.32/12a. In the earliest stages of pregnancy, certain diagnosis was recognized to be very difficult and mistakes common. For example, a physician might be misled if a woman's husband was not sufficiently clear in his description of her symptoms: Yan Shunxi, *Taichan xinfa* (New Methods for Pregnancy and Childbirth) (1739) (repr. Beijing: Renmin Weisheng Press, 1988), p. 170. In his critical treatise on diagnostic methods, the eighteenth-century physician Lin Zhihan cites various opinions, including one which claims to be able to distinguish between first-and second-month pregnancies: Lin (note 6), j.5/26a. Most authorities expected at best to be able to distinguish between a third- and a fifth-month pregnancy, and then between a boy, a girl, twins, or 'ghost pregnancies': Wu (note 16), j.3/9a–b.
23 Also known as 'Buddha's hand powder', *fushousan*. It consists of two parts of *chuanxiong* (*Ligusticum wallichii*) to three parts of *danggui* (*Angelica sinensis*), ground to a powder and boiled in water and wine. This prescription was considered very effective for treating stagnant blood: e.g. Wu (note 17), pp. 13–14.
24 Xu Dachun (note 22), j.32/12a.
25 See note 23 on Buddha's hand powder. *Xiaoyao* powder contains eight ingredients including the replenishing drugs peony and Chinese angelica.
26 These and similar formulae are still in wide use today. However, if a woman who wants a child suspects that she is pregnant, she will usually go to a Western clinic for a pregnancy test rather than using Chinese medicines.

skilled doctors than himself with extremely strong blood-vivifying drugs, and explains his objections:

A woman's menses stopped, she alternated between Cold and Heat symptoms, her mouth was dry and her forehead red, she could keep down little food and drink. At evening she would have two or three fits of coughing.[27] The doctors [she consulted] all used such types of drugs as gadfly, leech, dried lacquer[28] and [a range of purgatives and other drugs]. Only I said we shouldn't do so. 'Even if these prescriptions appear in the old collections, if the sick person takes them they will certainly have stomach-ache and be put off their food – and these are drugs that can kill ... We should not use gadfly and similar powerful drugs. If we do so then the menses will come, but they will be scanty, and urination on the other hand will stop, with other symptoms arising as a result. When Essence and blood are insufficient they should always be replenished. These dangerous and powerful drugs are unreliable and violent, and often result in damage.'[29]

These drugs were exactly the same as those used to procure abortions:

The wife [of a junior official]: her foetus was leaking, tai lou [slight but continuous bleeding]; doctors had treated her but the leaking did not stop. Her husband, given the circumstances, wished to have her abort and consulted me. I prescribed Buddha's hand powder so that if the foetus could be calmed it would, and if not it would abort, but in a natural fashion. She took the dose, but her husband was distressed and feared it would not work. A physician specialized in women's complaints sought out prescriptions to administer and told them to use one ounce of niuxi boiled in wine to dose her. The husband believed him and gave her the dose, and indeed the foetus was expelled.

At that time I was visiting my mother's relatives and did not hear about this, but as soon as I knew I rushed back, only to find her chamber overflowing with the smells of cinnamon and musk: since the placenta had not been expelled the women's physician had administered 'fragrant cinnamon powder'.[30] Thereupon her blood gushed forth like the Yellow River, and it was impossible to stop the flow. I hastily brewed a pure ginseng decoction,[31] but before it was ready she had died. Her husband never recovered from his grief.

I record this as a cautionary lesson.[32]

Many of the drugs used by physicians to treat menstrual irregularity, and by women themselves to prevent it, belong to the categories which strengthen or nourish blood or qi, or replenish deficiencies; among the

27 These are symptoms of a very serious disorder.
28 All powerful blood-moving drugs strongly forbidden to pregnant women, as were musk, cinnamon, Tibetan crocus, peach-kernels and niuxi (Acanthyrus bidentata).
29 Xu Dachun (note 22), j.32/3b.
30 'Fragrant cinnamon powder', xiangguisan, contains musk and cinnamon bark, and was commonly used to expel a dead foetus or the placenta: see Zhongyao xue (Pharmacology of Chinese Drugs) (Shanghai: Kexue Jishu Press, 1984), p. 304.
31 Dushen tang. This was an extremely strong yang-building tonic, not usually suitable for women. But this patient was on the verge of death, that is to say, complete depletion of yang.
32 Xu Dachun (note 22), j.32/20a–b.

most common ingredients are Chinese angelica, *danggui*, and peony, *baishao*, which nourish the blood, and ginseng and *baishu* (*Atractylodis macrocephala*), which replenish deficiencies of the qi. But it is noticeable that many of the prescriptions for amenorrhoea, listed in popular compendia and learned treatises alike, rely much more heavily on drugs to restore circulation, tong, by vivifying the blood and dispersing stagnation. Many of them are explicitly recognized as liable to produce haemorrhages or miscarriages; these include peach-kernels, Tibetan crocus, niuxi, leeches, gadfly and dried lacquer, which were all explicitly recognized in materiae medicae and other medical writings as being extremely powerful and requiring very careful use:

Peach kernels ... [are among] the most dangerous of all the drugs for breaking up and expelling blood. When a woman's menses do not flow there are two possible reasons. One is wind, cold, chill and damp, each of which can be transmitted to the ren and chong tracts [governing menstruation and fertility] to the point that blood and qi congeal and do not flow: in these cases the use of the aforementioned drugs is widely successful. But if the Sea of blood (*xuehai*) is dry and withered without menses to flow, then one should simply build up the three tracts of the Spleen, Liver and Kidney systems and thus nourish the origins of the transformation [of blood and qi]: this is the way of curing the depletion.[33]

It is interesting that although it categorizes all forms of amenorrhoea under the label 'blockage', Wu Qian's eighteenth-century rhymed gynaecology referred to earlier does not include any of the drugs known to cause miscarriage in its prescriptions for amenorrhoea, except in the case of nuns, virgins and widows, where presumably the possibility of pregnancy was not countenanced.[34] But other works include a number of prescriptions for amenorrhoea which include one or several drugs counter-indicated in pregnancy. The late Qing work *Nüke bijue daquan*, for instance, includes niuxi in several prescriptions to cure amenorrhoea due to the effects of cold, and crocus in most of the prescriptions to counteract stagnation.[35]

Conclusion

I have argued elsewhere, as has Charlotte Furth, that the ambiguities of the diagnosis of amenorrhoea permitted a woman who suspected she might be in the early stages of pregnancy to exercise control over her fertility in the name of her long-term health. Here I suggest that the

[33]   Xiao Jing, *Xianqi qiuzhenglun* (The Xianqi Book of Cures) (Ming) (repr. Beijing: Rare Books Press, 1983), j.3/62b–63a.

[34]   Wu (note 17), pp. 23–8.

[35]   Chen Lianfang, *Nüke mijue daquan* (Compendium of Secrets of Gynaecology) (1908) (repr. Beijing: Beijing Ribao Press, 1989), pp. 22–4, 65.

fear of blockage, of stopped circulation (bu tong) as a threat to health was so powerful that it influenced not only a woman suffering from amenorrhoea but also the physicians who treated her, inclining many who did not possess deep and subtle understanding of how symptoms were related and linked to profound causes to resort immediately to the use of dangerous drugs. To Chinese women and to their physicians amenorrhoea must have seemed doubly dangerous. It represented both the interruption of the most central of natural bodily cycles, fundamental to female health, and the blocked circulation of one of the most vital bodily fluids.

The cultural analysis of Chinese medical texts is not easy, for we have so little knowledge of the boundaries and overlaps between professional and popular knowledge and categories. However I think it is reasonable to suppose that the description in medical writings of amenorrhoea as 'the cycle does not come through', *jing bu tong*, and the use of 'menstrual blockage', jingbi, as the most usual heading describing its various forms (rather than some less directive term such as wujing, 'absence of menses') reflects the usual popular understanding of this symptom. This may well have influenced diagnosis, at least at the subconscious level. We find amenorrhoea was construed and treated at three levels: that of symptom, that of secondary cause, and that of primary cause. Although in Chinese medical theory the last was seldom justified, the emotive power of the notion of circulation, tong, and the vital role attributed to it in ordinary understanding, were likely to affect the level at which even learned physicians understood the problem.

12   Re-writing traditional medicine in post-Maoist China

Judith Farquhar

The field of 'Traditional Chinese Medicine' which caused such a stir in Western public health circles in the 1960s and '70s, and on which a few anthropologists and historians have commented since then, came into existence in its current institutional form only after the 1949 revolution that founded the People's Republic of China.[1] In the 1950s, within the newly organized or expanded colleges, research institutes, publishing houses, and professional associations, a rationalized 'traditional' medicine came into being as a discrete 'system of knowledge'. This essay emphasizes both the modernity and the historical continuities of systematic Chinese medical knowledge by examining a genre of autobiographical writing that emerged in the 1980s after the close of the Great Proletarian Cultural Revolution (1966–76). It sees writing medical knowledge and medical lives as a form of social labour that both modernizes and stubbornly resists full appropriation to either global bioscience or state development projects.

The practitioners and cadres who organized the profession of traditional Chinese medicine after Mao Zedong's 1955 proclamation that 'our motherland's medicine is a great treasurehouse' worked largely anonymously. Though they authored medical books and papers in technical journals, taught a great many students, and served on countless committees, their fame was largely propagated orally. It was politically inappropriate at the time to claim personal authority or draw attention to one's authorship. The masses were

[1]   Much of the argument of this paper is based on anthropological fieldwork conducted in the People's Republic of China (PRC) in the years 1982–4, 1988, and 1990–1. All of this research has been generously supported by the Committee on Scholarly Communication with China. Thanks are also due to the University of North Carolina Department of Anthropology for granting me leave during the academic year 1990–1; to the Guangzhou and Beijing Colleges of Traditional Chinese Medicine and the Medical History and Literature Institute of the Chinese Academy of Traditional Chinese Medicine for administrative support of my research; and to many helpful and stimulating friends in the world of Chinese medicine. I am also indebted to Don Bates, James Hevia, Dorothy Holland, Jia Huanguang, Tomoko Masuzawa, and Nathan Sivin for very helpful advice on versions of this paper.

taken to be both the source and target of traditional medicine's genius.

At the close of the Great Proletarian Cultural Revolution, after the death of Mao and the fall of the Gang of Four in 1976, this professional culture of selfless service suddenly changed. In mid-1980 the quarterly *Bulletin* of the Shandong College of Traditional Chinese Medicine began publishing a series of autobiographical essays under the title *Paths of Renowned Senior Chinese Doctors*. The journal's editors planned to include two or three of these personal histories each quarter, seeking to 'unearth the expert professional heritage [of Chinese medicine], introduce scholarly and therapeutic experience ... salvage precious research materials, and enrich research on medical history'. The editors also noted that 'the significance [of this project] lies in inspiring future scholarship; we can learn from the ways in which a generation of famous doctors has matured'.[2] In keeping with these goals, the essays focused particularly on recalling the formative experiences of study, clinical work, and (sometimes) political involvement of their authors, the 'paths' by which the senior doctors (*laozhongyi*) who had for several decades led the field of traditional Chinese medicine had reached their present eminence.

Reader responses to this feature were immediate and extraordinarily positive, catching even the editors by surprise; in each of the next few issues they published several pages of letters from medical luminaries all over China, lauding the project and offering to participate by writing personal memoirs. Most of the essays that appeared in the *Paths* series were eventually published in a three-volume anthology that appeared between 1981 and 1985.[3] The Preface to volume 1 suggests the special cultural weight this publication project developed by the time the *Bulletin* autobiographies reached anthology form:

Because of the passage of time and the ten years of turmoil, the famous scholars of Chinese medicine and renowned senior Chinese doctors who are still alive are few and far between. Moreover, according to our information, among these some are ill and in failing health ... Therefore we have from the very inception of this project cherished a pressing sense of urgency ... News [of deaths] has made it impossible for us to rest, and has led us to handle the revered authors' manuscripts as if we were protecting a flame. An unspoken imperative urged us to hasten the process of editing, making fair copies, and bringing this volume to

<hr />

2   Editors, *Shandong Zhongyixueyuan Xuebao* (Bulletin of the Shandong College of Traditional Chinese Medicine), no. 2 (1980), cover.

3   Zhou Fengwu, Zhang Jiwen, and Cong Lin (eds.), *Ming Laozhongyi zhi Lu* (Paths of Renowned Senior Chinese Doctors), 3 vols. (Jinan: Shandong Science and Technology Press, 1981–5).

the world; rescuing the work and realities of senior Chinese doctors' experience can brook no delays![4]

Readers seemed to agree about the importance of the project; these collections are now ubiquitous on the bookshelves of Chinese medical practitioners. The new biographical genre quickly expanded through the Chinese medical publishing world. In a literature survey I conducted in 1984, I found that all but one of the major monthly journals of traditional medicine published in the PRC had a regular section devoted to 'laozhongyi experience';[5] most of the essays adopted biographical conventions similar to those of the *Paths* project.

By reading two examples of medical autobiography with attention to the historical conditions in which they appeared and the controversies and wider concerns to which they refer, I hope to show that the author-subjects wrote their lives as a form of courageous and consequential action. This genre of writing about eminent persons[6] emerged as an important power in the forging of a new style of leadership and a new sense of the whole profession's agenda. The coherence and sense of purpose the authors and editors rather dramatically achieved may have been short-lived; but the social, political, and epistemological power of this inscription was for a time, I think, undeniable.

The strategies of the two author-doctors examined here are quite different, a fact that is partly due to their differential positioning in a professional speciality that both mobilizes considerable social power and considers itself to be under siege within Chinese modernization policies. As each of these authors constituted his own eminent personhood, he also generated a vision of traditional medicine's cultural specificity and historical necessity. Each of them also worked out a distinct style of argument and sought to show particular institutional developments in the field as natural and inevitable. Hence this paper is an exploration of personal story-telling as a mode of intervention in history and truth.

[4]   Ibid., vol. 1, p. 1f.
[5]   This convention of medical publishing is not completely novel, though it was never so widespread before the 1980s; Dong Demao, whose autobiography I take up in this paper, claims to have initiated the practice of publishing laudatory essays on the lives and significance of renowned *laozhongyi* in a journal he published in the early 1940s. But these earlier essays focus less on the personal histories of their subjects and more on the medical significance of their successful cases and preferred techniques.
[6]   It is difficult to clearly separate the genres of biography and autobiography in the world of Chinese medical publishing. 'Biographies' are usually authored by students or junior relatives of the senior doctors whose lives they recount, but they are also often chartered and guided by their subjects. And everybody in the field seems to know that the 'autobiographical' essays of the *Paths* project were 'actually written' by students and other juniors.

Historical considerations

Chinese medical people of the 1980s are living in a personal and professional world that has been deeply transformed both by the rise of a hegemonic scientism that far predated the 1949 revolution and by the rapid institutional modernization of indigenous medical practice that began in 1955.[7] Many traditional medical practices have now been modelled on the institutions and standards of allopathic medicine; medical schools, teaching hospitals, referral systems, and standard case-histories are, superficially at least, similar to those with which we are familiar. Modernization is an almost unquestioned positive value in terms of which even traditionalist arguments are advanced. Yet traditional Chinese medicine is still taught with constant reference to classic works of the latter Han period (the *Inner Canon* and the *Treatise on Cold Disorders* in particular), and clinical work mainly consists of designing and administering complicated herbal prescriptions the formulae for which are adapted from texts scattered through the two-thousand-year clinical and exegetical tradition of medicine.

In the intellectual climate of traditional Chinese medicine, Chinese and Western medical knowledge, practices, and technologies are constantly being compared; differences are analysed and reified, and analogies between the two 'systems' are advanced in efforts to point the way to an eventual unification or to assert the fundamental integrity and value of ancient medicine. In a context where 'scientific socialism' and a technology-based periodization of history drawn from historical materialism still rule at least the exteriors of intellectual life, there is nothing to be gained from suggesting that Chinese medicine is not scientific. If government support for traditional medicine is to continue, the essence of science and the essence of Chinese medicine must be constituted together in a way that can include the latter well within modernization programmes and a national health policy.

In such a context, writing an account of oneself or otherwise authorizing a biography in 1980 was a highly consequential activity. At the very least it was necessary to position oneself as politically correct relative to both the nationalist and socialist concerns that had ruled official discourses since the 1950s and to the renewed importance of modernization, expertise, and 'Science'. This was a somewhat delicate

[7] See Ralph Croizier, *Traditional Medicine in Modern China* (Cambridge, Mass.: Harvard University Press, 1964); D.W.Y. Kwok, *Scientism in Chinese Thought, 1900–1950* (New Haven: Yale University Press, 1965); David M. Lampton, *Health, Conflict, and the Chinese Political System*, Michigan Papers in Chinese Studies, no. 18, 1974; Nathan Sivin, *Traditional Medicine in Contemporary China* (Ann Arbor: Center for Chinese Studies, University of Michigan, 1987).

manoeuvre, as can be seen in other Chinese medical writing that appeared when publishing in 'expert' fields resumed in the late 1970s. (Scholarly publication ceased during the Cultural Revolution, 1966–76.) Everything from textbooks to case reports had to negotiate a sensitive politics of historical positioning. Prefaces to specialized textbooks like the following are emblematic:

Chinese medicine and pharmacy have a history many thousands of years long; they are a generalization from the extremely rich experience of the Chinese people's long period of engaging in struggle with disease, and they are an important component of the splendid people's cultural legacy of our country. Under the influence and guidance of a simple materialism and spontaneous dialectical thought, medicine slowly formed and developed a unique medical theory, a theory which has undergone a long period of therapeutic testing – this is a precious undertaking of the Chinese people and an increasingly established and flourishing major contribution of the Chinese race.[8]

In prefatory passages like this, assertions that Chinese medicine is informed by a fundamentally 'scientific spirit' (science here being understood as scientific Marxism) take their place beside arguments that the medical records of several thousand years include many discoveries since shown to have objective, clinical value. As is evident in the paragraph cited above, 'experience' (*jingyan*) is a constant touchstone for medical polemics. Definitions of science that are proposed within traditional Chinese medicine all ground the scientific on the concept of 'objective experience' (*keguan jingyan*). This privileging of one sense of empiricism (*jingyanzhuyi*) is strategically important for a field that can claim more than two thousand years of clinical records. Where recorded experience (hence empiricism, hence scientificity) is concerned, traditional Chinese medicine has a certain undeniable priority over all other medicines.

Given that Chinese historical materialist usage insists on a periodization of history oriented to mode of production, and tends to label as feudal every activity perceived to obstruct socialist modernization and scientization, Chinese medical people are faced with a complicated task if they wish their profession to continue with public support. They must find the 'simple materialism' and 'spontaneous dialectics' in their history and ally themselves with the labouring masses of China's long 'feudal' past if their knowledge is not to be denounced as itself feudal. This must be accomplished, moreover, without denying the dependence of all forms of knowledge on the historical state of development of the forces of production. In contrast, Chinese practitioners of a newly re-valorized 'Western [scientific] medicine' have a simpler ideological task (at least

8 Beijing College of Traditional Chinese Medicine (ed.), *Zhongguo Yixue Shi* (History of Chinese Medicine) (Shanghai: Shanghai Science and Technology Press, 1978).

since the Cultural Revolution) in justifying their (undoubtedly greater) academic privileges.

It is in this situation that senior doctors of Chinese medicine have crafted their newly vocal leadership. Though this group of men, and a few women,[9] led the field of Chinese medicine both intellectually and administratively from the mid-1950s, they did so during a time which was not conducive to taking personal credit for professional achievements.[10] The 'renowned' (*ming*) urban laozhongyi hold (and many have long held) multiple positions of power in the institutions of colleges, technical schools, hospitals, government bureaus, and/or medical associations. In the *Paths* anthologies, for example, each doctor's biography is accompanied by a list of his or her official titles. The importance and relative respectability of these positions reflect the role this generation played in assembling 'traditional Chinese medicine' into institutional existence in the mid-1950s. When Mao Zedong declared official support for 'our motherland's medicine and pharmacy', a 'traditional' medical profession could have been constructed only out of very diverse resources, mainly the many locally important practitioners, their libraries, and their small collections of apprentices and students. Whatever else today's ming laozhongyi may be, then, they are the major compilers of the very diverse body of knowledge that is today taught as Chinese medicine.

Working in committees along with cadres and a few doctors of Western medicine, ming laozhongyi wrote and designed textbooks, reference works, and college curricula. They were the experienced core around which the first colleges and hospitals of traditional medicine were formed, sites where they then developed larger cohorts of students and followers than most of them had had before, and where they engaged in intellectual struggle and exchange with newly proximate medical comrades.

Biographical and autobiographical materials on these venerable figures are therefore of interest as both more and less than factual accounts of this formative period (they are not, in any case, very detailed histories). As interventions in a continuing discursive struggle over the

---

[9] The three volumes of *Paths of Renowned Senior Chinese Doctors* include only one essay about a woman doctor.

[10] Much of the authorship claimed shortly after Liberation was collective; quite a few articles in professional medical journals between the mid-1950s and the cessation of publishing in 1967 were authored by work units or by large numbers of authors. Individual contributions varied but tended to confine themselves to narrowly clinical (i.e., not theoretical or historical) issues or assert what seem to me to be very conventional political views typical of the period. The sort of publishing that emerged in the late 1970s, emphasizing the integrated (both clinical and theoretical) contributions of individual doctors, was rare or non-existent before the Cultural Revolution. 'Expert' publishing in traditional medicine ceased in 1967 and there were many reasons to avoid 'sticking one's head up' during the period from 1967 to 1978.

nature of the field and its future in a modernizing China, they both constitute their authors and subjects and make strong claims to give form to the past and future of the Chinese medical field. Chinese medicine's historical situation demands a certain polemical stance, the maintenance of a state of struggle against the hegemony of Western scientific expertise. Moreover, considering the continuing vicissitudes of public life for intellectuals in general, these essays should be seen as courageously polemical: their authors have put themselves on the line, accepting responsibility as leaders in the field by placing the narrative of their lives at issue in professional controversies. Since ming laozhongyi are presumed to embody the essence of Chinese medicine, their lives could not be other than polemical. They take it as their natural task to constitute the future as they carry forward the past.

Two medical autobiographies

The autobiographies I take up below are those of Deng Tietao (vice-president of the Guangzhou College of Traditional Chinese Medicine, member of the Standing Committee of the National Council of Traditional Chinese Medicine) and Dong Demao (Honorary Editor-in-chief of the Journal of Traditional Chinese Medicine in Beijing, and also a member of the Standing Committee of the National Council). They were published along with thirty-five others in volume 2 of *Paths of Renowned Senior Chinese Doctors*. Professor Deng is a widely published theoretician, an influential teacher, a legendary clinician, and a devoted cadre; he has long been a Communist Party member. His son has also become a respected teacher and doctor. Dr Dong Demao has worked on textbooks since the 1949 revolution, but has published little in journals, and his scholarly activities before Liberation seem to have been chiefly confined to editing the work of others for a variety of journals. He has not been a leading Communist (he claims membership in the Chinese Peasants' and Workers' Democratic Party) or administrator, focusing his writing on technical insights gained from extensive clinical work rather than on medical policy. In my reading below I want particularly to indicate those gestures in which the authors and their field are situated in history and social practice.

'A long and clouded road' – the autobiography of Deng Tietao

Summary of essay

In his autobiography Deng states that he first learned medicine from his doctor-father and a few of the family's medical friends, then studied for five years at a small professional school of 'Chinese medicine and pharmacy' in Guangzhou, from which he graduated in 1937. Schools such as this began to proliferate in the 1920s. Histories of Chinese medicine emphasize efforts at the time on the part of nationalistic modernizers, in co-operation with the Guomindang government, to discredit traditional medicine,[11] and the academies were part of an effort by doctors both to preserve and to reform their practice and teaching.[12] Deng perceives these early years of his medical practice as embroiled in an 'intellectual quandary', in which there was 'devastating pressure' directed against traditional medicine and no satisfactory 'breakthroughs in scholarly research' to guide practice. 'In this kind of environment and under such conditions, when our scholarly seniors were unable to find any way, it goes without saying that we youngsters were even more without recourse.'

Deng fled 'the iron heel of [Japanese] imperialism' in Hong Kong; this is where he first encountered Marxism-Leninism, and where he first suspected that historical and dialectical materialism 'could be a great help to my study and researches into Chinese medicine ... Chinese medicine had a great deal in it that was consistent with dialectical materialism.'

The second part of the essay concerns Deng Tietao's intellectual formation. He says that although his father practised in the south, where 'Damp Heat is the most common illness type', he had no particular preference with regard to the two most prominent factions in Chinese medicine, the Warm Illnesses and Cold Damage schools of thought.[13] (Professor Deng has since become known for publications attempting to synthesize the two approaches.) He mentions by name the medical forebears and a few contemporary scholar-doctors who inspired his

[11]   See Cui Xiuhan (ed.), *Zhongguo Yishi Yiji Shuyao* (Essential Medical Records for the History of Chinese Medicine) (Beijing: People's Press, 1983); Beijing College (note 8); Shanghai College of Traditional Chinese Medicine, *Jindai Zhongyi Liupai Jingyan Xuanji* (Selected Writings from the Experience of Modern Factions of Chinese Medicine) (Hong Kong: Nantong Book Company, 1962); Xue Yu, *Zhongguo Yaoxue Shiliao* (Historical Materials on Chinese Pharmacy) (Beijing: People's Health Press, 1984); Zhao Hongjun, *Jindai Zhongxiyi Lunzheng Shi* (History of Modern Debates on Chinese and Western Medicine) (Hebei: Hebei Chapter of the Association for Research on the Integration of Chinese and Western Medicine, 1982).

[12]   Journals of Chinese medicine in the 1920s, '30s, and '40s reflect intense (but fairly small-scale) efforts to organize professional institutions as well as frequent defensive responses to proposed legal regulations that would limit the freedoms of traditional doctors to practise.

[13]   In this paper most technical terms of Chinese medicine are capitalized. This convention maintains a practice consistent with my published work on technical issues and also serves to remind the reader that the anatomical and pathophysiological referents of these terms cannot be directly inferred from the English word.

father, and discusses lessons he learned himself as apprentice to a senior practitioner, Chen Yueqiao.

Deng Tietao dates the beginning of his 'true scholarly research' after Liberation, when he had an opportunity to teach in a wide variety of Chinese medical subdisciplines and to 'test and temper' his clinical practice at the 157th People's Liberation Army Hospital. He argues in this context that traditional medicine can develop only if it is accorded full partnership with Western medicine in the management of cases ('control of hospital beds'). Unless the hospitals of traditional medicine where this therapeutic power can be exercised continue to expand and modernize, Chinese medicine as a practical means of relieving suffering will be in danger of gradual disappearance.

In the last section of his essay Deng mentions several allied areas of study – history and literature, medical and philosophical classics, acupuncture and massage therapy, and medical history – that he takes to be central not only to his own education but to the field of medicine as a whole. He concludes with an image of converging paths in medicine:

The centre of the path of development of Chinese medical scholarship has now been clearly indicated, and one can say that doctors on its margins have in recent decades been travelling the same highway. Just consider the hard work of other scientists on the modernization of Chinese medicine, the 'Let Western Study Chinese' movement, and the 'Research Chinese Medicine with a Will' movement. The future of Chinese medicine is like miles and miles of clouds, with a bright light far away; our responsibility, our burden, and our long-term task (*daoyuan*) is to take this 'long and clouded road' as our problem.

Some elements of Deng's life story are characteristic of the genre of medical biography. The fact that Dr Deng 'continued his family's studies', and that his medical lineage continues in this generation, is typical. It also appears to be important in the volume editors' eyes that Deng's reputation and influence have spread beyond China: they point out at the end of the biographical note that some of his works have been translated into Japanese. These continuities and extensions are made much of in the other essay we will consider here, but they are also predictable features of the biographical genre.

In addition it is a near-universal practice for doctors writing about their own lives and work to orient themselves to the field by naming their scholarly forebears and the living or recently dead elders with whom they studied or whose work they admire. These names are not themselves supplemented with biographical or scholarly details. Such renowned personages embody features of the field, its factions, and its history, and authors refer to them partly to situate themselves in relationship to controversies and schools of thought.[14]

Unlike some much revered ming laozhongyi, Deng Tietao has been actively engaged in politics; this is clearly the autobiography of a communist cadre. Deng's official influence is an important element of the essay and of his life. He concerns himself not only with Chinese medical knowledge, archival lore, practical techniques, and scientific evaluation, but also with the broad institutional life of Chinese medicine right up to the national level. When he speaks of Chinese medicine's long and clouded road, or of its 'mainstream', he speaks as a man who is engaged in constituting the field and its direction of development. His personal history is more than a metaphor of a 'deepening and developing' professional field; as one of the profession's leaders, his life is written as a synecdoche: he is *part* of this historic *whole*.

Deng's rhetorical tendency is to unify diverse elements, bringing them inward toward 'the main stream' and declaring them to be essential features of the field. His essay provides many examples of this strategy. The paragraphs on sub-speciality areas of study which make up most of section 3, for example, focus on subjects and subdisciplines – history, literature, art, acupuncture, and massage – that are considered by many to be outside Chinese medicine's mainstream. Showing how study of these subjects has formed his own thought and practice, Deng builds an explicit argument for their centrality to Chinese medicine. He calls this a reintegration of something that has been split, first quoting the *Complete Library of Four Branches of Knowledge*,[15] to the effect that 'the division of the scholars began in the Song (960–1278), the division of medicine began in the Jin-Yuan (1115–1333)', and then considering 'the present-day specialization of Chinese medicine'.

Specialities have indeed proliferated in Chinese medicine since reorganization in the mid-1950s. Some of these model the specialities of Western medicine and others have continued and institutionalized older foci of medical attention (examples of the latter are women's medicine and children's medicine). In his essay Deng argues that however productive the subdivisions within the field have been, and however inevitable the partial separation of medicine from a scholarly mainstream

---

[14]   See Wendy Larson, *Literary Authority and the Modern Chinese Writer: Ambivalence and Autobiography* (Durham, N.C.: Duke University Press, 1991), for a distinction between 'circumstantial' and 'impressionistic' styles of autobiography in modern China. All the biographies of *laozhongyi* I have read tend toward the former genre, in which the author-subjects locate themselves with reference to historical circumstances. The impressionistic literary styles studied by Larson have not appeared in the published discourses of traditional Chinese medicine.

[15]   *Siku Quanshu* (Complete Library of Four Branches of Knowledge) (1772).

must be, ignorance of such things as history, literature, and art nevertheless make it 'impossible to understand [medicine's] several thousand years of accomplishments and developments'. In the closing section of his essay, then, Deng places certain elements of medicine and culture within the medical mainstream, traces medicine's history back to its sources in early Chinese culture, and by emphasizing his own attempts to master these areas of knowledge looks toward the future as an embodiment of integration rather than fragmentation.

Deng's 'mainstreaming' project is not as conservative as this statement would make it seem, however. In his commitment to science and to dialectical materialist methods, Deng shows that his carefully con-structed 'centre of the road' or 'main stream' is not located precisely where previous Chinese medical roads have lain. He does this by referring to the divided path of Chinese medicine in his youth, when apprenticeship within the family and a small circle of independently practising doctors was usual. Older approaches to training and practice were in disarray as a result of the 'devastating pressure' of the Guomindang government, and 'modernizing' tensions were evident in the call by a few prominent scholars for the 'scientization of Chinese medicine'. But Deng says he felt at the time that such efforts to 'broaden and develop' Chinese medicine were hindered by the lack of a 'method and a large number of like-minded people engaged in a joint effort'.

These impediments are precisely those that were removed by the revolution. Deng's account of his early commitment to Marxism and his perception of commonalities between dialectical materialism and classic Chinese medical reasoning indicate his pre-revolutionary 'discovery' of the path that most Chinese medical people would later take. A heavy reliance on dialectical materialist modes of explanation and large-scale government support are the most prominent differences between the Chinese medicine of the Maoist period and all its social forms before 1949. Here as elsewhere in the essay, by forefronting his own central position and centrist politics, Deng forges a link between old and new directions of medical development. The direction Chinese medicine appeared to be taking as Deng wrote in the early 1980s is posited as a *natural* path that had in the past been obstructed by a short-sighted right-wing regime. The 1949 revolution is presented as the salvation of traditional Chinese medicine, that most crucial historical turn which allowed 'the profession' to realize its inner (dialectical) essence.

Another distinctive element influencing the location of Chinese medicine's path, according to Deng, is ideological and material competi-tion from Western medicine. Deng addresses this situation in a long account of his year of research on Spleen–Stomach theory at the 157th

People's Liberation Army Hospital. This dramatic portion of his essay renders the sense of mortal struggle that has informed a great deal of Chinese medical discourse:

Those were memorable days. There we had opportunities to join in the work of treating serious life-threatening diseases. Commissar Xie Wang completely supported Chinese medical treatments, and in the decision whether or not to do surgery he always sought and weighed the view of traditional Chinese doctors. This gave us an opportunity, together with the hospital's doctor and nurse comrades, to persevere with therapies that had Chinese medicine as their main component. This gave us all many anxious nights at bedsides tending seriously ill patients night after night and day after day.

In this part of the essay the joint practice of Chinese doctors and Western-style physicians is analysed in terms of their respective powers over case management, and it is strongly implied that any development of Chinese medicine requires a reduction of the powers of its Western counterpart.

Perhaps because of his disenchantment with early attempts to unify the two modes of medical practice that accorded too much power to Western medical explanations and techniques, Deng rejects unification on theoretical grounds alone.[16] He argues, ultimately, that both the validation of Chinese medical methods and the unification of Chinese and Western medicines for the greater good of all depend on practical exploration, 'testing and tempering'. If the Chinese medical profession is to prove itself clinically (which he suggests is the only way it can avoid 'gradual disappearance') it must be given more support and more control over case management.

Deng is here being remarkably explicit about not only his concern that Chinese medicine is dying, but also about the unequal power relations that may be hastening its death. This concern is tacit in almost every aspect of Chinese medical discourse. Consequently positions taken on the proper course for Chinese medicine as a field are far from being simple matters of taste, personal history, or traditional bias. Like Deng's, such positions are carefully considered and passionately argued strategies in a discourse that is at once scientific and political. The

[16] At the time Deng's essay was written, theoretical research exploring the logical grounds on which the two medicines could be combined (*zhongxiyi jiehe*) was fairly widespread. This sort of research has now lost some of its appeal as more practical combinations of Chinese and Western therapies are successfully put to use in clinical settings. In general the tendency of official research in the PRC is to pursue theory only insofar as it can 'guide' practical work 'in the service of the people'; theoretical programmes to find a common epistemological terrain for the combination of Chinese and Western medicine have not produced practical syntheses as fast as empirical experimentation in clinics has. Hence a slackening of intellectual interest in these (to me) rather fascinating problems.

conditions within which strategies of this kind take on coherence are seen as a collective dilemma differentially addressed; one way or another, Chinese medicine must prove itself, and many ming laozhongyi took responsibility not only for maintaining the struggle but also for determining its form.

The discussion of Chinese medicine's 'long and clouded road' with which Deng closes his essay is not only a clear statement of the rhetorical process that I have outlined, it is a completion of it. The 'centre of Chinese medicine's route of development' has been concretely embodied in Deng's own life and interests. Having in this personal account brought many major components of Chinese medical clinical and educational practice firmly into the centre, and oriented its future toward a certain form of 'modernization', Deng reveals some previously neglected Western medical and scientific comrades as having been 'travelling the same road'. The road is widened to accommodate those who come to Chinese medicine from a variety of directions; though the linear metaphors he uses are equally capable of connoting the ever-present possibility of diverging routes (many scientists see no point in medical history; many laozhongyi will have nothing to do with 'scientization'), only convergence and continuity are presented.

Convergence and continuity are also important concerns of the other autobiography I wish to discuss here, but as I will now try to show, these values are approached rather differently in the autobiography of Dong Demao.

'Emulate teachers and make friends, concentrate intensively and diffuse widely' – the autobiography of Dong Demao

Dong Demao's autobiographical essay, like that of Deng Tietao, self-consciously characterizes and positions both its protagonist within Chinese medicine and Chinese medicine in the world. In the first, personal, half of his essay Dong emphasizes his study under the master doctor Shi Jinmo, followed by his activities as an organizer and editor of Chinese medical journals. In the second, more technical, part of the essay he develops two lengthy didactic examples of medical work and study.

Throughout his essay Dong employs a structural device relating study and teaching (concentrated accumulation) to publishing and clinical work (wide diffusion); this relationship is schematized in Figure 1 as movement in 'vertical' and 'horizontal' dimensions. Though Dong does not himself employ a graphic device like Figure 1 to make his point, the neatness with which this trope organizes the whole essay is very marked.

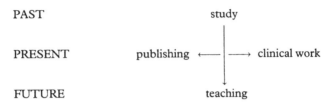

Figure 1: Accumulation and diffusion in Dong Demao's imagery

The essay's title condenses this spatial arrangement nicely: 'Emulate teachers and make friends, concentrate intensively and diffuse widely' (*congshi he jiaoyou, houji er bofa*). 'Emulating teachers' is parallel with 'concentrating intensively'; both phrases connote narrow or local accumulation. And both 'making friends' and 'diffusing widely' involve dispersion outward from a centre. Thus the second phrase restates the first in more abstract form, and the use of the strong conjunction '*er*' suggests a causal connection between the 'vertical' dimension of narrow accumulation and the 'horizontal' dimension of wide diffusion outward: concentrate intensively *in order to* diffuse widely.

Adhering to this structure throughout, the essay is divided into four parts. These four sections fall into two halves corresponding to the accumulation-diffusion couple. Parts 1 and 2 discuss social relations, i.e. vertical relations with teachers and horizontal relations with fellow students. Parts 3 and 4 cover vertical and horizontal dimensions, respectively, of the development of technical knowledge and skills.

In both the social and the technical halves of the essay, the vertical dimension is shown to cultivate the horizontal dimension: Dong's aunt, approving his filial interest in medicine, sponsored him to take the medical college examination, which 'was truly the beginning of [his] career in medicine'. His teacher Shi Jinmo approved and assisted the foundation of Dong's first journal, which was manned and written chiefly by Master Shi's other students. Both of these situations present the bestowal of help from a senior as the condition of possibility for extension of Dong's personal scope as well as for that of the profession.

Similar relationships hold for technical knowledge. In parts 3 and 4 of the essay, accumulated material from various locations in the medical archive is organized for ease of deployment in present clinical practice, diffusing medical powers outward to serve the people. This is traditional medicine's prototypical transformation of that which is passed down (the vertical-temporal dimension of Figure 1) into effective healing in the present (the horizontal-spatial dimension of Figure 1).

It is interesting that the examples Dong has chosen for parts 3 and 4 on accumulation and inductive analysis are Spleen–Stomach system research and Liver system physiology and pathology, respectively. By invoking complex physiological processes well known to Chinese medical readers, these examples literally embody not only the abstract social processes they are intended to illustrate but also the relationship that should hold between them.

Thus, accumulation is illustrated with reference to Dong's own 'gradual development' of expertise in Spleen system theory and practice. Just as the Spleen and Stomach systems process the nutrients that sustain life, managing up and down motion in the nourishment of the body, so orderly accumulation of medical understanding through study and clinical work maintain the substantive 'vertical' continuities of the nurturant medical heritage in individual lives.

Diffusion or knowledge is equally well figured by Liver system functions, which have more to do with collection (of Blood) and circulation (of Qi) within the whole body; the movement in question is one of ramification outward as well as upward and downward.

The parallel does not stop there; as with other writing in which physiological relationships are used to exemplify the connections between more abstract notions, there is a significant interdependence between Spleen and Liver systems. Dong's summary of Liver functions emphasizes their involvement with Blood storage and circulation. The Spleen, on the other hand, is presented as the source of Qi and Blood. This places the two visceral systems in an interdependent relationship, the Spleen being the source of the Blood and Qi which the Liver collects and circulates through the body.[17]

This, then, is an intimate interdependence capable of very suggestive metonymic extension. If it is superimposed on the basic vertical-horizontal structure of Figure 1, social past and present take on the organic relationship that should hold between substances and their proper circulating movement in the sustenance of life, as in Figure 2.

With this richly elaborated physiological example, Dong Demao seems to provide the field of Chinese medicine with a body in a way rather different from that adopted by Deng Tietao. Where Deng chooses to embody his profession as a human synecdoche, a centred part for a constructed whole, Dong assumes a certain organic historical existence

---

[17] In the complex visceral physiology of Chinese medicine, the Spleen is neither the only source of Blood nor is the Liver the only visceral system with a circulating function. Many points of view can be taken on physiology, and many points can be made with it.

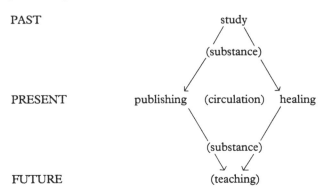

Figure 2: Substance and circulation in Dong Demao's imagery

for his field; the body of Chinese medicine requires not reconstruction in a new political terrain but merely wise maintenance of those long-standing social processes that have always nourished its autonomous existence.

This contrast reminds us that what Dong Demao wishes to present as self-evident is not universally acknowledged as such in the field of Chinese medicine. His ideas about education are old-fashioned, for example, and he makes few overt concessions to the radical scientizing and modernizing programmes that were so important at the time he wrote this essay. The dialectical materialist concerns of Deng Tietao are not in evidence, and the origins of Chinese medicine's institutional growth are located in a time well before the Communist triumph of 1949. Yet his rhetorical device of showing how conservative principles of filiality become smoothly embodied in practitioners and social institutions which successfully heal is powerful; it has the ring of natural (Chinese) common sense to it, and there is little doubt that many other doctors of Dong's generation appreciated his masterful presentation of this position.

In his essay Dong reproduces the 'publisher's manifesto' from the first issue of his first journal, the *Chinese Medicine and Pharmacy Monthly*.[18] Undoubtedly there is a sly manipulation here: a text written at a time when (all acknowledge) traditional medicine was in crisis and under siege is redeployed to refer to contemporary conditions. Perhaps Dong wishes to argue that the central tasks of Chinese medicine remain the

---

[18]   Dong Demao, 'Chuangkan Xuanyan' (Publisher's Manifesto), *Chinese Medicine and Pharmacy Monthly*, vol. 1, June (1940).

same as they have always been, and that the old-fashioned skills and social processes he advocates can respond quite as well to the challenges of the 1980s as they could to those of the 1940s. Is he also suggesting that the profession of traditional Chinese medicine, however radically transformed it is from the time the original preface was written, is still in crisis, still in need of a 'manifesto'?

In any case this small text serves as a concise statement of the purpose of his autobiography as well, and its structure neatly condenses the spatio-temporal organization of the essay as a whole:

From henceforth let us travel the same path. If we can work together, not admitting sectarian bias, taking scholarship as our cause, never diminishing Chinese medicine's strengths and never over-protecting its weaknesses, using scientific methods to seek the truth of therapeutics ... discarding the dross while saving the essence, eliminating idle chatter and going ahead with that which is practically useful, this will place the practical medical documents of our nation's past in the realm of world medicine, and advance and develop oriental culture. [Ellipsis in original.]

Past and future are here given their places vis-à-vis contemporary projects, placed in their proper relationship to each other in the new world of Chinese medicine. The predictions made in the closing lines are incontestable goals that, while conferring a certain necessity on Dong's proposals, also re-combine horizontal ('the realm of world medicine') and vertical ('oriental culture', which is to be 'advanced and developed') at a global level.

Writing and history

The above discussion of Dong Demao's autobiography has emphasized its formal qualities and its 'traditional' themes. This is partly because Dr Dong appears to have quite pointedly refused to acknowledge the historical moment of his writing, ignoring the many political and social upheavals he had lived through while emphasizing steady accumulation and continuity. Now, however, it is necessary to return to the questions with which this paper opened, and reconsider these two autobiographies as historically located gestures.

Both of these biographies can be politically located. Deng Tietao advocates scientific Marxism, and he takes a relatively separatist view of Chinese medicine's proper path while emphasizing clinical practice as the sphere in which it will be ultimately validated. He also foregrounds a strong sense of struggle with Western medicine, a struggle in which a unified profession of Chinese medicine is continually recreated through an active commitment to inclusion and expansion. Dong Demao emphasizes personal and collective experience and the orderly (filial) transmission of Chinese medicine's essence, relying on wide dissemination to ensure downward passage. His implicit enemies are the enemies of long historical continuity and of 'hundred flowers' eclecticism – presumably revolutionaries of many kinds imperil the project he advocates. He is very pointed in refusing to see the establishment of the PRC as a break of any kind, and seems to assume that it is not so much Chinese medicine's existence or continuity that is at stake as its health and stability. Put another way, Dong Demao seems content to be a component, even perhaps a marginal one, of the living body that is traditional Chinese medicine; Deng Tietao, however, constitutes his prominence by embodying the whole situation and struggle of the field in his own life and work.

Deng's 'progressive' stance can be contrasted with Dong's 'conservative' one, but the differences between their positions and texts are not fully clarified by such categorizations. In addition, certain preoccupations are common to both essays. These common concerns, to which we now turn, are shared with many other writers in the wider realm of contemporary Chinese medical discourse.

Continuity, unity, filiality

It appears from both of these essays, first, that a life in medicine is importantly concerned with forging continuities between the past and the future, and second, that the unification of elements that are scattered and diverse in the present is a process central to the achievement of such continuity. Deng Tietao uses the self-evident value of this process as a foundation for his valorization of the role of Marxism and the Chinese Communist Party, while Dong Demao attempts to trace the origins of the present vigour and democratization of Chinese medicine to a time prior to the Communist victory of 1949. Neither questions the necessity of medical continuity into the future from the most ancient recorded past; there is no romance with the radically new.

Rather, continuity is presented as the result of concerted human action. In both narratives, 'tradition' requires the committed involvement of specialists. It could hardly be perceived otherwise so soon after the close of the Cultural Revolution. Though the world of traditional Chinese medicine was criticized less than many 'expert' social groups during this divisive period, these authors surely witnessed and experienced much bitterness. They and most of their leading colleagues must have often wondered whether their profession and their skills had any future beyond the divisions and distrust that infected academic and clinical institutions for more than ten years. Surely the eloquent pleas for unity and continuity that were embodied in the biographies of Chinese medicine's senior generation in the early 1980s, and the intense affirmation with which such essays were received by a professional audience, arose partly as an attempt to heal and restore what had become a deeply compromised sense of community.[19]

But the means by which these authors exemplify the continuation of the field of traditional medicine under conditions of crisis are powerful in what I see as culture-specific ways; they are modes of filiality. This is clear in that both authors refer prominently to the point at which they chose to devote themselves to medicine. In each case this is presented as a personal choice: Deng Tietao 'was strongly inclined toward medicine' as a child and (lest we think he passively followed in his father's footsteps) during his exile in Hong Kong recommitted himself to Chinese medicine 'with even stronger confidence and resolve'. Spurred by his brother's illness, Dong Demao first sought to study medicine from his father-in-law.

These decisions reflect far more than simple filial obedience, in fact suggesting that filial virtue is far from simple. Dong Demao became a burden to his family when he turned to medicine, abandoning an apprenticeship through which he had been helping to support them. And Deng Tietao's Hong Kong resolve to struggle toward a 'way out' for Chinese medicine resulted from his individual rejection of his father's medical politics and his own subsequent attraction to dialectical materialism. In each case the choice described both diverges from any passive obedience to conventional expectations and seeks a higher and, if anything, more deeply filial road.

This pattern is ubiquitous in Chinese popular narrative, and should not surprise us. As in novels, the cinema, and opera, the filiality that characterizes these lives is one in which devotion is expressed through the courageous exercise of personal choice for the greater good. The commitment of lives to a heritage such as medicine is thus revealed to be far from automatic or passively obedient to tradition. Both authors emphasize that the achievement of continuity results not from rote repetition but from prudent evaluation and critical deployment of many elements of medicine.

This is far from being an individual undertaking. There is no

---

[19] Whether Chinese medicine ever constituted a community, much less enjoyed any 'unity', is a historical problem. Since there was no 'profession' of 'traditional Chinese medicine' much before this century (when modernizers began to assert the superiority and systematic nature of 'Western medicine' and doctors suddenly labelled traditional felt called upon to fight for the integrity and efficacy of their own expertise), appeals to a 'restored' community are more understandable as prescriptive than as descriptive.

autonomous self-creation posited here. Instead an interactive process is suggested in the images of gathering, centring, and unifying that describe the activities of these scholars in the 'horizontal' dimension of present practice: Dong Demao, for example, includes detailed descriptions not only of the way in which he has learned from his own and other doctors' cases, but also of the slow cumulative process of sorting among diverse and contradictory items in the medical archive. And Deng Tietao emphasizes teaching and emergency hospital practice, in addition to routine clinical work, as modes of practice that fostered his medical judgement. These are processes of self-formation as a doctor undertaken in dialogue both with the social world of healing and the recorded experience of medical ancestors (who are presented – especially these days – as having maintained their own clinical practices).

Good medical judgement must consult the teachings of the past, since the experience of forebears is the only reliable guide to successful healing. But it must also respond sensitively and appropriately to contemporary situations, to each illness manifestation, otherwise it would hardly be judgement at all. It follows, then, that it is the skill accumulated in the continuing exercise of clinical judgement that constitutes that experience which, in all its complexity and final inexpressibility, should be passed down to doctors of the future.

These accounts make no effort to reduce the conditions of medical practice to biological states in abstract bodies that can be observed across a distance by the medical or intellectual gaze.[20] The conditions of practice are always social: Deng Tietao asserts that the degree of power a Chinese doctor has over the management of cases profoundly affects what can be learned from therapeutic practice. Dong Demao holds that wide communications networks are necessary to 'create the conditions for good scholarly and democratic practice'. Conditions in the present also limit the scope of innovation and judgement, and contingency appears here to be as central to the life courses of the laozhongyi as it is to their daily practice – they continue medicine downward and outward, but it is a medicine that, unified by the centrality of practice and experience, lives in them as much new as old, as much theirs as their teachers', colleagues', and patients'.

It follows that, if the continuation of traditional medicine was felt as an acute problem in 1980 (under pressure from 'science' and the four modernizations, debilitated from years of internal and external struggle), personal biography might have been received as a particularly suitable arena in which to address this crisis. These essays assert an integrated

[20] Michel Foucault, *The Birth of the Clinic: An Archaeology of Medical Perception* (New York: Vintage Books, 1975).

and effective personhood for their author/subjects, they show how medicine's past, future, and present reach is embodied in its leaders, and they achieve a rhetorical force based on healing and the recovery of a rich national past. Writing of this kind could be seen as manipulative and self-serving, but I suspect that its appeal went deeper, speaking to an assumption that medical knowledge is nothing apart from its realization in clinical work, and that the field of Chinese medicine has no future separate from the fate of its leading exemplars.

Directionality and dispersion

Amidst all this talk of unification, there is a marked tendency to orient all activities in very specific political and technical directions. Deng's dialectical materialism, and Dong's democratic 'hundred flowers' idealism, are rather different, but equally marked, gestures toward directing the flow of medicine along a certain course. 'Bias' of this kind is not only, I think, essential to the genre of biography but also to the social and pedagogical life of the field. Doctors who avoid clear political coloration in their published works nevertheless take a position on physiological and pathological processes at every level of professional work. They argue for their own interpretations of which aspects of the body's holistic and resonating functions are most basic, and they found their practice on these views.[21] Deng Tietao's self-characterization includes several such 'purely medical' positions. He refers in his autobiography to his own synthetic approach to the problems of exogenous Heat illnesses with which the Cold Damage and Warm Illnesses factions have concerned themselves, and he emphasizes in addition his well-known experimentation with the Chinese medical treatment for 'serious life-threatening' illnesses. He has elsewhere published his controversial argument that ancient Five Phases theory remains important for understanding the physiology and treating the pathologies of the visceral systems of function.[22]

In Dong Demao's exploration of archival materials on Spleen–Stomach theory, he lists a number of differing viewpoints, some of

[21] See also Judith Farquhar, 'Time and Text: Approaching Chinese Medicine through Analysis of a Published Case', in Charles Leslie and Allan Young (eds.), *Paths to Asian Medical Knowledge* (Berkeley: University of California Press, 1992), pp. 62–73.

[22] Deng Tietao, 'Zhongyi Wuxing Xueshuode Bianzhengfa Yinsu', and 'Zailun Zhongyi Wuxing Xueshuode Bianzhengfa Yinsu' ('Dialectical Factors in Chinese Medical Five Phases Theory', and 'A Reconsidering of Dialectical Factors in Chinese Medical Five Phases Theory') in *Xueshuo Tantao yu Linzheng* (Theoretical Inquiries and Clinical Encounters) (Guangzhou: Guangdong Science and Technology Press, 1981), pp. 4–15.

them contradicting each other, on the physiology and pathology of the Spleen–Stomach visceral system. Having 'traced the wellsprings' and 'investigated the flow' of this area of medical concern, he takes a position himself, locating Spleen function as a common root of many illnesses.[23] In doing so he opposes the famous Ming Dynasty scholar Zhang Jingyue, among others, who emphasized 'treat[ing] all five viscera in order to regulate Spleen and Stomach'. In this account Dong seems to take for granted a certain imperative to declare himself; but there is no requirement that contradictions in theory be reconciled or errors eliminated or vigorously opposed. At issue, rather, is the epistemological requirement that a particular stance be taken on body (physiology) and history (the medical archive), both of which are infinitely complex. In other words, unlike the anatomical body that has for a long time grounded the logic of biomedicine, the body of Chinese medicine offers no stable point of view on its physiological and pathological dynamics and pretends to no structural totality. Doctors place themselves and their learned judgement in relation to specific illnesses and specific traditions of practice. In contrast to a history of science that valorizes development toward an increasingly good 'fit' between scientific representations and the natural world, Chinese medical history offers itself as a vast array of useful clinical resources and exemplary teachers. Never becoming completely obsolete, it is rather continued through being embodied in particular combinations by each doctor.

The point to be taken here is not that Chinese medicine deviates in practice from some neutral theoretical totality. Rather it is important to ask why differences of perspective are placed right at the centre of medical signification. Amidst all these biases and facets, directions and arguments, one searches in vain for a unitary, standard, or impersonal level of 'traditional Chinese medicine'. The social convergence sought by Drs Deng and Dong is not and could never be a consensual knowledge foundation. In contemporary China, only Western science appears to offer such a totality. Within Chinese medicine, many doctors and their biographer-students continue (nostalgically?) to orient themselves and their hopes for medicine to distinctions among specificities and to the unique positions taken by each laozhongyi. Differences may be, indeed should be, encompassed within a profession, but in the traditional

[23] See also Dong Demao, 'Congshi he Jiaoyou, Houji er Bofa' (Emulate Teachers and Make Friends, Accumulate Intensively and Disseminate Widely) in Zhou Fengwu et al. (eds.), *Ming Laozhongyi zhi Lu* (Jinan: Shandong Science and Technology Press, 1984), vol. 2, pp. 329–42.

Chinese medicine that many still imagine today they cannot be reduced to unity.[24]

Agency, embodiment, writing

I have elsewhere shown that in the course of the clinical encounter in Chinese medicine the doctor's personal judgement plays a crucial role in diagnosis and treatment determination.[25] In methodological literature, much is made of the adeptness of the therapeutic virtuoso, whose artistry has been forged ('tested and tempered', in Deng Tietao's words) through long years of both study and clinical experience. The turning points in illnesses are delicately negotiated without the aid of codes, rules, handbooks, or impersonal systems. Codified and rationalized medical knowledge brings the doctor only so far; it delimits the space within which he must make the really consequential diagnostic synthesis and design a subtle and effective therapy.

A clinician of this kind is not made overnight, nor is he graduated whole from a modern college of Chinese medicine. Rather his powers and his unique presence are assembled or accumulated over a long period of time, and he slowly comes to embody 'the essence' of medicine. Even in the PRC today, Chinese medicine is not primarily learned from books, but must still be learned from teachers; it is only in continuing practical relationships with teachers that the inner synthesis of medical practice can be sought. Here we glimpse a social process and a matched epistemological ideology that may still bolster 'gerontocracy' in the world of traditional Chinese medicine, at least for a while yet. Where 'essences' cannot be spoken of but must be acquired through obedience and emulation, there are no short cuts; becoming a person of substance is a long, slow process, and junior doctors seeking to master forms of knowledge that are still being brought forward from the medical past – the cryptically recorded observations of doctors whose experience always

[24] The field of traditional Chinese medicine is, however, increasingly influenced by the work of radical scientifizers who seek to produce a body of internally consistent, uncontested, and impersonal knowledge that could be called Chinese medicine. An example of this problematic effort was the project of mechanizing the art of pulse-taking: see Hu Qingyin and Wang Wande, 'Maizhen Qiantan' (Comments on Pulse Diagnosis), *Heilongjiang Zhongyiyao*, no. 2 (1983), 15–20 and no. 4 (1983), 10–15. A widely acknowledged problem with such a project was that the only pulse readings that could be considered correct were those done by experienced doctors; when they disagreed (and they often did) there was no external standard with reference to which a choice could be made between readings.

[25] Judith Farquhar, *Knowing Practice: The Clinical Environment of Chinese Medicine* (Boulder, Co.: Westview Press, 1993).

exceeded the verbal – cannot claim expertise in the way that their laozhongyi teachers can.[26]

The idea that an ancient form of medical practice should be more embodied than recorded, more evident in its practices than in its lavish written discourse, is not new in anthropology. It is interesting to note, however, that there are still voices in China, not all of them elderly, who assert that this embodied medicine, the 'precious learning and rich experience' of the laozhongyi,[27] *is* Chinese medicine's essence.

This may be a short-lived bulwark against the tide of scientization and institutional rationalization that seems to threaten older social forms on every front in contemporary China. Yet embodied knowledge has a way of ramifying into many domains of everyday life. Changes in this form of knowledge will take time.

Conclusion

I have argued here that a personal genre of writing emerged within the technical field of traditional Chinese medicine in the early 1980s in response to a number of particular conditions. Credit was overdue in coming to leaders who had laboured for decades to institutionalize the work of traditional medicine and systematize its expertise in teaching and publishing. Students wished to acknowledge the personal greatness of their teachers while recovering respectable intellectual genealogies for themselves. This re-establishment of filial continuities in the field was a gesture of healing after the many painful rifts of the Cultural Revolution had been declared inappropriate. A new kind of memory was required, one that could valorize service and experience over any sort of political correctness.

Moreover, there was a new policy regime to which a concerted profession-wide response was required; a national commitment to modernization of science and technology, the constant refrain of

[26] 'Western' science and medicine of course operate on quite a different epistemological ground in the PRC. As opportunities have expanded for Chinese medical professionals to study bioscience, younger people have seized these chances to challenge a 'traditional' knowledge which can be embodied only in elders with one which seems to promise an 'objectivity' available through assiduous study of impersonal texts and the conduct of laboratory research. This rising generation of practical scientifizers, whose commitment to the clinical effectiveness and scientific validation of traditional medicine has little to do with the aesthetics of an ancient heritage, may increasingly dominate the field as the generation of the *laozhongyi* dies off. A parallel hiving off of young 'traditionalists' is also apparently in progress in some institutions.

[27] Deng Tietao, 'Wanli Yuntian Wanli Lu' (A Long and Clouded Road), in Zhou Fengwu et al. (eds.), *Ming Laozhongyi zhi Lu* (Jinan: Shandong Science and Technology Press, 1984), vol. 2, pp. 1–8.

'seeking truth from facts' (which meant not only no more politics but also no more 'superstition'), placed traditional medicine in an ambiguous position. It was necessary not only to rectify the status of Chinese medicine in keeping with new scientistic priorities but also to ensure that national support for its work would continue. This new articulation of the field's nature and future had to be rhetorically powerful in the face of a strong government commitment to an epistemological regime quite foreign to traditional medicine's 'essence'.

The ming laozhongyi risked much as they wrote both themselves and their profession in their autobiographical essays. In the face of possible later reprisals against clear political positions taken in these prominently authored works, they claimed a special authority and centrality as leaders and teachers; but they also offered their own lives as examples of indebtedness to the past and as hope for future success in many unfinished tasks. In this writing they drew on filial social relations, irrefutable archival knowledge, and personal histories of effective healing to argue for an alternative epistemology and practice (clinical, pedagogical, and literary) for traditional Chinese medicine, one which could both stand apart from Western biomedicine as a legitimate profession in its own right and support national projects of modernization and improvement of 'the people's health'.

Yet this articulation may have come a little late. It was possible for the field and its leaders to be constituted as such only when a certain end was in sight, only when a position outside the old social relations of the field could be contemplated by some of its members. Young, scientifically trained researchers who saw pharmacological and therapeutic potential in a scientifically legitimated traditional medicine, and clinicians who had abandoned canonical theory in favour of many practical combinations of biomedicine and herbal medicine, were beginning to dominate publishing and win increasing amounts of research money. Purists who still insisted on the epistemological inconsistency of traditional Chinese medicine with Western biomedicine were being classified into the increasingly isolated subdisciplines of medical history and philosophy.

Hence the air of urgency, regret, and ambivalent affection in the preface cited in the opening section of this paper. The generation of ming laozhongyi whose passing is mourned by the editors of the *Paths* volumes embodied medicine in a way that may soon become impossible. Actualizing and unifying so many diverse strains of history, healing practice, and scholarship in their contingently assembled and adept personages, this generation of doctors brought a precious medical heritage through half a century of crisis and renewal. Must 'our motherland's medicine' now be fragmented into Westernized subdisciplines? Must its 'precious learning and rich experience' be reclassified as bits of scientific knowledge legitimated under rubrics provided by a hegemonic world science? All this is now under contest.

Part 3

Āyurvedic medicine

13 Writing the body and ruling the land: Western reflections on Chinese and Indian medicine

Margaret Trawick

Like all history, this paper is fiction. It is not a lie, it is an honest account of things the author has seen. In the act of seeing, each seer creates an image; in the act of telling, each teller creates a story. As stories go, this is a bad one, being static and having no characters in it. The badness of this story is not my fault, it is the fault of the things I must look at (some texts) and the conventions I must follow (some rules) which preclude my making a really good story to put in this edited volume.

There were two main texts I looked at when I first composed my bad story. The first was a book by Paul Unschuld called *Medicine in China*.[1] I employed it because I am ignorant of China and Unschuld's book was the most comprehensive scholarly work on the history of Chinese medicine accessible to me at the time. The second was a Master's thesis written some time ago by a graduate student in Chicago.[2] I was that graduate student and therefore I know most of what is worth knowing about her. I know nothing about Paul Unschuld, and I hope he will forgive me for setting his book on a par with my first effort at interpreting Indian medicine.

These two texts – one and two decades old, respectively – remain the basis of my story. Any reader who would dismiss them as dated had better stop here, for we are talking in terms of millennia. Objections concerning interpretive styles, social and linguistic theories, and choice of translations may also be raised. How valid will be this essay, or the objections raised to it, two thousand years from now? I address a general audience, that neither knows nor cares about academic disputes. If we wish to construct something lasting, we had best take the interests of non-academics into account. They are smarter than we think. The initial draft of this paper was one of fifteen chapters of a study guide I wrote for

---

[1] Paul Unschuld, *Medicine in China: A History of Ideas* (Berkeley: University of California Press, 1985). All references to Unschuld in the text of this chapter refer to this book.
[2] Margaret Trawick (Egnor), 'Principles of Continuity in Three Indian Sciences: Psychology of Samhkya and Yoga, Biology of Āyurveda, Sociology of Dharmashastra and their Concentric Domains', unpublished Master's thesis, University of Chicago (1974).

279

undergraduate students in New Zealand. My aim was to introduce students to literature about systems of healing worldwide. When I came to discussing medicine in India and China, I noticed a gap. I could not find a simple, straightforward description of Chinese and Indian medicine generally as they related to one another. Indologists spoke to Indologists and Sinologists spoke to Sinologists and neither camp spoke to undergraduates at all. For the sake of undergraduates, Maori and Pakeha, Chinese and Indian, Anglo-Euro-American and Other, I have tried to begin to bridge that gap.

Perhaps Asian medicine too is a fiction. Perhaps the images we have of it have been projected by British, American and European scholars onto a blank screen which they see as exterior to themselves. Perhaps we are all Orientalists and perhaps we have created Oriental medicine along with the Orient as a whole. But surely we have not created it out of nothing all by ourselves. It would be both arrogant and insane to believe such a thing. There are people living in Asia and they far outnumber, out-think, and outproject all us scholars of Anglo-European descent. They out us by exceeding us and they in us by encompassing us. Let us remember these thoughts, and let us, for the sake of discussion, assume that not all perceived reality is projection. Much introjection also occurs. Strong forces on the other side of fantasy shape our thoughts.

Granted all the above, and using materials from a few selected modern English-language accounts, I will draw, in what follows, a sketch of my vision of some parallels between the history of medical thought in India and the history of medical thought in China. For the sake of simplicity, I will talk as though the statements I have read in history books were facts. I will take it as true that two text-based medical systems – one in Sanskrit and one in Chinese – became hegemonic in South and East Asia over the last two millennia. I will give examples of the ways in which these hegemonic medical systems were, as I see them, moulded to suit the ideologies of statehood that developed in India and China during the last centuries BC and the first centuries AD. I will argue that Indian and Chinese principles of control of the body through medicine came to be modelled in large part upon Hindu and Confucian principles of control of the land through cultivation. Not only was the body seen to be governed in the same way that the kingly state was governed, with different categories of agents providing different goods and services through the centre to the whole, but the flow of materials through the body was regulated in a fashion that mirrored the flow of materials over the landscape ruled by the king. The economy of the body was an agrarian economy.

Unschuld points out that there are many systems of healing in China. Therefore, to refer to a single one of them as 'Chinese medicine' is something of a misnomer. The single system that Westerners think of as 'Chinese medicine' was first codified, according to Unschuld, in a text called the *Huang-ti nei-ching*, 'The Yellow Emperor's Inner Classic', by a series of medical scholars working from the second century BC onwards. This text, Unschuld says, was compiled at the same time that various warring states in China were in the process of being organized into a centralized polity governed (in principle) according to Confucian doctrines of morality. The medical system that developed out of this text was the most authoritative medical system in China for many centuries, right up until the (re)introduction of Western medicine to China in the late nineteenth century.

Unschuld refers to this authoritative Confucian medical system as 'the medicine of systematic correspondences'. Because Unschuld's term is rather cumbersome, and because I wish to distinguish the authoritative, state-supported literate Chinese medical system from non-state-supported Chinese medical systems, I will henceforth refer to Unschuld's 'medicine of systematic correspondences' as 'Confucian medicine' – always bearing in mind, however, that the texts of this system incorporated many elements that were not strictly speaking Confucian.

Indian medicine, like Chinese medicine, is not homogenous any more than Asia is homogenous, but becomes, when one goes there and looks, a veritable ocean of ideas and activities. Like Chinese medicine, Indian medicine is permeated by multiple religious ideas and practices, such that it is often futile to try to distinguish between 'religious' ideas and practices and 'medical' ones. For a scholar trying to sort out different religious and medical systems in India and China, the situation is further complicated by the fact that Hinduism, unlike Confucianism, is a widely varied set of ideas and practices with no central dogma that all people we would call 'Hindus' adhere to.

Confucianism is a philosophical school of thought founded by one man, Confucius. However, there is really no such thing as Hinduism. The word 'Hindu' is not a Sanskrit word, but a word affixed to the South Asian world by Persians who wanted some way to label the religions that newcomers to the sub-continent found there. Thus the term 'Hinduism' covers every indigenous religious practice in India from drinking the blood of chickens to avoiding the touch of non-vegetarians, from singing bawdy wedding songs to writing abstruse treatises on the nature of the cosmos. When I refer to 'Hindu medicine' here, I am really referring to only one kind of healing connected with one kind of Hinduism, viz, the system of healing called Āyurveda, 'The Revealed Truth of Long Life', which is connected with the form of Hinduism commonly known among Western scholars as Brahmanism.

The central ideas of Āyurveda were expounded in a set of Sanskrit medical texts beginning with the text called *Caraka Samhita* dated somewhere between 200 BC and 200 AD. During the same period of Indian history, people called Brahmans (members of the caste of teachers, priests, and scholars) working within the context of kingly states developed a series of treatises concerning the moral and natural structure of human society. These treatises are called *Dharmashastra*, which means (very roughly) 'the science of morality'. The texts of Dharmashastra are considered by Western scholars and many Brahmans to embody the fundamental principles of Brahmanism. According to these texts, there is an appropriate mode of behaviour, or *dharma*, for every different kind of creature and every different kind of human being in the universe, as well as for every stage of life through which a man of high caste passes.

The Brahmanic concept of dharma roughly corresponds to the Confucian concept of *cheng-ming* or 'rectification of names': the doctrine according to which there is an appropriate form of behaviour for every different social status, from the king down to the ditch digger. The name 'king', according to this doctrine, should be given only to someone who acts as a king should act. Both the philosophy of Dharmashastra and the philosophy of Confucianism comprised attempts on the part of scholars to impose limits on what kings should be allowed to do.

Confucian medicine and Āyurveda are two distinct traditions which nevertheless have many attributes in common. For instance, both Confucian medicine and Āyurveda are founded upon certain ancient books whose essential verity is held to be beyond question. A second shared attribute of the two traditions is their exponents' construction of elaborate and comprehensive systems of classification of bodily and environmental phenomena. These systems posit orderly and symmetrical patterns of relations and processes of transformation underlying the apparent messiness of the phenomenal world. The patterns and processes so described are considered to be eternal and invariant: life is presumed always to proceed in accordance with the rules of order expounded in the texts. Diseases and other misfortunes result from infractions of the rules, but the disturbances themselves follow regular rules and can be corrected through ruled procedures. The rules disclosed in the texts thus render temporal events predictable and controllable. Nothing is random, nothing is inexplicable, nothing is left to chance. By the same token, animistic explanations of well-being and disease are discredited or ignored in the classical Confucian and Āyurvedic texts. Gods, demons, ancestors and other capricious and self-willed agents are accorded at most a very small place in either medicine.

A third shared attribute of the two traditions is their stress on physiology at the apparent expense of anatomy. There appears to be also in classical Chinese and Indian medicine, when viewed in comparison with modern Western medicine, more interest in the subjective experience of the body than in the objective observation of it. No Chinese or Indian Leonardo has ever appeared. From a Western point of view, both Confucian and Āyurvedic medicine suffer from an absence of realism; they seem to show a certain lack of interest in what most Westerners would consider the empirical realities of the body. Organs, substances, and structures are described in the Confucian and Āyurvedic medical texts that cannot be found by dissection. Neither system attributed any significance whatever to the brain or the central nervous system, though there must have been ample opportunity to observe that a blow to the back of the head can be paralysing or fatal. (Tantric medicine, by contrast, mapped a whole geography of mystic experience from the base of the spinal column to the crown of the skull.)

Some Western scholars attribute this seeming ignorance to religious prohibitions upon the handling and dissection of corpses. Others have suggested that Indian and Chinese physicians ignored the details of anatomy because they were more interested in function than in structure or because they thought of the body as a surface upon which things happened rather than as a container within which things happened. In my view, such explanations beg the question – but we will return to this issue presently.

A fourth attribute held in common is that the classificatory patterns of both systems are built upon a fundamental polarity between two types of land: wet, dark and low on the one hand; dry, light and high on the other. In Āyurvedic thought, as Zimmermann shows us,[3] this polarity derives from the distinction between open grassy land, called in Sanskrit *jangala*, and marshy tree-filled land, *anupa*. Eating meat from the jangala was considered to produce a dry and hard body; eating meat from the anupa was believed to produce a body that was soft and 'given to fluxes'. These two types of land with their associated body-types, in turn, fit into the general cosmic distinction between *agni*, the fiery power of the sun, and *soma*, the watery power of the moon.

In Chinese thought, a similar polarity developed between *yin*, the dark side of a hill, and *yang*, the bright side of a hill. In Chinese medicine, yin

---

[3] Francis Zimmermann, *The Jungle and the Aroma of Meats: An Ecological Theme in Hindu Medicine* (Berkeley: University of California Press, 1987).

and yang came to be generalized, like the Sanskrit soma and agni, to signify all that was dark, moist, cool and soft on the one hand and all that was bright, dry, hot and hard on the other.

Likewise, in both Chinese and Āyurvedic medicine, the notion of 'wind' occupied a prominent place. In Āyurvedic medical texts, a whole set of 'winds' moved through the body, pushing things around as it were. Not only was there the wind of the breath (*prana*), often assimilated with the idea of life force (for when the breath ceases, life ceases), there was also a wind fanning the flame of digestion (digestion was considered to be essentially a cooking process), a wind going up through the stomach and another going down through the bowels, a wind blowing through the uterus shaping and hollowing out the developing foetus, a wind which caused tremors, and so forth. In general in Āyurvedic thought, wind was considered responsible for the animation of the body, for in the world outside the body, wind is a power that moves things. Similarly, the wind in the body like the wind in the world was the force that was considered to dry things out and cool things down. Āyurvedic medicine regards just three substances in the body to be responsible for all processes, good and bad, occurring there. These three substances are *pitta* or 'bile' which provides the body with heat and luminosity; *kapha* or 'phlegm' which provides the body with moisture and cohesiveness; and *vata* (also called *vayu*) or 'wind' which performs all the functions that wind in the world performs. Heat, moisture, and wind thus constituted the climate of the Āyurvedic body, and of these three wind was the most variegated in its functioning, the most powerful and the most dangerous (see for example Car. I, XII).[4]

Unschuld (pp. 68–70) argues that in Chinese medical thought a gradual transition occurred from the notion of demons (*kuei*) as a source of disease, through the notion that wind (*feng*) could bring disease, to the notion that subtle influences or emanations or essences (*ch'i*) from various sources inside of and outside of the body could cause disease. The character for ch'i, Unschuld says, literally means 'vapors from cooked grain'. Ultimately, ch'i acquired a more abstract meaning, something like 'life essence': it was considered to be a vital, subtle fluid coursing through the vessels of the body, whose loss or disharmonious functioning could lead to death. The transition from demons to wind to

---

[4]   For convenience, I have abbreviated some of the references to English translations of Sanskrit texts that appear frequently in this chapter. Car. I, XVII, 75 should be read *Caraka Samhita*, Sthana I, chapter XVII, verse 75; Su. I, 109 should be read *Susruta-Samhita*, vol. I, p. 109; M. VI, 57 should be read *Manavadharmashastra*, chapter VI, verse 57. The full references for all these works are given in the list of abbreviations at the end of this chapter. The translations cited there are not reliable, but were the best available ten years ago.

food vapours to subtle essences reflects a slowly changing set of ideas and associations concerning the nature of life. For Chinese as for Indians, the concepts of 'spirit' and 'wind' appear to have been in many contexts interchangeable.

It is easy to see how people could think that the wind is something alive. The wind brought the weather, for good or for bad, and with changes in weather came changes in people's bodies. Hence diseases were thought to be wind-borne. Moreover, in an agrarian society, what kind of weather the wind brought in determined the success or failure of crops in any given year. If the wind misbehaved, people could starve. Food was necessary to life, as much as breath. Hence, the leap from wind (feng) to grain (ch'i). Perhaps the 'vapors from cooked grain' were identified by Chinese people with the energy they derived from this grain when they ate it. In India, such an idea is often expressed. What seems sure in any case is that in the agrarian worlds of both China and India, the earth equally with the body was seen as a food-processing plant, and both body and earth were animated by wind.

Yet another detail common to the Confucian and Āyurvedic medical systems was their elaboration of theories of transportation of the substances of the body through networks of channels and vessels. Regulated fluidity was evidently regarded by the compilers of both medical systems as the key to human health. The body was seen as a vast circulatory system, with the heart at the centre, though the various vessels and junctions described in the Āyurvedic and Confucian medical texts do not correspond either with each other or (for the most part) with anything found in Western anatomical texts, and the mechanics of blood circulation (including the recognition that the heart is a pump) was never actually worked out. Instead, the role assigned to the heart by both the Confucian and Āyurvedic theoreticians seems to have been something analogous to the role of the king's capital as military command-post, centre for the collection and redistribution of foodstuffs, and regulator of commerce within the kingdom.

In the Āyurvedic texts, the heart is called *mahat*, which means 'the great one' (Car. I, XXX, 3). It is regarded as the seat of consciousness in the body. The mind, dwelling within the heart, is said to be ever-active: its major function, says Caraka, is control (Car. IV, I, 21). Two sets of organs (*indriyas*) issue from the mahat: the organs of action (hands, feet, mouth, organs of generation and excretion) and the organs of sensation (eyes, ears, nose, tongue, and skin). The organs of action receive orders from the mahat via their respective channels, and the organs of sensation send information back to the mahat via theirs. All the constructive substances of the body (*dhatus*) are joined to each other via a complex chain of derivations, beginning with food in the belly and culminating in the finest and 'hardest' constructive substance, semen, which is 'like gold a thousand times purified' and which is stored within the heart. Semen in turn contains *ojas*, which means 'light', and is said in the Āyurvedic texts to be the essence of consciousness and vitality (much like the Chinese ch'i).

Each of the three active forces (wind, bile, and phlegm) in the Āyurvedic body, each of the senses, each of the constructive substances, and each of the waste products (*malas*) has its own channels (*nadis*) through which it is supposed to flow. Absolutely everything in the Āyurvedic body from bones to sneezes flows through channels (Car. II, VII, 4; Su. II, 210). Channels are said to spread all over the body, like veins in a leaf, sustaining and nourishing every part (Su. II, 210). Every sense organ and every pore is the termination of a channel. At the same time as they connect all the points on the body, channels also differentiate distinct substances from each other; for instance, they separate each succeeding constructive substance from the cruder material that serves as its 'ore' (Su. II, 210–11). Disease is caused by the blockage and overflowing of channels; if one substance overflows into the channels of another, then the 'invaded' channels become diseased (Car. III, V, 24). Every disease, ultimately, is caused by an excess or deficiency of some substance flowing in channels. When a substance is excessive, it overflows its own channels and makes troubles in other channels; when a substance is deficient, its channels dry up, provoking other substances to enter and make troubles there.

As in the Confucian medical texts, so also in the Āyurvedic texts constant references are made to things filling up and going dry, to cycles of repletion and depletion. The polarity between full and empty, wet and dry, has both temporal and spatial extension. Not only are there wet and dry lands, there are also wet and dry seasons, during which the whole earth becomes filled up or dried out. So Caraka writes:

The year has six seasons. The first three seasons are the time of absorption (*adana*), when the sun follows its northward course; the last three seasons are the time of release (*visarga*), when the sun travels southwards. In the time of release, the wind is not rough as it is in the time of absorption; the moon is strong and replenishes the world continually with its cool rays; thus the time of release is moist (*saumya*). But the time of absorption is fiery ... [At that time] the sun soaks up the world's moisture; the wind is sharp and rough; bitter, astringent and hot flavours predominate; and human beings are weakened. In [the time of release] the sun faces southwards and its strength is tempered by time, direction, wind, clouds and rain; then the strength of the moon is unobstructed and the world is cooled by rain; sweet and smooth flavours predominate; and human beings grow strong. (Car. I, VI, 4–7)

The vital importance of the rains to the growth of food and the consequent health of human beings is obvious in this passage.

At least three models of organization seem to be involved in the Āyurvedic theory of channels: first, the economic model of commerce and redistribution of foodstuffs; second, the social model of everybody following the dharma allotted to him (*sic* – the texts we must work with are androcentric), doing his own job, and not trying to usurp the place of others; and third, the agrarian model of an irrigation system, in which the flow must be carefully monitored so that each field gets its proper share of water, no field gets too much or too little, and no farmer breaks the irrigation ditch and steals another farmer's share of the water – an event which happens all the time in rice-growing regions of India. Like many theoretical constructs, the Āyurvedic construction of the body is a hybrid of multiple images drawn from various realms of experience.

The model of the body developed in the Confucian medical texts attributes, if anything, even greater importance to channels of communication and transport within the body than do the Āyurvedic texts. The recently discovered Ma-wang-tui medical manuscripts, which are considered to predate the *Huang-ti nei-ching* by about a century, describe eleven separate 'vessels' (*mo*) permeating the body. 'Each of the eleven vessels is associated with a list of specific symptoms or illnesses', Unschuld tells us, which 'represent a deficiency or surplus of the contents of these vessels' (p. 74).

The *Huang-ti nei-ching* 'consistently refers to twelve vessels – now called "conduits" (*ching*) or "conduit vessels" (*mo-ching*) – which are linked to each other and which are passed by a continuous circulatory flow of specific substances' (Unschuld, p. 75).

'The flow in the conduit vessels never stops', says a sage quoted in this classic text, 'it moves in an annular circuit without a break. When influences of cold enter the conduits, [the flow] is retarded. [The contents of the conduits] congeal and do not move' (Unschuld, p. 75). It seems clear to me that the author of this passage is thinking in terms of water pipes freezing. This is an all-too-familiar phenomenon to those of us (including northern Chinese) who live at higher latitudes, but it would be an experience infrequently suffered by Indians living in the Gangetic plain or Deccan peninsula. The latter are more concerned, as we have seen, with the prospect of the sun drying everything up.

Just as in *Caraka Samhita* the heart is considered to be the 'root' of all the vessels (Car. I, XXX, 8), so in the *Huang-ti nei-ching*, the heart is considered to be the 'master of the vessels'. Although the heart is the chief, there are altogether twelve principal organs recognized in Confucian medicine, each organ being associated with one particular

vessel. The twelve organs are divided into two groups, called respectively
'storage facilities' or 'depots' (*tsang*) and 'grain collection centres' or
'palaces' (*fu*). The 'depots' are the kidneys, liver, heart, spleen, lung, and
heart-enclosing network. The 'palaces' are the stomach, small intestine,
large intestine, bladder, gall, and something called the Triple Burner –
an organ which was supposed to transform raw materials of the body
into useful products by means of heat at three locations. (Āyurvedic
medical theoreticians imagined a similar organ, which they named
grahani, burning like a stove beneath the stomach, cooking the food
mixed there.) The 'depots' of the Confucian body were considered to be
'interior' and yin; the 'palaces' were considered 'exterior' and yang.

Unschuld suggests that the body described in Confucian medical texts
is in large part a mirror of the centralized grain transportation system
developed during the Ch'in and Han dynasties in China of the last
centuries BC. Grain was not only food, it was currency for the early
Chinese kingdoms as it was for the Indian kingdoms. During the Ch'in
dynasty, great urban population centres were created, and large
numbers of people were moved into them. To feed all these people,
granaries (tsang) were built in the urban centres to store grain brought
in from outlying agricultural districts, where it was temporarily stored in
collection centres (fu). The granaries and collection centres were
connected by a network of roads and waterways. The maintenance and
protection of these roads and waterways was essential to good management of the empire. The great vessels of the body were evidently seen as
analogous to the Grand Canal built by the founder of the Ch'in dynasty,
Shih Huang-ti (Unschuld, pp. 75–80).

The same emperors who built these cities and transportation systems
also developed major hydraulic projects. Consequently, in conjunction
with its use of the terminology of grain transport, we find the *Huang-ti
nei-ching* also borrowing the terminology of irrigation systems to describe
processes occurring in the interior of the body. Hydraulic terms applied
to the body included the words for 'gutter' (*hsu*), 'drainage ditch' (*lo*),
'underground passage' (*sui*), and so forth (Unschuld, p. 82).

Reading such contextualized accounts, we begin to understand how
early Chinese and Indian medical theoreticians saw things in the human
body that Westerners cannot see. In their efforts to create rational
explanations of the mysteries of bodily processes, they drew upon what
they witnessed in the world around them, and reasoned by analogy from
there back into the body. Where there were blanks in the picture, they
interpolated into those blanks what their theories predicted should be
there, just as Western scientists do. The difference in theories, I would
suggest, accounts for the difference in visions. But the objectives were

quite similar. The Āyurvedic and Confucian medical scholars, like their modern Western counterparts, were trying to make sense of the body, and, in this way, to gain control of it.

The idea that a territory can be controlled through rational governmental policy must certainly have lent impetus to the idea that the body can be controlled through rational medical action. One is tempted to hypothesize that the Chinese therapeutic procedure known as acupuncture was simply a projection onto the body of governmental policies of police intervention at trouble spots in the kingdom. According to Chinese medical texts, through insertion of an acupuncture needle at a precise location in the body, a doctor could correct the flow of influences through the particular vessel that the needle entered, and thus correct systemic disturbances whose symptoms might show up far from the site of intervention. How did Chinese medical scholars get this idea? Perhaps they observed that by protecting the flow of goods from the depredations of bandits at particularly vulnerable points along trade routes, a king could protect the welfare of his kingdom as a whole. Perhaps the medical scholars incorporated this observation about government into their medical theories.

However, I believe it would be a mistake to consider the general theoretical structure of Confucian medicine to be simply a reflection of Chinese political economy. If there are similarities between Chinese models of the kingdom and Chinese models of the body, this is in part because both kinds of models were developed in accordance with certain basic cultural templates whose origins predate either the system of government Unschuld describes or the system of medicine that emerged together with that system of government.

What do I mean by 'basic cultural templates'? I mean approximately the same thing that Victor Turner meant when he coined the term 'root metaphor'.[5] A template is a mould that gives shape to the contents you pour into it – like a mould that you pour muffin batter into. A root metaphor is a kind of conceptual mould in this sense: a basic idea or image that people use, generally unconsciously, to give shape to their world, and to unify all the different domains of their experience. For Americans, to give an example, the automobile is an important cultural template or root metaphor. When a person says, 'My marriage is not running smoothly', or 'The stock market crashed', or 'This economy is going nowhere', they are (probably unconsciously) using the automobile root metaphor. In South India, where most people are directly dependent on agriculture for a living, plant-growth is an important root

5   Victor Turner, *Dramas, Fields, and Metaphors: Symbolic Action in Human Society* (Ithaca and London: Cornell University Press, 1974), pp. 28–9.

metaphor: people talk about faces 'blossoming' and businesses 'bearing fruit' and marriages 'rotting' and so forth. Of course a culture and especially a large civilization may have more than one root metaphor, but some such metaphors are outstandingly persistent and pervasive. Sometimes they are clearly derived from the natural environment but more often they are what I have referred to above (following the philosopher of science Ernest Nagel) as 'hybrid' models – i.e. they are derived from a merger of experiences in a number of different domains.[6]

According to the reports of such scholars as Unschuld, Farquhar, Kleinman and others, one gathers that an important root metaphor in Chinese medicine – indeed, in Chinese civilization as a whole – is the idea of pattern. 'Far-flung and numberless move the Great Patterns, Returning in sequences that never cease', wrote the fourth-century Chinese poet Wang Shijy, quoted by Mark Elvin.[7] 'The parts and the whole together form a relationship, in which they oppose one another, yet at the same time constitute a homogenous entity. If there are no parts there is also no whole, and if there is no whole there are also no parts', wrote a Maoist medical theoretician cited by Unschuld (p. 256). 'Chinese scientific and philosophical discourses have been characterized by forms of holistic participation in which no isolated observer standpoint has been fostered,' writes Judith Farquhar,[8] arguing that an order of dynamic relationships between knowledge and practice and among different forms of knowledge and practice characterize Chinese as opposed to Western medicine. Throughout her article, Farquhar stresses relationship as essential to the holistic quality of Chinese medical thought. Arthur Kleinman likewise employs such terms as 'pattern', 'holistic' and 'interrelationship' to capture in words the order of the medical scene he witnessed in Taipei.[9]

What do Unschuld, Farquhar, Elvin and Kleinman – all of them careful analysts who choose their words carefully – mean by such terms? The image that comes to my mind as I read their descriptions is the image of an elaborately designed rug or tapestry. Such a tapestry is a total picture: it does not make sense if you look at just pieces of it; to

[6]   Ernest Nagel, *The Structure of Science: Problems in the Logic of Scientific Explanation* (New York: Harcourt, Brace and World, Inc., 1961).

[7]   Mark Elvin, 'Between the Earth and Heaven: Conceptions of the Self in China', in Michael Carrithers, Steven Collins, and Steven Lukes (eds.), *The Category of the Person: Anthropology, Philosophy, and History* (Cambridge: Cambridge University Press, 1985), pp. 156–89, esp. p. 163.

[8]   Judith Farquhar, 'Problems of Knowledge in Contemporary Chinese Medical Discourse', *Social Science and Medicine*, vol. 24, no. 12 (1987), 1013–21. Quote cited on p. 1015.

[9]   Arthur Kleinman, *Patients and Healers in the Context of Culture* (Berkeley: University of California Press, 1980).

comprehend it, you have to look at the whole thing at once. Perhaps the most accurate term for such an image is 'Gestalt' – like a human being's face or like a constellation of stars, it is something that is apprehended in its totality, all at once, or not at all. Chinese written characters are total pictures in this sense: they are not like English written words which you can spell out letter by letter, they are constructed upon stylized pictures of things, such as a tree, or a man standing under a roof. A single brushstroke by itself means nothing (unlike a single English letter, which does mean a particular sound). A Chinese character is a visual image whose meaning is related in some way to the meaning of the word it denotes.

In the same way, the Chinese body, Unschuld et al. tell us, is apprehended as a totality. You cannot just look at the hand or the appendix and if something is wrong with it fix it and ignore the other parts. You must perceive the whole thing as a system of relationships, where disease consists of disarrangement or disruption of the pattern, and treatment is proper rearrangement of the relationships so that they form an orderly pattern once again. Similarly, the Confucian kingdom was conceived as an orderly pattern of relationships: father to son, ruler to subject, and so forth. Disruption of one or more of these relationships led to disruption of the kingdom as a whole. The landscape, meanwhile, seems to have been imagined as something which, if it could not all be seen at once, could at least be visualized in the imagination as a single picture. The *Huang-ti nei-ching* at several places describes the symmetry of the empire by referring to the complementary attributes of the four cardinal regions (east, west, north and south) in turn: thus uniting the whole conceptually into a balanced totality.

The notion of the body/kingdom as a whole bound together by patterned relations was strengthened, as we have seen, by the notion of vessels running through from one end to the other, like the warp and woof of a tapestry. It was further strengthened by the concept of uniformity: the same pattern repeated throughout the whole tapestry, the same rules followed by all who occupied certain roles and entered into certain relations with others. In government, this concept materialized in the form of standardized weights and measures used throughout the whole empire, bureaucratic officials who were granted offices throughout the empire on the basis of certain standardized tests they had to pass, massive public works projects – such as the Grand Canal and the capital city of the Ch'in Empire – that were planned in whole in advance, and laws rendering all public officials solely and directly responsible to the central government instead of to local feudal lords (Unschuld, p. 63).

The holistic Confucian images of kingdom and of body were what Pierre Bourdieu would call totalizing visions.[10] Michel Foucault notes the intimate connection between vision and control in European medico-political thought.[11] Both Bourdieu and Foucault underline the point that neither a holistic philosophy nor an all-encompassing gaze is necessarily always benign. With a strengthening of the whole often comes disempowerment of the parts. When the parts are individual human beings, this can be a problem. Similarly, one man's all-embracing vision can be another's loss of autonomy. Thus, we should be careful not to be blinded by the beauty of the concepts of harmony and pattern. In practice, they do have their costs.

In India, in the Brahmanic thought of Āyurveda and Dharmashastra, another kind of holism prevailed. In the world view of these texts we find all things conjoined, not by patterns of relations, but rather by processes of generation. Whereas in Chinese medicine, events at different sites on the body are considered to be linked by reason of their places in the pattern, in Indian medicine different events in the body are considered to be linked by reason of their origins. Thus, while Chinese medical and social theory are dominated by patterns and configurations, Indian medical and social theory are dominated by derivations and births.

In the Āyurvedic medical texts, one indication we have that the process of birth was of great interest to the compilers is the amount of attention they devote to theories and descriptions of embryogenesis. In *Caraka Samhita* the entire section entitled 'Sarirasthanam', 'Section on the Body', is really about how the body comes into being. There is a discussion of the migration of the soul (*Purusa*, literally 'The Man') into the womb where a body will grow around it until it is ready to be born; a set of precise instructions for the conception of a high-quality child; instructions for prenatal and postnatal care of mother and child; a discussion of the contributions to the foetus of the father and the mother, respectively; an argument over which organs develop first in the growing embryo; and so forth.

Not only is the process of birth itself the subject of considerable discussion and speculation, but this process forms the theoretical template for many other bodily processes. The psychological apparatus of the human body as well as the set of constructive substances are described in the Āyurvedic texts as emerging via a set of generative

10   Pierre Bourdieu, *Outline of a Theory of Practice*, trans. Richard Nice (Cambridge: Cambridge University Press, 1985).
11   Michel Foucault, *The Birth of the Clinic: An Archaeology of Medical Perception*, trans. A.M. Sheridan Smith (New York: Random House, 1985).

processes. The mental faculties are constituted as a lineage is con-stituted; so also are the constructive substances.

According to the Samkhya school of philosophy upon which Āyurveda is founded, the human person consists of two components: Purusa ('The Man' or soul) and Prakrti (matter, literally 'she out of whom it is made'). When the soul or Purusa enters the womb, it becomes involved in matter, or Prakrti. Then a series of births take place. From Prakrti is born mahat ('the great one'), also called buddhi ('intelligence'). From mahat is born *ahamkara*, 'the sense of self' or 'ego'. From ahamkara is born *manas* or 'mind'. From manas are born the five *tanmatras* or 'subtle elements' (sound, light, smell, taste, and touch). From these are born the five *bhutas* or 'gross elements' (space, air, fire, water and earth). From these are born the five *jnananendriyas* or 'sense organs' (ears, eyes, etc.) and the five *karmendriyas* or 'organs of action' (hands, feet, etc.). Through this series of generations, the psychological apparatus – the machinery of the body through which the soul knows the world and acts upon it – becomes complete. In Yogic meditation, the whole process is reversed, and the Purusa or soul becomes liberated from Prakrti or matter, as it was in the beginning before the soul (blindly and foolishly, so it would seem) was attracted to the womb, entered there, and became embodied.

The constructive substances (dhatus) of the body are created by means of a similar series of generative processes. From the food in the stomach, blood is derived, with faeces as a waste product. From blood, flesh is derived, with urine as a waste product. From flesh, fat is derived, with perspiration as a waste product. From fat, bone is derived; from bone, marrow is derived; and from marrow, semen is derived. At each derivation, a waste product is emitted, and each derivative substance is considered purer and 'harder' than its precursor. Thus through seven generations or derivations, the seven constructive substances of the body are formed. Once again, as with the liberation of the soul from the body, we find the derivation of a pure male essence from its mixed female substrate.

The root metaphor of birth and the associated interest in origins, generations, derivations, and purifications may be found not only in the Āyurvedic texts but also in Dharmashastra, the texts describing ideals of human society and behaviour that were compiled in northern India around the same time that the Āyurvedic texts were compiled. The most famous of the Dharmashastric texts, *Manavadharmashastra* ('The Laws of Manu'), is concerned with explaining the origin and proper ranking of the kin-based social groupings which had proliferated in India by the time the book was written, about 2000 years ago, and which are still active today.

This system of social groupings is known to most English-speakers as 'the caste system'. Every living thing in India belongs to a caste, or *jati*. The word jati means 'birth group'. The jati that a person or animal or plant belongs to is the jati of its parents. So a cub born to a tiger belongs to the jati of tigers, a plant grown from a millet seed belongs to the jati of millet, and a person born to a leather worker belongs to the jati of leather workers. Every human jati has a particular function or job to perform. This job is the dharma of that jati. Every jati is endogamous – i.e. one should marry only a person belonging to the same jati as oneself.

Furthermore, all the jatis are ranked, from the highest to the lowest, in accordance with how close they are considered to be to the gods (and also, in real life, in accordance with how much wealth and power they have). Brahmans, the literati, were ranked highest in the Dharmashastric texts because Brahmans were the people who – being born to the priestly and verbal arts – best knew how to communicate with the gods (and also because Brahmans wrote the Dharmashastras!). In many kingdoms, the jati system was organized around the king, who was treated as a kind of god. The same rituals that are performed for gods in modern Hindu temples were once performed for Hindu kings in their palaces.

The king in his kingdom was considered to be like the soul in the body. 'As the souls of living creatures are tormented by tormenting their bodies, even so the lives of kings are destroyed by oppressing their kingdoms', writes Manu, author of the *Manavadharmashastra* (VII, 112). Caraka also writes, 'Like the lord of a city in the affairs of his city, so should a wise man be ever vigilant in the care of his own body' (Car. I, IV, 105). In the philosophical text *Samkhya-karika* we find, 'Since the intelligence with the other two internal organs [ego and mind] advert to all objects of sense, these three are said to be the warders [of the city], and the others [the organs of sense and action] are said to be the gatekeepers.'[12] The metaphor used here is again that of the city, where the soul (Purusa) is the king, and the three internal psychological organs are his ministers, for they act on his behalf and are closer to him than the others. The king, like the soul, stands at the head of an outgoing hierarchy of agents of command and an incoming hierarchy of agents of information. He receives information and materials from his villages through a set of intermediaries, and, similarly, distributes wealth and gives orders (M. VII, 115–18).

Manu divides human social groups into four classes or *varnas* ('colours'). He says that these four varnas are as they are because they were born from different parts of the body of the original creator, called (like the soul) Purusa, 'The Man'. Brahmans were born first and came out of the mouth of The Man. *Kshatriyas* (warriors) were born next and

---

[12]   Gaudapada, *The Samkya-Karika of Iswara Krishna with the Commentary of Gaudapada*, trans. Henry Thomas Colebrook (Bombay: Tookaram Tatya, 1887).

came out of The Man's arms. *Vaishyas* (farmers and merchants) were born next, out of the thighs of The Man; and *Shudras* (servants) were born last, out of The Man's feet.

Both the social groups of the Hindu kingdom and the constructive elements of the Āyurvedic body are ranked not only according to how close they are to The Man (king/creator/soul), but also according to how pure or free of dirt they are. The lowest of the constructive elements of the body, food in the belly, has all kinds of dirt mixed in it. The next element, blood, has had some of this dirt removed. The next element, flesh, has had more dirt removed, and so forth, until one comes to the purest element of all, which is semen. In the same way, high-caste Hindu men who have undergone initiation are called 'twice-born' (*dvija*) because through their initiation they have been purified of the ignorance beclouding the minds of ordinary people. Birth, in short, is a kind of purification, a derivation of the purer from the less pure, and all the different substances and organs of the body as well as all the different kinds of people in the world became differentiated from each other through such processes of birth, derivation, and purification. So say the texts of Āyurveda and Dharmashastra.

Just as the Chinese root metaphor of pattern is displayed in its system of writing, so the Brahmanic root metaphors of purification and origination are displayed in the ideas held about language by people of Caraka's time. The Sanskrit language was the *lingua franca* of Hindu literati until the British took over India and the English language became the language of power. Sanskrit is an old language: the earliest written texts composed in India were composed in Sanskrit. These texts are the Vedas, the sacred texts of Brahmanism. By the beginning of the first millennium AD, Sanskrit was no longer anybody's native language; the spoken vernaculars had all evolved in their own directions. Sanskrit, however, remained the sacred language. It was called, for that reason, 'the language of the gods'. The name Sanskrit literally means 'purified' or 'refined' or 'perfected'. All other languages were considered inferior to Sanskrit; they were thought to be corrupt and impure, and they were called Prakrits, a term related to the Āyurvedic word for body, Prakriti. Vernacular languages were 'derived' in a negative sense.

Conclusion

The choice of the term 'literate' to characterize the epistemologies under discussion in this volume implies the existence of 'non-literate' epistemologies also. Nagarjuna, the Madhyamika Buddhist logician and physician, discusses the nature of such implication at length, so I will not go into it here. Suffice it to say that 'discursive thought', as it is called in early Buddhist texts, is founded upon delusions concerning what is and what is not. Discursive thought is words running through our heads. This inner discourse must be silenced, Buddhists say, if true vision is to find a place in consciousness. I invoke Buddhism because its influence upon both Chinese and Indian medico-religious thought is well documented. Had I been granted more word-space here (how ironic!) I would argue that the textualization of medical knowledge throughout Eurasia exacerbated the obstructions placed by discursive thought in the way of medical vision. Foucault, if I may again mention him, surely supports what I try to say here, by way of his silence concerning non-text-based medical traditions, and his verbosity in respect of medical texts. For nineteenth-century French pathologists, Foucault would have us believe (and I believe him), the body was a book. For present-day Euro-American academicians such as ourselves, this same metaphoric conflation of body with text remains in effect.

But non-text-based forms of medical knowledge also continue to thrive, trance-healing being the most prominent among them. These extraliterate epistemologies, though barely acknowledged, have always informed the literate ones. Perhaps it is just as well that we not write too much about the unwritten, but from time to time stop the flow of words, and silently heed the unwritten as closely as possible. East and South Asian medical thinkers long ago chose this strategy, and many follow it still. Perhaps Western medical thinkers will learn in the next millennium to do so, too. With these words of cautious hope, I end my essay.

[13] ' "It is" is a notion of eternity. "It is not" is a nihilistic view. Therefore one who is wise does not have recourse to "being" or "non-being".' Nagarjuna, *Mulamadhyamikakarikas*, chapter XV, verse 10, translated in Frederick J. Streng, *Emptiness: a Study in Religious Meaning* (Nashville: Abingdon Press, 1967). Nagarjuna is said to have lived during the first century AD.

ABBREVIATIONS

Car.   *Caraka Samhita.* English translation: *Caraka Samhita,* Shree Gulabkunverba Āyurvedic Society (Jamnagar, India, 1949)

M   *Manavadharmashastra.* English translation: *Manu, The Laws of Manu,* trans. George Buhler (Oxford: Clarendon Press, 1886)

Su   *Susruta-Samhita.* English translation: *Susruta, Susruta Samhita,* trans. and ed. Bhishagratna (Calcutta, 1907)

14   The scholar, the wise man, and universals: three aspects of Āyurvedic medicine

Francis Zimmermann

Our approach in this volume is both epistemological and comparative. We are raising two types of questions. Since we are historians working on textual sources written in different languages, we are first of all engaging in comparisons, and raising questions about the validity of a comparative approach to classical medicine: 'What are the relevant intellectual parallels and the possible historical connections between, for example, Āyurvedic medicine in India and Galenism in the West?' This contribution to the debate is based on the historical evidence we have of extensive intellectual exchanges between India and the West in the first centuries of the common era. Although the detailed evidence must be kept in the background, the following pages will expose two features that relate Āyurveda with Galenism. The first section, which deals with stylistic and rhetorical features of medical Sanskrit texts, will describe an Indian version of scholasticism, comparable on many points with medical Galenism. Another feature common to both scholarly traditions is humoralism. But a comparative study of the humoral theory is dependent upon a second type of question that bears upon the ways knowledge is established and put into practice: 'What are the criteria for regarding a given aetiology, diagnosis, or prognosis as valid in Āyurvedic medicine, or any other scholarly tradition for that matter, and, in therapeutics, what are the criteria for efficacy?' I shall first address the question of knowledge and experience in the context of a classical tradition, emphasizing the role of language. Then, pursuing one concrete example, the aetiology and therapeutics of epilepsy, I expound some key concepts of Āyurveda that revolve around the themes of rationality, truth and efficacy. Classical medicine, since its practical value is based on confidence, is *wisdom* as much as *scholarship*. The title of this essay aims to characterize the three different faces of an Āyurvedic physician: the scholar, the wise man and, so to speak, the naturalist.

Clearly, the Indologist is at a disadvantage in comparative studies, due to the drawbacks of Sanskrit philology and the lack of appropriate translations. We can only test the ground, and we must keep textual references to a minimum, because we have to provide our own translations, and to retrieve concordances from our own personal files. Therefore, I shall here concentrate upon a well-documented sample of the classical doctrine of Āyurvedic medicine on which I am currently working, the place of passion as a malady in Āyurvedic medicine. The portions of the classical system that are directly relevant to the theme of passion revolve around the aetiology of seizures and madness. Psychical disorders are divided into two main categories, deliriums (*unmāda*) and convulsions (*apasmāra*). Epilepsy is the prototype of convulsions, and I have selected one very short passage from the *Carakasaṃhitā* expounding the aetiology of epilepsy, upon which to base our reflections.[1] A most striking feature of this scholarly tradition is the multi-perspectivalism of Āyurvedic concepts like apasmara,[2] a syndrome within which epilepsy is only one facet among many others, including hysteria, eclampsia, and so forth. Since the word *epilepsy* in Greek and Latin nosology carries the same complexities and represents a similar cluster of nosological entities, this example seems to be an appropriate touchstone for comparison. Sanskrit texts are much more coded and formulaic than the Greek and Latin. Indian pundits have resorted to all kinds of stylistic devices: the alternation of prose and verse, ellipsis and parallelism, listings of signs and names, metaphorical terms, the interplay of synonyms, circumlocution, and redundancy. These devices have been systematized in the form of *tantrayukti*s appended to the medical compendia, that is, 'combinatory rules' (*yukti*) to be applied in the interpretation of 'scientific texts' (*tantra*).[3] I can try to present only one or two examples of these figures of speech in this short essay, and I thought the presentation would be more consistent if they were all excerpted from the same text. We shall be digging, so to say, beneath the rhetorical surface of the Sanskrit text, in order to delineate in turn the

[1] *Carakasaṃhitā* by Agniveśa, revised by Caraka and Dṛḍhabala, *Āyurvedadīpikā* commentary by Cakrapāṇidatta, Jādavajī Trikaṃjī Ācārya (ed.), 3rd edn (Bombay: Nirnaya Sagar Press, 1941). The *Carakasaṃhitā*, 'Corpus of Caraka', is one of the most celebrated compendia of Āyurvedic medicine. The recension available nowadays in printed editions dates back to the beginning of the common era.

[2] Etymologically, *apasmāra* means 'the state of being off one's memory'. 'Epilepsy' is a conventional interpretation, warranted by the possible connections of Āyurveda with Galenism. On the multi-perspectivalism of Āyurvedic concepts, see Francis Zimmermann, *The Jungle and the Aroma of Meats. An Ecological Theme in Hindu Medicine* (Berkeley: University of California Press, 1987) and his *Le Discours des remèdes au pays des épices. Enquête sur la médecine hindoue* (Paris: Payot, 1989).

[3] A specific bibliography is to be found in Zimmermann (note 2, 1989), and the presentation of a few combinatory rules in F. Zimmermann, 'Terminological Problems in the Process of Editing and Translating Sanskrit Medical Texts', in Paul U. Unschuld (ed.), *Approaches to Traditional Chinese Medical Literature* (Dordrecht: Kluwer, 1989), pp. 141–51.

three layers of Āyurvedic knowledge: (1) the scholarly tradition as a text, (2) the medical praxis as wisdom, and (3) the rationalistic pursuit of knowledge which comes close to natural history.

At each of the three levels, I shall focus on epilepsy, which reflects upon the mixture of rationalism and 'folk', or 'mystic', or magic views on possession and demons in ancient medicine. This is precisely the gist of my argument: I would like to show that Āyurvedic medicine is neither a folklore nor a mystique.

The scholarly tradition as a text

There is a fundamental ambiguity in the word 'scholarly', when applied to ancient medicine. Whenever we emphasize the Great Divide between 'scholarship' and 'science', whenever we call Galenic medicine, or Āyurveda for that matter, a 'scholarly medical tradition' in the narrow sense of the phrase, we implicitly deny it any scientificity, and we have to bear the burden of the proof, we have to justify this implicit distinction between scholarship and science. It is this presupposition, firmly established in the dominant paradigm of Western epistemology, which we may want to question.

The following pages aim to show that it is not enough to describe Āyurvedic medicine as a scholarly tradition. It is much more than that; it is a rationalistic pursuit of knowledge, synthesizing important observations on culture-bound realities of physiology, disease and environment. Where exactly should we draw the demarcation line between scholarly and scientific knowledge? We can find elements of an answer to this question in the Āyurvedic doctrine itself, which combines two paradigms of knowledge, namely, textual studies and diagnosis. Let us first concentrate upon this definition of ancient science as made up of 'classical texts'. When we say the Āyurvedic physician is a scholar, we mean he[4] is the student of a literate tradition laid down in authoritative texts called *śāstra*, 'the Texts'.

We used to conceive of India, Hinduism and the Sanskrit texts as constituting a culture. Insofar as each culture is free to define its heritage in its own terms, we cannot but accept the characterization of Āyurvedic medicine that is offered in India itself. To an English-speaking Indian practitioner, sastra means 'science', and Āyurveda is a 'science', that is, part of the scientific tradition of India, just as 'allopathic medicine' (i.e., the one we, Westerners, call scientific) is part of the scientific tradition of the West. There is an ambiguity in this formulation which merges

---

[4] I am using 'he' advisedly, because, in principle, there are no female pundits, and consequently no female physicians.

science with tradition. I shall address this ambiguity from a linguistic point of view.

In India with Sanskrit, as in the West with Latin, science evolved in a linguistic situation of *diglossia*: a learned language was superimposed upon the vernaculars. By focusing upon diglossia, we shall be able to examine the place of textual sources and textual authorities in medical practice.

The Āyurvedic physician speaks to patients in the vernacular, but he quotes Sanskrit phrases extensively, and furthermore, he devises diagnoses and therapeutic schemes in Sanskrit. Sanskrit still is an ethnographic reality in India, as Latin was in Europe down to the turn of this century. Both learned languages used to be spoken in a situation of diglossia whenever the classic texts provided the canvas of conversation.

This is the case, for example, in specific medical contexts where humoral explanations are resorted to. In India, as in the West, scholarly medical traditions have revolved around the theory of humours. Humoralism, however, is a mode of thought more than a theory; the dialectic of the humours entails a rhetoric intertwining passion with malady.

Here we must keep our distance from medical anthropologists working on what they improperly call humoralism, and we must emphasize the indissoluble link between humoralism and classical rhetoric. Anthropologists collecting data on the folk classification of everything into categories of hot and cold have tended to assimilate this 'Hot–Cold Syndrome' to humoralism. This is most misleading, and I shall try to show that the scientific tradition of humoralism clearly separates itself from folklore. The learned language precisely is the instrument of this distancing. The Āyurvedic physician is a professional trained by a teacher. Nothing is seen with the eyes which has not been said in the texts. I shall try to describe the connection, from the classic texts to the practice of diagnosis, in the case of epilepsy. The sample text translated below is self-contained and will be cited in full, to convey the flavour of Sanskrit rhetoric.[5]

[1] We shall now expound *The Aetiology of Epilepsy*
[2] as propounded by Lord Ātreya.
[3] There are four types of epilepsy respectively caused by wind, bile, phlegm or the conjunction of the three.
[4] Epilepsy arises quickly in the following types of predisposed living beings:
– when the mind is hurt [or seized] by *rajas* and *tamas* [the two mental humours],
– when the humours are agitated, abnormal, overabundant,

---

[5]   *Carakasamhitā*, 'Nidānasthāna', chapter 8, sections 1–15. Numbers follow the printed edition. I have attempted a literal translation, but I felt it necessary to add a few glosses in parenthesis.

– when one takes food that is impure [*aśuci*], or prepared from unwholesome or damaged ingredients, and observes dietetic rules improperly [*vaiṣamyayuktena*],
– when one practises unwholesome Yoga techniques and other bodily postures,

then, the humours, unsettled, in those whose mind is hurt by rajas and tamas, spread over the heart, this most excellent abode of the inner self, and settle there as well as in the sense organs. The humours staying there, when excited by desire, anger, fear, bewilderment (*moha*), exhilaration, grief, anxiety, agitation, etc., suddenly overflow, and the patient falls a victim to epilepsy.
[5] Epilepsy is defined as an entrance into unconsciousness [tamas], an episode accompanied with loathsome gestures [vomiting of froth, convulsions] due to the ruin of memory, intellect and *sattva* [the purity component of mind].
[6] Its premonitory signs are the following:
throwing aside of eye-brows, constant abnormal movement of the eyes, hearing of non-existent sounds, excessive discharge of saliva and nasal mucus, lack of appetite, anorexia, indigestion, cardiac palpitation, distension of the abdomen [with borborygmus], debility, tearing pain in bones, body-ache, bewilderment [moha], vision of tamas [the murky depths of unconsciousness], swooning, giddiness, dreaming of being drunk, of dancing, of being pierced, of aching, shivering or falling. Epilepsy follows immediately.
[7] Specific features of each type of epilepsy.

Signs of epilepsy due to wind:
Repeated fits, instantly regaining consciousness, protruded eyes, violent vociferations, froth from the mouth, neck excessively swollen, puncturing pain in the head, fingers abnormally contracted, hands and feet constantly moving, the nails, eyes, face and skin are red, rough and blackish, vision of unstable, fickle, coarse and dry objects, indisposition (*anupaśaya*) to windy substances and disposition (*upaśaya*) to their contraries.

Signs of epilepsy due to bile:
Repeated fits, instantly regaining consciousness, groaning sounds, one strikes the ground, the nails, eyes, face and skin are green, yellow and coppery, vision of things wet with blood and of bodies agitated, fierce, in flames, irritated, indisposition to bilious substances and disposition to their contraries.

Epilepsy due to phlegm:
Delayed fits, delayed recovery of consciousness, falling down, gestures not so abnormal, saliva from the mouth, the nails, eyes, face and skin are white, vision of white, heavy, unctuous objects, indisposition to phlegmy substances and disposition to their contraries.
The one due to the conjunction of the three humours combines all these signs; incurable.
[8] Such are the four types of epilepsy.
[9] Sometimes a sympathetic,[6] adventitious disorder comes along with them,

6   In ancient medicine, a *deuteropathy* is a secondary affection, *sympathetic* with or consequent upon another. The technical Sanskrit term for this is *anubandha*, 'sympathetic; sympathy, deuteropathy'. The same word means 'companion' in common parlance, and 'concomitance' in ancient logic.

which will be described later. Its particularities can be known from the predominance of its own signs over the signs described above, and from some sign indicating a non-humoral origin.

[10] Beneficial to epileptics are:
acrid (*tīkṣṇa*) substances, evacuants (*saṃśodhana*) and calmatives (*upaśamana*),[7] selected according to the patient's humoral condition, and magic formulas (*mantra*) when an adventitious disorder intervenes.

[11] In ancient times, during the destruction of Dakṣa's sacrifice,[8] while humans were fleeing in all directions, dropsy sprang from the agitation of their body due to their fleeing, swimming, running, jumping, leaping, etc.; diabetes and leprosy sprang from their eating ghee; madness [or delirium, unmada] sprang from fear, torture and grief; epilepsy [or convulsion, apasmara] from impure (asuci) contact with various creatures; fever from the forehead of Lord Siva; internal haemorrhage from the excessive heat of fever; and consumption sprang from Lord Candra's excessive indulgence in sex.

[12] Memorial verses[9] –
Epilepsy is due either to wind
or bile or phlegm
or the conjunction of the humours,
and this fourth is incurable.

[13] Wise physicians treat the curable ones
cautiously,
with acrid substances, evacuants
or calmatives according to the humoral condition.

[14] If an adventitious disorder
comes along with the humoral aetiology,
wise physicians will prescribe
the general treatment (both magic and humoral).

[15] One who knows the particularities of all diseases
and the properties of all medicines,
such a physician will cure all diseases
and will never fall into bewilderment.

My reasons for translating this passage in full stem from both its content and form. First, the disorders described under the name of epilepsy clearly go beyond the limits of humoral pathology and provide us with an example on which we can raise the issue of 'supernatural

---

7   Diets, evacuants and calmatives constitute a fixed set of three therapeutic methods. *Sodhana* and *samana* are often rendered as 'purifying' and 'pacifying' measures, following their etymology and common meaning in Sanskrit, but I would like to insist on their technical meaning in medical terminology, which is accurately rendered as 'evacuants' and 'calmatives' in technical English.

8   Celebrating a great sacrifice to obtain a son, Daksa omitted to invite Siva, who punished him by spoiling the sacrifice.

9   The following sections are composed in the *kārikā* style, that is, as summarizing and memorial distichs, each of them divided into four hemistichs. I am starting each hemistich on a new line, and references are alphanumerical: hemistich 15d means the fourth hemistich of section 15.

causes', and of the place of 'spiritual' realities like sattva (the purity component of mind) in an overall rationalistic system of thought. Then the mix of a humoral aetiology, references to Hindu mythology and a sententious conclusion in verse is quite indicative of the spirit of the system. Lastly, it is only through our reading lists of clinical signs like those given above that we become aware of the highly coded and abbreviated style of scholarly medical discourse.

Let us come back, for example, to the signs of epilepsy due to wind: 'Repeated fits, instantly regaining consciousness, protruded eyes ... the nails ... are red ... indisposition to windy substances ...' Clearly words are missing, and the sentence is grammatically disjointed; furthermore, the listing of clinical signs shifts from physical symptoms to abstract notions. These are medical notations jotted down, as it were, by clinicians in their files. Some time ago Jackie Pigeaud studied what he called 'l'écriture d'Hippocrate', that is, a set of figures of speech, first of all ellipsis, that were turned into scholarly techniques of information retrieval in the Hippocratic texts.[10] This sample of Sanskrit medical text exemplifies the same stylistic devices.

A common trope in Āyurvedic texts is the reduction of everything to a three-fold division, sometimes to a set of three plus one. This extract is patterned on this model. Four types of epilepsy are reckoned, because there is a closed set of three humours, 'wind, bile, phlegm', plus the conjunction of the three. The same scheme appears in section 10, which displays a closed set of three plus one, the three modes of therapy, 'diets, evacuants, calmatives', plus mantras or magic spells. But an epistemological interpretation of these kinds of texts cannot restrict itself to their rhetoric in the narrow sense of the word. Rhetoric, the conceited use of tropes, is a means of constructing a multi-faceted system of diagnosis. Whenever a given concept – here, the humours – presents a fixed number of facets, the diagnosis plays upon their various possible combinations.

The foregoing extract plays upon another closed set of three, the three strands of Nature, sattva (see section 5), rajas and tamas (see section 4). As already indicated, psychic disorders are divided broadly into deliriums (unmada) and convulsions (apasmara). Rajas, the principle of passionate activity and mania, is associated with deliriums, and tamas, the principle of stupor and collapse, is associated with convulsions. As a couple, they are defined elsewhere as 'the two mental humours'. Thus, tamas is the pathogenic principle responsible for epilepsy at large, and

---

[10] Jackie Pigeaud, 'Le Style d'Hippocrate ou l'écriture fondatrice de la médecine', in Marcel Détienne (ed.), Les Savoirs de l'écriture. En Grèce ancienne (Lille: Presses Universitaires de Lille, 1988), pp. 305–29.

there is a play on the various connotations of the word tamas all over this text (sections 4, 5 and 6): first darkness, then unconsciousness, then principle of stupor, a depressant humour which is the mental correlative of bile. From this example we can see that the trope of closed sets is combined with another figure of speech, named 'catachresis' in Western classical rhetoric,[11] in which a word is diverted from its proper meaning to be given a new, technical meaning. The medical concept of tamas is constructed by means of a series of catachresis. The word tamas itself undergoes successive shifts of meaning, through which descriptions (darkness, swooning) are replaced by explanations (a depressant humour which stupefies the patient).

Tamas (darkness, bewilderment) is to be contrasted with sattva (a principle of lucidity and serenity). The phrase 'memory, intellect and sattva' (section 5) denotes a closed set of three mental functions. When the three words are mentioned in a row, they constitute an implicit reference to the doctrine of the three functions of the mind, so that, in order to understand this extract fully, we must criss-cross it with other parts of the scholarly corpus. The scholar physician, for example, will cite the following verses:[12]

> When someone, whose application of mind is out of balance,
> mistakes the non-eternal for eternity, the unwholesome for
>   wholesomeness,
> one can say that his intellect is perturbed,
> because the intellect normally sees things in balance.
> When the sattva is infatuated with an object of the senses,
> owing to the perturbation of the will, it is impossible
> to keep away from the unwholesome object,
> because only the will has this power of restraint.
> When memory, in the reminiscence of true things, is perturbed,
> in someone whose self is blocked by rajas and bewilderment (moha),
> that is perturbation of memory, since
> the true things to be known through reminiscence reside in memory.

This is an elaborate philosophical statement and one can hardly imagine that a practitioner will bear all this in mind in the course of his routine consulting hours. But we are dealing here with the basic tenets of the scholarly tradition, and our approach to the classic texts comes closer to the pundit's than to the practitioner's attitude. The verses just

[11] See Pierre Fontanier's definition reproduced in Zimmermann (note 2, 1989), p. 135, and translated in Zimmermann (note 3), p. 146. This is not by any means a Western idea that is here being tacked onto the Indian texts, since catachresis has its own place among the *tantrayuktis* under the Sanskrit name of *svasaṃjñā*.

[12] *Carakasaṃhitā, Śārīrasthāna*, chapter 1, verses 99–101 (I am starting each hemistich on a new line).

quoted above have displayed the triad of mental functions, 'intellect, will, memory'. This is equivalent to the 'memory, intellect and sattva' set in the text on epilepsy (section 5).

The comparison gives a clue to the interpretation of the word sattva, which physicians borrowed from philosophy and theology where it first meant purity and spirituality. As a medical concept, it must be construed in the perspective of humoralism. Sattva, rajas and tamas, the three strands of Nature, when acclimatized to the medical domain, are conceived as fluids or energies that fill or besiege the heart, before being discharged into the channels of thought and sensibility. Sattva is a mental fluid, in medical parlance, although it is devoid of any negative connotation and cannot be called a humour. Sattva represents a measurable quantity of 'high spirits', so to speak, a measurable power of volition, will and fortitude of mind. As far as the word comes to be integrated into medical terminology, its meaning shifts from 'purity' and 'spirit' to 'lucidity' and 'will', which is exactly what I meant by catachresis. The word is the same, but the conceptual tenets are different. Thus it would not be fair to say that Āyurvedic medicine is deprived of its own First Principles.[13] On the contrary, I would like to suggest that it has always been a full-fledged, autonomous scientific tradition.

In comparing it to scholasticism, I have three specific features in mind: (1) the central position of language and rhetoric not only in the Sanskrit texts but also in practice, (2) the pundit-like profile of the practitioner who comments and debates upon the classic texts, and (3) the philosophical and theological spirit of the classic texts, in which medical arguments are co-ordinated with philosophical and theological themes. This raises the question of the status of experience, of the relationship of texts to practice, and of the place of medicine in the division of sciences. The foregoing comments on diglossia and figures of speech have partly addressed these issues. We must skip further remarks on the construction of experience. An allusion was made already to the brahminic statement according to which nothing can be 'seen' that has not first been 'said' by an authority. Perception is shaped by the word of a teacher citing authoritative texts; this is the way experience is constructed. But we shall now focus on the relationship of medicine to philosophy and theology. Another fundamental catachresis will make a suitable transition to the second part of this essay.

[13] In the course of our debates in Montreal, Professor Amos Funkenstein argued that medicine, in the mind of some medieval scholars in the West, was not a full-fledged science but only a *scientia media*, deprived of its own 'first principles'. Be that as it may in Europe, Āyurveda in India did enjoy a much higher epistemological status.

In the text just mentioned above, the ruin of memory was described as a blockage, of the atman, or self, 'by rajas and bewilderment (moha)'. Moha is obviously here a synonym for tamas. The two mental humours, rajas and tamas (or moha), have blocked or besieged the self, or soul or atman, in the heart or cardiac orifice of the stomach, which is the physiological abode of mental functions. Let us now come back to the text on epilepsy. The word moha, rendered as 'bewilderment', appears in sections 4 and 6 where it means exactly 'coma', a pathological condition, an accident, a symptom. But when it appears again in section 15 (hemistich 15d), it denotes a moral and philosophical principle, bewilderment as illusion, the opposite of wisdom.

Medical praxis as wisdom

That humans fall victims to cosmic illusion is one of the tenets of religious Hinduism, and the Āyurvedic doctor does partake of this cosmology. Medical scholarship is rooted in the culture at large and Indian scholars are, so to say, continuists. Their presupposition is that there exists a continuity from cosmology to learned practice to folklore. Take, for example, the basic ideas of humoralism. There is a cosmic dualism of the Sun and the Moon, underlying the dialectic of bile and phlegm in medicine, and again the hot–cold syndrome in popular belief. Westerners are prone to take this continuity for granted, although it is actually sheer ideology. In today's collective sensibility, Āyurvedic medicine, an oriental learned tradition of healing and well-being, is associated with holism, mysticism, environmental activism, anti-science populism and other romantic or postmodern mottos.

This is a deplorable misunderstanding, prompted by the ambiguities of Sanskrit rhetoric. If we study only the texts without relating them to practice, the texts seem to fall squarely within the realm of the religious Hinduistic tradition. Therefore, we must break the glassy surface of their rhetoric and reach for the traces of medical observations and practice. The way tamas (unconsciousness) and moha (bewilderment) are described offers an appropriate example for such an analysis.

So, let us come back to the two passages where tamas or moha, conceived as fluids, are said to block or besiege the heart. Two readings are possible, a physiological and a moral reading. In physiological terms, some fluids or spirits of a phlegmatic nature, cold and wet, producing drowsiness and stupor, are blocking the channels of thought and sensibility that originate in the heart or cardiac orifice of the stomach. (The functional ambiguity regarding these two regions is the same in India as in Greece.) In moral terms, illusion, allurement or passion is besieging the soul, and 'the heart' then denotes the ontological centre of the human person. The Āyurvedic physician acknowledges the validity of the two readings, although they do not bear the same relation to practice. Insofar as a given case of epilepsy can be explained in physiological terms, as an epilepsy due to unbalanced humours, it will be treated by acrid foods, evacuants and compound medicines of the kind we shall describe in the third part of this essay. However, when epilepsy cannot be explained by natural causes, it is labelled as adventitious. Adventitious maladies are said to be inflicted by the gods and demons, and the physician will refer his patient to an exorcist, a *mantravādin* (see sections 10 and 14 in the text above). But the physician will also disclaim all responsibility for the religious and mystical beliefs underlying this course of action, by invoking a principle of human responsibility:[14]

[a] Neither the gods nor the Gandharvas
[b] nor the Pisacas nor the Raksasas
[c] nor any other demons will ever afflict a human
[d] who has not first afflicted himself.
[a] When they go after someone
[b] already afflicted by his own misdeeds,
[c] obviously that affliction is not caused by them,
[d] since deeds already done are no longer to be done.
[a] When a disease is produced by a breach of wisdom,
[b] born from one's misdeeds, inflicted by oneself,
[c] the wise man should not blame
[d] the gods, ancestors or demons.

The key concept is that of 'breaches of wisdom' (*prajñāparādha*), which are one of the three causes of disease. This is one of the most essential doctrines of Āyurvedic medicine, and it should not be dulled or flattened. It is sometimes interpreted in a pragmatic perspective, and 'breaches of wisdom' are then equated with 'errors' or 'mistakes' in behaviour and diet, as if only menial things were at stake. On the contrary, I think that we should acknowledge its philosophical and metaphysical tenor. It is a principle of human responsibility, which has close parallels and possible connections with the Stoic philosophy of action in the West. '(1) The inappropriate conjunction of the sense organs with their objects, (2) a breach of wisdom, and (3) the maturation of time: here are the three causes of disease.'[15] An important epistemological question is whether these three causes are operating jointly, each

---

[14] *Carakasaṃhitā, Nidānasthāna*, chapter 7, verses 19–21.
[15] *Carakasaṃhitā, Sūtrasthāna*, chapter 11, section 43; the same phrase recurs dozens of times in the classic texts. An occurrence close to the text cited above (note 12) is in *Carakasaṃhitā, Śārīrasthāna*, chapter 1, verse 98.

and every disease having three causes, or separately, some diseases being due to inappropriateness, others due to a breach of wisdom, and the rest due to the maturation of time. We have some good reasons to think that Āyurvedic doctors will take it both ways according to the context. I shall restrict myself here to the second interpretation, because it suits the example on which this presentation is based, and I deem that humoral cases of epilepsy are due to the patient's inappropriate connections with the sensible world, while adventitious epilepsy is due to a breach of wisdom.

Medical truth, as we shall see now, is a matter of subjectivity. The causality of disease is not to be found inscribed in the cut-and-dried, objective facts of biology; it is grasped through the subjective experience of clinical symptoms, just as the efficacy of a given therapy is assessed through the subjective experience of an improvement. (I situate the debate here, of course, outside the realm of modern, positivistic biomedicine). Therefore, the ambiguity of catachresis mentioned earlier on the level of language will be met again on the level of principles, namely, the implicit substitution of reasons or causes for an initial observation, in the course of a medical argument. The status of the three mental functions in the description of epilepsy is an example of this ambiguity. A breach of wisdom is a misdeed resulting from the perturbation of intellect, will and memory:[16]

> An impure (or shameful) deed
> committed by someone whose intellect, will, memory are perturbed:
> this is what is known as breach of wisdom;
> it provokes all the three humours.

Thus, the perturbation of intellect, will and memory is the cause of a disease. But in section 5 of the text on epilepsy, the very same perturbation was reckoned among the symptoms of the disease: 'An entrance into unconsciousness ... accompanied with loathsome gestures due to the ruin of memory, intellect and sattva' (which means will, as we have seen). We are engaged in a circular argument, as it were. The impairment of intellect, will and memory, the three mental functions, is, in turn, the cause and the symptom. A moral cause and a psychological symptom, since, as a cause, it is defined as a misdeed and a breach of wisdom, while, as a symptom, it is described as the ruin of mental functions. Similarly, moha, 'bewilderment', as we have already mentioned, is in turn a symptom, when it means a beclouding of the mental functions, and a cause, when it is equated to tamas, a depressant humour which blocks the channels of thought and sensibility. The

[16] *Carakasaṃhitā, Śārīrasthāna*, chapter 1, verse 102.

diagnosis goes to and fro between the subjectivity of illness experience and the objectivity of causal inferences.

The circularity of cause and symptom is explicitly recognized in Āyurvedic medicine. Diseases are, in turn, causes and symptoms of one another. There is a relationship of mutual entailment – the technical name for it is *anubandha* in Sanskrit and 'sympathy' in English – which connects one disease to the next in a chain. This is explicated in the *Book of Questions Relative to the Body*:[17]

[a] The chain of sympathetic (anubandha) maladies
[b] [which bring about one another] can be broken only by
[c] a regimen of life that respects the reasons for well-being,
[d] and then only will well-being come forth.
[a] Humours in balance do not go to imbalance without reason,
[b] unbalanced ones are not restored to balance without reason,
[c] bodily humours always evolve
[d] in accordance with due reasons.
[a] It is by paying this principle of reason (yukti)
[b] the utmost attention, that the physician cures
[c] all maladies, past, present and future.
[d] But the definitive cure is by eliminating allurement (*upadhā*).
[a] For, allurement is the ultimate cause
[b] of maladies and of the body, receptacle for maladies,
[c] and the repudiation of all allurements
[d] eliminates all maladies.

In other words, medical thought and practice are based on a consistent system of first principles evolving from one another: illusion (upadha) is the root cause of diseases; diseases are diagnosed according to a principle of rationality (yukti); which helps deconstruct the chain of sympathetic (anubandha) diseases. Let us recall the last few words of the text on epilepsy, which remained somewhat obscure at first reading. The competent physician is one 'who will never fall into bewilderment'. This now makes sense in the light of what we learnt of 'allurement'. Bewilderment and allurement are names for the concept of cosmic illusion in religious Hinduism. Illusion is the root cause of reincarnation, and of misdeeds that will produce maladies in later lives. The Āyurvedic physician must address himself to this metaphysical dimension of disease and healing. However, he always proceeds according to a 'principle of reason' (yukti), which says that there is no erratic event in the physiological and medical domains. Bodily humours always evolve rationally. There is always a reason, a rational causality, to all changes observed in humoral physiology.

[17] *Carakasaṃhitā, Śārīrasthāna,* chapter 1, verses 92–5.

This principle of reason calls for a few comments. Yukti, in the foregoing text, means (the art of making) rational conjunctions. In other words, it is the art of diagnosis, logical inferences based on a realistic and rationalistic conception of causality. 'Humours in balance do not go to imbalance *without reason*', that is, without an assignable cause. This statement is directed at the Buddhists. The Buddhist doctrine of momentariness, according to which all links of causality are sheer illusions, allows for the definition of meditation and ascesis as a religious path to healing. But there is no such dispassionate idealism in Āyurvedic medicine. The physician is a man of action, who actively manipulates the network of causes and clinical signs which constitute 'the chain of sympathetic diseases'. We saw that yukti commonly means 'a rule'; to proceed *yuktyā* means to proceed 'according to the rule'. It also means 'a conjunctive proposition',[18] establishing the 'conjunction', or 'conjuncture', of factors or events. Then, it means 'reason', or 'rationality', as opposed to *daiva*, 'destiny', or 'the supernatural'. Physicians make inductions by observing, for a given disease, the alternation of fits and relapses through time: this is rationality. Now let us come back to the example of epilepsy. In India as in Greece, epilepsy is a malady that goes far beyond the boundaries of humoral determinism. The 'sympathetic, adventitious' forms of epilepsy (section 9 in the above text) are sacred diseases. Āyurvedic doctors will say that they escape the reach of yukti (rationality) and belong with seizures and passions in the realm of daiva (destiny). It is just because doctors make this epistemological distinction, that their art is both a wisdom and a science.

The question of universals

In describing one of the common tropes of Āyurvedic discourse, which consists in reducing the whole world to a number of closed sets of items, we touched upon a basic feature of the scholarly tradition which will now be elaborated further. This is a pattern of thought somewhat akin to the Chinese system of correspondences. An accurate formulation of the correspondence concept has already been given above, in section 7 of the text on epilepsy. For each and every type of humoral epilepsy, that is, epilepsy due to wind, or bile, or phlegm, one of the clinical signs to be taken into account was 'indisposition to [respectively] windy ... bilious

[18] A book in preparation will explore the parallels and probable conceptual exchanges between Indian and Stoic logic. We are touching upon such parallels, here, between *anubandha* (companionship) and Greek *akolouthia*, or else, between *yukti* (conjunctive proposition) and Greek *sumpeplegmenon*.

... phlegmy substances, and disposition to their [respective] contraries'. At first sight, this phrase is to be understood in a Galenic sense, as an Āyurvedic equivalent to the well-known Latin phrase, *contraria contrariis curantur*, contraries are cured by contraries. It indicates which kinds of medicines are appropriate for a given case.

Phlegmatic epilepsy, for example, is aggravated by phlegmatic substances, and cured by their contraries, namely acrid substances (see the first word of section 10). Disposition to contraries means the mutual compensation of contraries. However, the mention of indisposition and disposition to foods and drugs amounts to saying that the good or bad effects of a medicine on a given disease are part of the diagnosis of that disease. Clinical observations made on unfavourable and favourable responses to medicines constitute, so to say, a therapeutic diagnosis. In other words, therapeutics is encompassed within aetiology, and vice versa. This relationship of mutual implication between aetiology and therapeutics is formalized both in the composition of the compendia and in the formulas of compound medicines. I would like to expose this particular pattern of thought.

The *Book of Aetiology* (*Nidānasthāna*) and the *Book of Therapeutics* (*Cikitsāsthāna*) are symmetrical in all compendia. Thus, the chapter on the aetiology of fever, or haemorrhage, or epilepsy, etc., announces a corresponding chapter on the therapeutics of fever, or haemorrhage, or epilepsy, etc. Semeiotics (rules for the interpretation of symptoms), which is treated in full in the Aetiology chapter, is repeated in concise form in the Therapeutics one. Furthermore, Therapeutics is essentially comprised of a formulary of compound medicines. Recipes often are very long and complicated, but their structure is always the same: a first part gives the list of ingredients with directions for processing them, and a second part gives the indications of the remedy, that is, a list of diseases which it is supposed to cure. Each recipe is based on a polarity of malady and remedy, since its two parts – ingredients and indications – exhibit opposite humoral qualities. For example, acrid drugs are used in a compound meant to cure phlegmatic diseases, etc.

Part of my ethnographic research in South India has been to collate some four hundred ancient recipes, culled from Caraka and other classic texts, that are still processed and prescribed today. I used a computer to retrieve the thousands of names which constitute the materia medica on the one hand, and nosology (the list of diseases) on the other hand. This is the kind of material on which we can try to evaluate the 'scientific' content of Āyurvedic medicine, by which I mean the proportion of botanical and pharmacognostic knowledge which was transmitted by pundits to the Western natural historians.

For modern natural history was born from a combination of field studies and indigenous scholarship.

Before concluding this essay with some reflections upon the relationship of natural history with scholarly medical traditions, let me come back to the epilepsy example and elaborate upon the network of humoral connections around tamas (unconsciousness) and moha (bewilderment). Apart from their philosophical and cosmological connotations, these two words designate essential qualities of phlegm. The overflowing of phlegm brings about cold and depression, torpor and unconsciousness, and the predominance of tamas and moha in the semeiotics of epilepsy points to an overflow of phlegm as its principal cause. This is confirmed in section 10 of the text on epilepsy, already mentioned, which says, 'Beneficial to epileptics are: [1] acrid substances, [2] evacuants and [3] calmatives.'

These three modes of therapy administered to epileptics constitute a closed set of three basic methods parallel to the three-fold division of medicine expounded by Celsius in the *Prooemium* of his *De Medicina*:[19] (1) dietetics, (2) operative medicine, since the administration of evacuants belongs with blood-letting and surgery in the category of manipulations, and (3) Galenical medicines, that is, compound medicines made essentially from vegetable materials. Let us consider the first division, dietetics, with respect to the use of 'acrid substances' in epilepsy. I interpret 'acrid substances' as referring to diet and food, the kind of food which is good in general against the humoral basis of epilepsy. Acridity is the quality which specifically counteracts the excess of phlegm.[20] A therapeutic statement such as 'Acrid foods are good against epilepsy' is indirectly an aetiological statement on the humoral nature of epilepsy in general, and it amounts to saying 'Epilepsy is essentially a disorder caused by excess of phlegm.' It is clear that the three-fold division of humoral epilepsy into wind-, bile- and phlegm-epilepsy is artificial. We must pursue our investigation beneath the rhetorical surface of the text to reach some more realistic observations and, then, we shall discover that epilepsy is fundamentally related to phlegm. In Āyurveda as in Galen's theory, epilepsy is a 'cold' disease.[21]

Diseases and drugs are both ascribed specific complexions, charac-

---

[19]   A detailed comparison was published in Zimmermann (note 2, 1989), pp. 168–72, and F. Zimmermann, 'Gentle Purge: The Flower Power of Āyurveda', in Charles Leslie and Allan Young (eds.), *Paths to Asian Medical Knowledge* (Berkeley: University of California Press, 1992), pp. 209–23.

[20]   Zimmermann (note 2, 1987), p. 147.

[21]   Galen's views are expounded in Owsei Temkin, *The Falling Sickness. A History of Epilepsy from the Greeks to the Beginnings of Modern Neurology*, 2nd edn, revised (Baltimore: Johns Hopkins University Press, 1971), p. 63.

terized in terms of humours, saps and sensible qualities – hot or cold, moist or dry, bilious or phlegmatic, torpid or delirious, etc. – on the basis of subjective experience. Within the framework of a scholarly tradition, the subjective experience of pathological symptoms is, so to say, culturally constructed. In other words, humoral complexions represent cultural categories or universals. Maybe we should differentiate between *categories* and *universals*, from an anthropological point of view, according to whether we focus on a particular society, seen from within and described in its own terms, or comparatively on various cultures, seen from afar, in order to reveal invariants. On the basis of this distinction, categories are culture traits shared by most members of a particular society, while universals would be patterns of sensibility existing in all cultures. The question of universals in its philosophical dimension, that of the ongoing debates on cultural relativism and comparativism, is far beyond the scope of this essay. What is of interest to us here is the construction of humours as Hindu categories, and possibly universals, since universals, if any, presuppose the cultural construction of categories.

Āyurvedic medicine provides two kinds of data on maladies as subjective experiences in the context of culture: (1) clinical observations and (2) elements of pharmacognosy, that is, descriptions of the medical properties of crude drugs and plants. If there are patterns of sensibility, the knowledge of which is concealed in the classic texts, they are to be found at the interface of clinical and pharmacognostic observations. This is the reason why recipes are central to our epistemological inquiry. The format and structure of Āyurvedic recipes are precisely those of an interface. They bring together two semantic areas, materia medica and nosology, the names of ingredients and the names of diseases. They provide the required connections between the knowledge of the proper ingredients and the knowledge of the appropriate therapeutic indications. Let me illustrate this pattern with a few examples related to epilepsy.

Acrid substances like *brahmī*, that is, leaves and roots of a fresh young plant of *Bacopa monnieri*, are the best remedies against epilepsy. Therefore, one compound medicine still very popular nowadays is 'The Brahmi-Based Ghee', *Brahmīghṛta*, whose recipe in verse appears in Caraka:[22]

---

[22] *Carakasaṃhitā, Cikitsāsthāna*, chapter 10, verse 25. I selected Caraka's version of the *Brahmī*-Based Ghee for its clarity and brevity, although, strictly speaking, it is not the one you find in Āyurvedic shops, where Vāhaṭa's version is in use. The *brahmī* and *śaṅkhapuṣpī* pair is common to both versions. Ghee (a semifluid clarified butter) is cooked in a plant decoction; it is to be taken internally.

In the juice of brahmi, with a paste of *vacā, kuṣṭha*
and *śaṅkhapuṣpī,*
old ghee should be cooked: it will cure insanity,
inauspiciousness, epilepsy, and sin.

I selected a short recipe (one distich) so as not to pad out this essay,
but the format would remain the same in longer ones: there is a list of
names, ingredients and diseases. The question whether 'inauspiciousness' and 'sin' are diseases will be discussed below. But it is clear that an
Āyurvedic recipe provides two points of departure for research on the
universals of sensibility. One is the list of diseases, which should be
interpreted as forming one *syndrome*, that is, a set of concurrent maladies
forming a specific pattern. The other one is the list of drugs which
constitute a mix of synergic drugs. In the foregoing example, there is a
polarity between a syndrome 'insanity, inauspiciousness, epilepsy, sin',
and a synergism '*brahmī, vacā, kuṣṭha, śaṅkhapuṣpī*'.

From these two points of departure, we may now proceed step by step
along the double network of humoral correlations. We can draw up the
concordance of all recipes mentioning apasmara, 'epilepsy'. It amounts
to listing all syndromes in which epilepsy concurs with other maladies,
and to pinpointing the most characteristic associations of subjective
clinical observations. Note that, in accordance with what has been said
of medicine as a wisdom in the second part of this essay, 'inauspiciousness' (the evil eye) and 'sin' (fateful misdeeds) are diseases clinically
observed; they are passions as maladies. But a comparison with other
recipes would yield some more common syndromes like delirium,
cough, epilepsy and blood poisoning, for example. We can also make
out recipes in which a synergism between two or more ingredients, like
brahmi and sankhapuspi, is resorted to as a cathartic in mania,
convulsions and blood poisoning. The association of these two drugs
will be explicated below.

Another typical synergism is '*paṭola, nimba, kaṭukā*', which constitute
the base in processing the celebrated 'Ghee with the Bitter Plants',
Tiktakaghṛta.[23] These are only three out of sixteen ingredients used to
prepare the Ghee with the Bitter Plants, theoretically prescribed in case
of mania and some thirty other bilious ailments including epilepsy. But,
in practice, the base of the compound is the patola, nimba, katuka set,
which develops a particular synergism and turns the whole compound
into a very efficacious disinfectant to be taken internally for skin diseases,
chronic ulcers, fistulas, etc.

The medicinal plants in question will be identified below. At the

[23] Vāhaṭa's *Aṣṭāṅgahṛdayasaṃhitā, Cikitsāsthāna*, chapter 19, verses 2–7. An analysis is
offered in Zimmermann (note 2, 1989), pp. 261–2.

moment I wish to emphasize the presence of numerous synergisms in Āyurvedic recipes. It is not easy to trace them, because many synonyms are used in Sanskrit and a given pharmacognostic pattern has many variants. I confess some of the most important synergisms were pointed out to me orally by Vayaskara Moos, my teacher, years ago in South India. I would not have spotted them without the help of an experienced practitioner. But this is precisely the kind of ethnographic material, or field data, on which we can build, to expose categories of collective thought and patterns of collective sensibility.

This approach to Āyurvedic medicine through Hindu categories is akin to the 'ethnosociology' project developed by McKim Marriott in Chicago,[24] although we must spare for another occasion a discussion of ethnosociology and the concept of categories. There is a circular argument in the cultural process through which categories of collective thought are constructed. Categories are culture traits characteristic of a good number of people, a number of people significant enough to make these traits appear as universals in the mind of people who share them, as seen from within the community which adheres to them; they are ideological artefacts. The humours, for example, are categories in the eyes of an Āyurvedic physician, because they are shared by all patients, which means implicitly all adult, male, twice-born Hindus, who represent patients *par excellence* in Āyurvedic medicine.

The humoral framework of Āyurvedic pathology thus is quite artificial and biased. A more detailed presentation would include an analysis of the consequences of male domination on the scholarly traditions of India, which keeps women, children and other minorities at the edge of the scholarly discourse and promotes a masculine world view in which the humours are construed as fundamental principles of life and raised to the status of cosmic forces. Nevertheless, the humours can be of use to us, at a much more realistic level, as mere labels applied to *patterns of sensibility* that have been clinically observed and recorded by the scholarly tradition.

The humours are diffracted into various syndromes and synergisms, and they can be marked out by comparing between them the humoral qualities of these syndromes and synergisms. This is done with the help of a very rich apparatus of secondary texts, in Sanskrit and in the vernacular, which provide glosses of the Sanskrit names of diseases and drugs. In that respect, the most important literary genre is the *nighaṇṭu*, or dictionary of materia medica. Some of these dictionaries played a

---

[24] Āyurvedic categories play an important role in McKim Marriott's seminal essay, 'Constructing an Indian Ethnosociology', in McKim Marriott (ed.), *India through Hindu Categories* (New Delhi: Sage, 1990), pp. 1–39.

fundamental role in the development of tropical botany, as we shall see below.

Let us come back to the examples of Ghees prescribed for epilepsy. We mentioned the association of brahmi, the juice freshly expressed from the leaves and roots of a fresh young plant of *Bacopa monnieri*, with a paste made by crushing on the curry-stone with small quantities of water vaca, the dried rhizomes of *Acorus calamus*, kustha, the dried roots of *Saussurea lappa* (a well-known aromatic spice, the Costus of Latin authors), and sankhapuspi, the leaves and roots of a fresh plant of *Clitoria ternatea* (according to South Indian doctors). I must skip the detailed analysis of this association between an Acrid (brahmi), a Bitter (the Acorus), an Aromatic (the Costus) and again a Bitter (sankha-puspi), which yields an anti-bilious and anti-phlegmatic compound, while cooking transforms the naturally anti-bilious ghee into an anti-phlegmatic, to fight both rajas and tamas, deliriums and convulsions, mania and epilepsy.[25]

For brevity's sake, I shall focus on the brahmi and sankhapuspi pair. Both are Bitter plants, but they develop a typical synergism because they share another property: they are nervine tonics that strengthen the intellect. The Āyurvedic practitioners in Kerala, the southern province of India where I studied the scholarly tradition, used to recite by heart a dictionary of materia medica named *Guṇapāṭha*, 'The Recitation of the Virtues [of Simples]'. This is a Sanskrit text in verse, with glosses in Malayalam, where they learnt the humoral properties of drugs. According to the *Guṇapāṭha*:[26]

> Sankhapuspi is purgative and bitter,
> a vermifuge, an antidote, it strengthens intellection
> . . .
> Brahmi cures oedema, anaemia and fever,
> it is acrid, hot and purgative,
> it strengthens intellection,
> bitter, it cures bile and phlegm.

These formulas are to be compared with the recipe for the Brahmi-Based Ghee. In both texts, two semantic areas are brought together: the recipe juxtaposes drug-names and disease-names, and the dictionary

[25]   On ghee shifting properties from anti-bilious to anti-phlegmatic, when cooked, see Zimmermann (note 2, 1989), pp. 63–4.
[26]   Since this text is unpublished, except in local editions in Malayalam characters, a transliteration of the relevant verses may be appropriate: *śaṅkhapuṣpī sarā* [purgative] *tiktā* [bitter] *medhyā* [strengthening intellection] *krimiviṣāpahā* [vermifuge, antidote] *śophapāṇḍujvaraharī* [cures oedema, anaemia, fever] *tīkṣṇoṣṇā ca* [acrid, hot] *viśodhinī* [purgative] *brahmī prajñābalakarī* [strengthening intellection] *tiktā* [bitter] *pittakaphā-pahā* [cures bile and phlegm].

interweaves sensible qualities (bitter, acrid, hot, etc.) with disease-names. The medicine and its ingredients are described in the light of an encompassing syndrome or set of concurrent signs and qualities: the medicinal plants in question are purgative *plus* bitter *plus* nervine tonics *plus* ... and they cure mania *plus* epilepsy *plus* oedema *plus* ... A wealth of pharmacognostic and clinical observations is thus laid down in the form of what is called by taxonomists a polythetic system.[27] A polythetic system of classification is a multi-faceted network, along which we can proceed step by step, from a given syndrome to a neighbouring one, and so on. The above-mentioned Ghee with the Bitter Plants will give us a good example of this procedure.

Epilepsy is one of the therapeutic indications of the Ghee with the Bitter Plants, but it is no longer a central one. This Ghee is more commonly prescribed for blood poisoning. Therefore, the emphasis is put upon bilious ailments and anti-bilious drugs. Of patola, for instance, which is the Bitter Gourd *Trichosanthes cucumerina,* only the leaves are used in processing this Ghee, because 'the leaves of patola are anti-bilious', while the stems are anti-phlegmatic, etc.[28] *Nimba,* the Neem, the dried bark of *Azadirachta indica,* and katuka, the Hellebore, the dried rhizomes of *Picrorhiza kurroa,* are both anti-bilious and anti-phlegmatic, but the Neem is more precisely a vermifuge and an antidote, while the Hellebore is a cathartic and a depurant.[29] All these details are recorded either in the classic compendia or in the *Guṇapāṭha* and other dictionaries of materia medica. Although I have to break the analysis here for the sake of brevity, I hope these examples will suffice to reveal the existence of a complex and sophisticated system of pharmacognosy.

An indirect proof of its scientific value is adduced by the early history of tropical botany in the seventeenth century. I can only make an allusion to the role played by the celebrated *Hortus Indicus Malabaricus* (12 vols., Amsterdam, 1678–93) in the development of Linnaean binomial nomenclature.[30] This herbal was compiled in Cochin, under

---

[27] This is the central argument in Zimmermann (note 2, 1989).

[28] *Guṇapāṭha: paṭolapatraṃ pittaghnam* ('leaves of patola are anti-bilious'), etc.

[29] *Guṇapāṭha:* the Neem is *śleṣmakrimipittaviṣāpahaḥ* [cures phlegm, worms, bile, poison], while the Hellebore is *stanyaśuddhikarī sarā* [depurant of mother's milk, purgative], etc. For all its ethnographic value, the *Guṇapāṭha* is a later apocryphal piece of secondary literature; I am skipping the question of its classic sources, but most of the foregoing phrases appear in Vāhaṭa's *Aṣṭāṅgasaṅgraha.*

[30] The story of this early encounter between Āyurvedic doctors and Western botanists has been told by J. Heniger, *Hendrik Adriaan Van Reede Tot Drakestein (1636–1691) and Hortus malabaricus. A Contribution to the History of Dutch Colonial Botany* (Rotterdam: Balkema, 1986). See p. 147 about the role played by an unspecified *Mahānighaṇṭa,* or 'Grand Dictionary' of materia medica.

the authority of the Dutch Governor, with the help of local pundits whose expertise relied upon a nighantu – an Āyurvedic dictionary of materia medica – to establish the Sanskrit and Malayalam identity of collected specimens. This is a landmark in the history of botany, but the Western botanists retained only the names and morphological descriptions of plants. The most precious part of local knowledge was missed in the development of Western studies on tropical plants. There is a misunderstanding of the concept of ethnobotany in that respect, since ethnobotanists working in India studied the plant lore of local people but ignored the scholarly tradition of polythetic pharmacognosy laid down in the nighantus. Local pundits would have been able to teach the Dutch things infinitely more precious than simply plant-names. They would have been able to arrange them according to *families* of plants having the same pharmacognostic properties, and to devise syndromes and synergisms.

The Āyurvedic dictionaries of materia medica resemble what we call natural history, insofar as they record a wealth of empirical data on the vegetable world (and other natural substances, minerals, animal products, etc.), but they differ from natural history in style and spirit. First, the texts, often in verse, are composed according to the rules of a scholastic rhetoric. Then, empirical observations are couched in humoralistic terms. Plants and other crude drugs are mirrors of men, since the prescription of compound medicines is based on a polarity of malady and remedy. In the context of humoralism, the human inhabitants of a given soil are said to share with the surrounding natural resources the same humours and saps. Therefore, the Āyurvedic equivalent of natural history – dictionaries and sections of the compendia dealing with realia – presents itself as a *prima facie* knowledge of Nature, but soon reveals its true character, namely, its being indirectly a knowledge of human susceptibilities.

An attempt has been made in these pages to present three aspects of Āyurvedic medicine that were likely to incite a comparison with other classical traditions of medicine. The first two sections of this chapter dealt with the more contextualized ones, I mean, those aspects of Āyurveda that were essentially context-dependent. For scholasticism evolves through the practice of a learned language – here, Sanskrit – and wisdom establishes itself on the basis of a religious world view – here, Hinduism. On the other hand, the polythetic system of aetiology and therapeutics described in the last section raises the question of universals, because the syndromes and synergisms recorded in the classic texts and pointed out to students by learned practitioners might remain valid beyond the boundaries of a particular culture. However, such universals, if I may use the word with all the necessary qualifications, do not belong with the natural sciences but with the social sciences. I introduced the word *susceptibilities* in the last paragraph, as a gloss on the concept of humours, to suggest that what is at stake in the scholarly traditions of humoral medicine is the discovery of collective patterns of sensibility.

15 The epistemological carnival: meditations on disciplinary intentionality and Āyurveda

Lawrence Cohen

I started by talking about knowledge, the better to be understood: the French philosophy with which we've grown up deals with little but epistemology. But for Husserl and the phenomenologists our consciousness of things is in no sense restricted to knowledge of them. The knowledge or pure 'representation' of it is only one of the possible forms of my consciousness 'of' this tree; I can also love it, fear it, hate it; and the way 'consciousness' goes beyond itself, which we call 'intentionality', is also to be found in fear, hatred and love. To hate someone is another way of breaking out toward him, it's suddenly finding oneself confronting a stranger and experiencing, above all suffering, his objective quality of 'hatefulness'. And all at once those famous 'subjective' reactions of love, hate, fear and sympathy, which were floating in the rancid marinade of Mind, are removed from it; they are just ways of discovering the world.[1]

Apparent determinacy, in the guise of regularities of classification, symbol, and of form, may veil fundamental instabilities and changes of content.[2]

We used to imagine all of Āyurveda as a 'system', and now that the formalism, coherence, and synchronicity of a system do not seem to map well on to medical knowledge and practice *in situ*, we isolate that which appears most structured and coherent as the epistemology of the thing and trace it backwards and forwards to give ourselves back time. As in the work of the French sociologist of India Louis Dumont, structure here requires a residuum, a category of that which does not fit into the beautiful passivity of the object of inquiry.[3] Still, for all their false dualisms between knowledge and the rest, our epistemogenic labours produce beauty, and understanding; the mar-

---

[1] J.-P. Sartre, 'Intentionality', trans. M. Joughin, in J. Crary and S. Kwinter (eds.), *Incorporations* (New York, 1992), p. 390.
[2] S.F. Moore, *Law as Process: An Anthropological Approach* (London, 1978), p. 49.
[3] L. Dumont, *Homo Hierarchicus: The Caste System and its Implications*, trans. M. Sainsbury, L. Dumont, and B. Gulati, revised English edn (Chicago, 1980), pp. 38–9.

320

inade of structuralist practice is not as rancid as Sartre would have us believe, or rather sense.

And yet there is a soupçon of something unpleasant, an epistemological anxiety which dogs our efforts. For it may be, against the grand theoretical debates of French sociology and American anthropology, that the relevance of the unabashedly local – structure and epistemology and knowledge and culture – against the universal contingencies of political and material forces is not an either/or sort of thing, to be debated by the proponents of structure or of practice or of a negotiated settlement, *pace* Bourdieu.[4] Against those who would reduce knowledge to a totalizing politics and those who would reduce politics to a totalizing knowledge, or culture, it may be that the relevance of 'knowledge' to totalities and to practice is in itself a contingent one. This contingency is known by another name, the missing piece in all grand theoretical debates between structure and practice: it is the body.

For the lived and mindful body is not the stable universal which both cultural and practical accounts tend to assume in offering it a rather passive presence in grand theory. It resists its reduction to any one totalizing frame. This conception of the body as resistant juncture of the individual, the symbolic, and the political or material, from Scheper-Hughes and Lock's already classic discussion,[5] problematizes the monoglot coherence and stability of any medical inscription of the body. For as the body and its afflictions are rooted in and between these multiple frames, the meaning of bodily knowledge is slippery. Apparent continuities in a medical tradition, in articulating knowledge of and relationships to bodies in shifting symbolic and political contexts, disguise points of deep disjuncture and conflict.

There are of course multiple bodies – in the polysemic sense of Scheper-Hughes and Lock – in any complex social space, splayed across axes of social difference, gendered and class and colonial – not just multiple individual bodies, but multiple social bodies and bodies politic. The construction of a unitary epistemology of '*the* body' is dependent on the possibility of the routinization or erasure of this multiplicity of claims by the makers and redactors of esoteric knowledge. This possibility is *political*, that is, is dependent on the power to reduce the body to an uncontested meditative or laboratory space. To the extent that such reductions are possible, structure, system, and epistemology may be

<hr/>

4   P. Bourdieu, *Outline of a Theory of Practice*, trans. R. Nice (Cambridge, 1977), pp. 91–5. 'The body' is often the site of this negotiated settlement of habitus, for Bourdieu, but it remains a somewhat passive signifier subsumed by the logic of practice.

5   N. Scheper-Hughes and M. Lock, 'The Mindful Body: A Prolegomenon to Future Work in Medical Anthropology', *Medical Anthropology Quarterly*, N.S. 1 (1987), 7–8.

useful and coherent abstractions in the analysis of practice. But they are more coherent at some times than others, with some healing practices than others, and for some bodies than others. This essay is about a conference which recognized the plurality of epistemologies but not of bodies, and which presumed dialogue between epistemologies as useful and even possible while ignoring the internal dialogics constituting and often convulsing epistemologies-in-themselves. It is about Āyurveda, about a contemporary moment in Āyurveda when at least two bodies – the national body and the cosmopolitan body – are superimposed, rendering the analysis of normative epistemology a challenge. In questioning, near its conclusion, a particular erasure in the Euro-American construction of contemporary Āyurveda, this essay points toward other moments in an Āyurvedic genealogy, other superimpositions of splayed bodies and other challenges to the meaningfulness of totalizing conceptions of medical practice. The carnival it recounts may not just be a feature of contested knowledge in colonial and post-colonial settings, but may characterize the limits to epistemological coherence in other times and in other sorts of political engagement.

Bombay

In 1990 the International Association for the Study of Traditional Asian Medicine (or IASTAM) held its third International Conference on Traditional Asian Medicine (or ICTAM-III) in the elegant Oberoi Towers Hotel in Bombay. IASTAM was founded by the Australian Indologist A. L. Basham to bring together diverse professions with an interest in the understanding and utilization of Āyurveda, traditional Chinese medicine, Unāni, and other Asian traditions of healing. By the late 1980s, the organization had expanded significantly; historians and philologists, sociologists and anthropologists, traditional and biomedical professionals, and public health and other state officials periodically gathered to debate what Traditional Asian Medicine (TAM) had been, was becoming, and might in future be. The vision of IASTAM involved a dizzying compression of time, in which ancient texts, current institutions and bodies, and future epidemiological predictions and policy needs were superimposed onto the figure of TAM.

I arrived an hour late. My train from Varanasi had been held up. I was finishing two years of research on senility, and was travelling to IASTAM to give a paper entitled 'The Marketing of Weakness'.[6] I

---

[6]   L. Cohen, 'The Marketing of Weakness', paper presented at IASTAM–ICTAM-III (Bombay, 1990).

wanted to suggest that modern Āyurveda might fruitfully be reconcep-
tualized – not only on the level of practice but of structure and
epistemology – in terms of its most ubiquitous contemporary intervention, the newly mass-commodified longevity or *Rasāyana* tonic. I arrived
grimy and breathless and went in search of a more affordable hotel than
the Oberoi. I found one not too far from the conference venue, an
elegant flophouse where budget travellers, middling Saudi princes, and
Churchgate Station cheap tricks mingled. Quickly cleaned up and with
paper in hand, I strode along the seawall to the Oberoi. Outside the five-
star hotel, I saw dozens of *vaidyas*, Āyurvedic doctors, milling about
along with several foreign scholars of Āyurveda. As ICTAM-III was
being held in India, many local Maharashtrian vaidyas had the
opportunity to attend; the traditional 'T' in TAM here clearly stood for
Āyurveda. Excited by the promise of multiple exchanges, I entered the
hotel.

My reflections here on the models medical historians and anthropologists often use to frame the object of study in TAM come out of the
following four days at the Oberoi, and I use the hotel itself here to
reconstruct my experience as an argument. At the time I was studying
the relationship between the commodification of weakness, *kamzorī* (in
particular the kamzorī of old age), in contemporary Āyurvedic practice
and the abstract models of life, the person, the ageing body, and time
used by practitioners. I came to ICTAM-III as a fieldworker, not only to
share with and learn from other scholars but to pay attention to the
sociology of knowledge at the conference in regard to weakness and
Rasāyana. A veteran of numerous smaller Āyurvedic conferences in
north India, I found myself drawn at ICTAM-III to its internationalism,
to the articulation of local Āyurvedic and global sociologies of knowledge, and to the commodification of larger geo-political weaknesses.
The conference was a carnival of post-colonial delights.

But what of it? Large conferences are often carnivals, colossal events
where academic proceedings are overshadowed by professional politics,
ritual enactments of disciplinary boundaries, sexual liminality, tourism
and trade, personal and national rivalries, the care and feeding of
professional kinship, and the sheer enormity of discourse. Yet the
carnivalesque at ICTAM-III represented more, rooted as it was in an
absolute disjunction between the knowledge of discursive bodies – the
Indian national body represented by both practising Āyurvedic and
scholarly researchers as being the signified object or beneficiary of their
inquiries – and real bodies, those of other persons in Bombay, not
attending ICTAM-III, for example, as well as those of the varied
researchers themselves. Through the reiteration of carnival here, I want

to raise two questions. Why is the relationship between knowledge and practice so troubling for the study of Āyurveda? And what is the relationship between the lived body of the scholar and the ways in which he or she approaches the study of medicine?

Varanasi

I begin with excerpts of the paper I travelled to Bombay to give, both to locate my discussion of contemporary Āyurvedic practice, the intent of that initial paper, and to re-read that paper's discussion of the tonic in terms of the broader epistemological concerns of this essay. Thus I start with a Hindi film dance number, not only to introduce the language of bodily weakness and its relation to failed economic circuits but as a metaphor: the figure of a woman's body within a patriarchal field of signifiers, through which I want to link the constructed seductiveness of an epistemological system to the erotic repression of scholarly disbelief. What sorts of processes underlie the objectification of the unruly body of the medical as discrete and coherent epistemologies which can be said to generate inquiry and practice?

In Varanasi, a relatively poor city in north India and a classical and contemporary centre for Āyurvedic research and practice, a local Bhojpuri term *jhandū* means all used up, without any more potential. Many Banarsis are proud of the term and its uniqueness to the region. They define jhandū specifically as a lottery ticket after the lottery. Not only is a jhandū thing all used up, it probably would have been no good anyway. During the 1989 Hindi film hit *Chandni*, India's then top-drawer movie star Sridevi did a Bombay version of a classical dance routine, dressed in silvery white and dancing in a timeless mist. Audiences, composed mostly of young men, went wild during this number. In Varanasi, a brief fad was to throw handfuls of jhandū lottery tickets in the air while Sridevi danced, and have them, so many pieces of spent and unattainable ambition, sparkle in the projected mist as they gently fluttered down through the stale air of the cinema hall.

Jhandū is the all-but-unattainable, and that after the fact. Men in Varanasi cinema halls no more believe in the fantasy of Sridevi than many European and American scholars of medicine with whom I have talked over the years believe that much within the Asian medical systems they study actually works. I do not say that they *should* 'believe' in their efficacy or not believe, but it seems worthy of reflection that they often *don't*. Other scholars have advocated the efficacy of various TAM practices, and invoke TAM as narrative protagonist in critiques of biomedicine, science, and state hegemony. Yet their (and my) intellectual versus embodied practice – To which doctors does one subject one's body, and for what? – often presents a contradiction. Again, I am not interested in accusations of bad faith. The problem is not that one cannot say interesting things about Āyurveda unless one is a patient. It is, rather, that *of the relationship between one's embodied and one's theoretical practice*. Does a lack of bodily engagement influence the forms through which practice is embodied? Thus my question: Whence the seduction? Do the forms through which we embody our interest – medicine as bounded and ultimately hermetic systems or, more recently, epistemologies – offer us clues?

Jhandū in Varanasi is frequently said jokingly by the young about the old. They are all used up; they are not worth the expenditure. In the untouchable Chamār slum of Nagwa where I worked for two years, jhandū was used by the young and particularly by young men more reflexively: they too, by virtue of their class position, were jhandū. There was a pun I heard in Nagwa, jhandū *cyavanaprāśa*, which, to explain, I need to offer some brief background on Rasāyana tonics. Rasāyana is one of the *aṣṭānga*, the eight traditional limbs of classical Āyurveda. It connotes alchemy or the radical transformation of ageing bodies into all but ageless beings. The Rasāyana sections of many Sanskrit texts, including the *Suśruta* and *Caraka Samhitās*, offer series of formulae, each followed by the promised results of one hundred to several thousands of years of youthful existence: freedom from old age and death, enhanced memory, lustre, sexual vigour, and intelligence. The administration of these drugs is often encompassed by other therapies which involve the literal destruction of the old body in the creation of the new. Through the confinement of the body and its separation from the world, followed by violent purgings, sweatings, enemas, or other radical purifications, the body is reduced to its skeletal essentials and then rebuilt.

Given the violence of its therapeutics, Rasāyana, many texts inform us, is not always for the old.[7] Several Rasāyana tonics are exceptions, most notably Chyawanprash, the administration of which in *Caraka* is explicitly allowed for old people.[8] Cyavana was a sage who cursed a king whose daughter had accidentally poked out his eyes. To win back the saint's affections and avoid the curse, the king married his offending daughter to the venerable man. She remains the villain of the narrative, quickly wearing down the old sage's vitality. He became decrepit. When the divine physicians, the Asvins, gave him the secret of what subsequently becomes known as Chyawanprash, Cyavana was rejuvenated.[9]

---

[7] *Suśruta Samhitā: Cikitsāsthānam* 27:3–4; 27:8; 33:11; 33:19.
[8] *Caraka Samhitā: Cikitsāsthānam* 1:1:62–74; 1:4:42–5.
[9] J. K. Ojha, *Chyavanaprasha: A Scientific Study* (Varanasi, 1978).

Chyawanprash is big business in India today. Long a staple tonic given by parents to children and taken by old people, it is increasingly being marketed to a young male market, with more macho sounding names like Chyawan*shakti* (*shakti* is energy or power). Unlike more explicit Āyurvedic sexual tonics, which draw on the aphrodisiac tradition of *Vājīkarana*, the neo-Chyawanprashes offer a more generalized power. Advertisements offer images of successful businessmen 'on the go'; the language of the ads weaves together mental, sexual, and economic indices of strength. Chyawanprash ads dominated one of the most watched time-spots in television history, the few minutes before the weekly national telecast of the serialized *Mahābhārata* epic from 1988 to 1990.

In the middle-class residential colonies in Varanasi where I worked, young men and women took neo-Chyawanprashes for building up their bodies and particularly for memory power and disease resistance, all linked together in the taking of competitive exams. For many of them, particularly men but many women, their projected future rested on the taking of such exams, allowing them to enter civil-service training programmes. Economic success, peak alertness, and physical shape all went together in the preparation of an examinable body. Even more than Chyawanprash, which despite its recommodification still smelled of an old person's or a child's tonic, young men in the residential colonies tried preparations with saffron or Korean ginseng. The ginseng preparations were explicitly sexual: usually red capsules, they drew on the repeatedly elaborated connection in daily Hindi newspaper advertisements between capsule size and phallic girth.

Perhaps not surprisingly, young men in the slum of Nagwa felt such tonics were useless. The space between the slum body and the examinable body was usually too vast to be signified by a tonic. The smart young men in the advertisements with stores of memory, money, and semen in the bank were fantasy objects. Tonics – represented by the ubiquitous Chyawanprash – were jhandū. Thus the pun: the Zandu company is a major Āyurvedic pharmaceutical house in India, one which has put several neo-Chyawanprashes on the market and advertised them heavily. Zandu, in Varanasi, is pronounced *jandu* and sounds like Jhandū, and thus: 'jhandū Chyawanprash', the tonic as lottery ticket. The *jouissance* of the pun comes in the irony that the successful young Chyawanprash-eating businessmen in the ads were clearly successful to begin with. Chyawanprash's effectiveness as a Rasāyana for urban élites is no great medical triumph. Within the Chamār ideology of caste in Nagwa slum, caste and hierarchical differences are structured as embodied states of weakness, kamzorī. I argue elsewhere that in Nagwa, subordinacy is experienced as bodily pathology, as a form of starvation for which no medicine – save the restitution of political and symbolic capital – could ever be effective.[10]

Bombay: the lobby

This subaltern discourse on the tonic and its relation to the commodification of Rasāyana and of 'Āyurveda' itself were the topics of the paper I had planned to give in Bombay. When I entered the cool lobby of the Oberoi, I received a briefcase filled with IASTAM–ICTAM-III materials. The briefcase, I wryly noted, was stamped with the imprimatur of the Zandu company. Zandu, it turned out, was among the principal sponsors of the conference. At the opening session, a Vote of Thanks was offered from the dais, on which were seated an impressive array of assembled international experts: 'I propose a Vote of Thanks to the Zandu Pharmaceutical Works, because it is the Big Brother.'

I use the *location* of conference events to approach the epistemological anxiety of the conference. The Oberoi is the epitome of 'five-star culture' in Bombay, a powerful sign of life in 'the West' frequently elaborated – in ridicule or awe – in newspapers and film. Five-star space is hermetically sealed, creating through air-conditioning and subdued colour schemes an anti-tropical space 'which could be anywhere' (the complimentary remark of a visiting relative of mine), anywhere, that is, except here. The internationalism of such space is thin. Nodes of cosmopolitan privilege and the frequent sites of international meetings, Indian five-star hotels offer the illusion of dialogue within a space putatively erasing cultural and political difference. When such difference appears, it then must be as a disruption, the incursion of the disgusting: the rat or the fly or the native-looking Indian. From the point of view of Management, then, the *problématique* of IASTAM–ICTAM-III within such a space becomes: how to air-condition the natives? Or, to place the ecology of the hotel lobby in Āyurvedic terms, how do you make bodies that are hot and wet (as young bodies are supposed to be) cold and dry (as old bodies are)? How do you, in short, make the natives grow up?

Yet the most powerful disruptions are not those of local smells but of global noises. Three years after the conference, in the aftermath of the Bombay riots, powerful explosives set by mysterious saboteurs – linked variously, by journalistic cognoscenti, to Dubai-based smugglers, Pakistani spies, Latin American cartels, and European arms suppliers – attempted to rend irreparably the Oberoi's façade of hermetic moder-

---

[10]   L. Cohen, *No Aging in India: Alzheimer's, The Bad Family, and Other Modern Things* (Berkeley, in press).

nity. The five-star hotel was targeted as the vulnerable nexus between a cash-hungry state and potential global investors. The putative cool hermeticism of the Oberoi in which all bodies are relaxed and equal disguises the permeability of local control and the dependence of Third-World five-star space on heavily weighted circuits of exchange.

I linger in the lobby for two reasons. First, it is the site of obvious local exclusions which mirror some of the global politics of knowledge in the conference rooms within. Second, regarding my parodic framing of air-conditioning in 'Āyurvedic' terms – hot/cold, wet/dry, and windy/still – the oppositions operant in the construction of five-star conference bodies are simultaneously cultural structures pervasive in and character-istic of Indian society *and* markers of social distinction and the everyday politics of who can best utilize these structures to advantage. Before we leave the lobby and rejoin our TAM conferees, this critical point needs underscoring. Āyurvedic epistemology and practice are indeed rooted in some sense in such structures, and yet their invocation by scholars seldom reflects the irony and contingency with which they are often utilized, their constitution through as well as of practical and embodied reason. Here again I have in mind Sartre's rancid marinade.

The parody in my use of hot and cold in diagnosing the lobby is thus not directed at the appropriateness – particularly or in general – of the opposition, but at a logic which all but fetishizes distillations of structure or system or epistemology as adequate ways into ideologies and practices of healing in local or global contexts. I juxtapose the three sets of oppositions at the Oberoi noted above in reference to another box-like structure, McKim Marriott's 'cube'. Marriott draws on classical Samkhyan cosmology in relating Āyurvedic physiology to a more general Indian 'ethno'-epistemology,[11] foregrounding three Āyurvedic opposi-tions – wet/dry, windy/still, and hot/cold – as isomorphic with other polarities structuring society, the person, space, and time. Marriott's representation of these three structural dimensions through the heuristic of a cube upon which he is prepared to graph all South Asian ethnographic data is exemplary of the most brilliant and most frustrating in structural anthropology. The growing number of cubes which he has drafted display careful attention to the ethnographies, traditions, and texts he has analysed, opening exciting possibilities for data analysis and offering a fruitful scheme for combining Indian philosophical and social theory. And yet, despite their heuristic value, the cubes like the Oberoi remain edifices of misplaced concreteness. Non-Hindu, non-upper-caste, and antinomian experience is discounted; the messiness of life is

[11]   M. Marriott, 'Constructing an Indian Ethnosociology', *Contributions to Indian Sociology*, N.S. 23 (1989), 1.

neglected to fit it to a triune model; and the projected desire of the theorist – like the tourist, bureaucrat, and investor – for a coherent, predictable, and rule-bound universe remains unquestioned.

Bombay: the Big Rooms

Let me leave the lobby. On the conference floor: four large meeting rooms, seating from one to five hundred each, ranged along a long foyer from where the frequent and elaborate buffets were served. At one end of the foyer: two far smaller rooms, seating comfortably forty to fifty. After the initial plenary session in which the integrative promise of IASTAM was re-enacted through appeals to Zandu largesse, the distinction between Big Room events and Small Room events became critical.

The meetings were dominated by hundreds of Āyurvedic practitioners, primarily from Western India, and the Big Room events were by and large presentations of Āyurvedic clinical research by and for vaidyas. Everyone else – medical historians, sociologists, anthropologists, public health professionals, traditional medical healers from non-Indic traditions, allopathic doctors and psychiatrists – were crammed into the Small Rooms. The segmentation was not the result of poor planning nor a misguided set of organizational aims: it reflected contemporary politics of knowledge. For the Big Room participants, the international set in the Small Rooms validated the cosmopolitan quality of their own practice. For Small Room participants, the presence of 'local healers' validated their claims to be authentic speakers of and for traditions which were not their own.

The extent of local Indian domination – the sheer numbers of vaidyas – alarmed some of the international set and in degree surpassed previous ICTAMs. It reflected the enormous symbolic capital for vaidyas of membership in IASTAM and of attendance at its sessions. The existence of IASTAM linked Āyurvedic practice with global authority, moving Āyurvedic claims to state and multilateral patronage into the possibility of five-star space. The globalizing legitimation of the international meeting as a social form was rooted both in its ever more routinized acceptability as a source of authentic knowledge[12] for Indian autochthonous science and in the practice of the reinscription of such meetings in counter-hegemonic, non-'Western' terms.

Meetings such as ICTAM-III are framed within contemporary Āyurvedic representational practice as latter-day extensions of the

---

[12] In the Indian epistemological tradition of Nyāya, authentic or valid sources of knowledge are termed *pramāna*s; the international meeting has all but achieved the status of a new *pramāna*.

archetypical symposium whereby Āyurveda was first promulgated. Many contemporary Āyurvedic texts or conference programmes display an image of a group of bearded sages being taught by a venerable physician – a *rsi* or seer – in the open air with the mountains as backdrop.[13] The picture suggests the early transmission of Āyurveda to its initial redactors from the rsis, recipients of Āyurvedic knowledge from the gods and its primary teachers in this world. It places the exchange in the cool shadow of the Himalayas, a different form of air-conditioned knowledge. Against any internalized orientalist opposition of Western critical rationality versus Indian lineal and convention-bound tradition,[14] the appropriation of ICTAM-III through the image of the primordial symposium claims the forms of cosmopolitan communicative practice as classically and even originally Āyurvedic. That appropriate medical knowledge is rooted in the specific sensuality of a given terrain is central to any Āyurvedic epistemology; the ecology of discovery has been developed at length in Zimmermann's path-breaking work.[15] The Āyurvedic question here would seem to be: What forms of knowing, what modes of tasting and compounding and pulsing, are appropriate to symposia located not in timeless mountains but in timebound metropolises? What happens to Āyurvedic knowledge and practice when they articulate themselves less through any engagement with clinical reality[16] but primarily through the oppositional dialogics of internationalist legitimacy?

By dialogic, I mean that Big Room panels rarely ever addressed themselves to the body of the suffering patient but rather to a contest for that body with a straw-man form of biomedicine. Healing was reduced to the rhetorical strategies of the successful contest. Biomedicine was omnipresent, a 'dialogic third' in Bakhtin's sense which stood behind each medical utterance by the vaidya about the suffering body. Biomedicine was signified in a variety of ways, from its usual depiction as the antithesis of traditional holism to the use of the pornographic. The provocative Bombay sexologist Kothari – an allopath – was, as expected, provocative. I sneaked out of the beginning of my own panel to hear him. Showing explicit slides of heterosexual couples copulating and pictures of various elaborate dildos, Kothari offered a spectacularly indecent presentation which seemed all of a piece with an afternoon at

13 See, for example, the jacket covers of *Caraka Samhitā*, trans. and ed. P.V. Sharma, 3 vols. (Varanasi, 1981–5).
14 A. Nandy, *The Intimate Enemy: Loss and Recovery of Self under Colonialism* (Delhi, 1983), pp. 112–13.
15 F. Zimmermann, *The Jungle and the Aroma of Meats: An Ecological Theme in Hindu Medicine*, trans. J. Lloyd (Berkeley, 1987).
16 A. Kleinman, *Patients and Healers in the Context of Culture: An Exploration of the Borderland between Anthropology, Medicine, and Psychiatry* (Berkeley, 1980), p. 41.

the Oberoi and the international 'values' one might expect from a collection of foreigners. The audience, composed of middle-class, primarily male Āyurvedic physicians and their wives, was titillated and shocked. As expected. Sex, the West, and scientific modernity are linked in a semantic network which is continually rehearsed in popular texts and cinema. Down the street from the hotel, the film that would become the year's big hit was opening, *Maine Pyār Kiyā*. In it, the hero and the naïve heroine, a good Indian girl, attend a party held in the ultra-modern high-tech mansion of the 'Westernized' villainess, a Kothari-esque den where couples are seen silhouetted behind rice-paper walls engaged in sexual acts while a menacing soundtrack conveys the violence and inauthenticity of the moment.

Kothari has had a well-known column in the Indian men's soft-porn magazine *Debonair*, in which he responds to letters from readers. The most common theme of his responses is that semen loss is harmless, against the concerns of his readers and the semen-conserving male physiology of Āyurveda. Kothari offers a world of unlimited free exchange, without costs, the sexual analogue of five-star fantasy space. Like the management of Indian five-star hotels,[17] he is also known to be highly concerned about whether he is up to Euro-American standards. Sexologists from the United States and Europe have received frequent unsolicited manuscripts from Kothari in Bombay, seeking their feedback and approval.[18] Yet at ICTAM-III Kothari offers his Āyurvedic audience a different narrative, one which roots his state-of-the-art seminiferous appeals not in international sexology but in the primacy of Indian tradition. He makes what is by now a classic counter-hegemonic argument, often heard at Āyurvedic conferences: whatever new sophistication the West dangles before us as the latest necessity for any socially or scientifically mature society, ancient India has already produced it. Sexual surrogates? We had 'em. Marital aids? You name it. Kothari's slide show – dildos, positions, courtesans – is offered to demonstrate the diversity of Asian sexology.

[17] Five-star hotels' offering of 'free exchange', albeit within their restricted and vulnerable internal spatialization, is continually under challenge by foreigners citing the porousness of the hotel walls which fail to keep the real India out. In 1993, the touring British cricket team and management blamed a string of test failures on the diarrhoea and gastroenteritis some members allegedly got from five-star hotel food. Fair and equal exchange, the hallmark of cricket and civilization, was for the British sportsmen impossible in the tropics (see A. Nandy, *The Tao of Cricket: On Games of Destiny and the Destiny of Games* (New Delhi, 1989), on why cricket is a revealing marker of post-colonial exchange). As long as no Indian team can claim legitimate victory because such a victory has to be attributed to parasites and India's failure to be adequately air-conditioned and authentically five-star, 'fair' exchanges are impossible.

[18] Paul Abramson, personal communication, 1993.

Recall *Maine Pyār Kiyā*, the popular Hindi film where heroines and villainesses constitute an axis of authentic national identity but heroes and villains wear their sartorial nationalism loosely, without any clear correlations between traditional *desi* Indianness and male heroism. That the woman's body is narratively structured as the repository for authentic national identity in colonial and post-colonial engagements is a point which has been made powerfully by Partha Chatterjee in his discussion of nineteenth- and twentieth-century Bengali male nationalist expectations of the female body as the site of preserved and protected Indianness,[19] and by Ann Laura Stoler in her discussion of nineteenth-century Dutch male colonial expectations in colonial Indonesia of the female body as the site of preserved and protected Europeanness.[20] Men must engage in messy exchanges, of appropriation, adaptation, control, and resistance, in ways which often blur or distort an increasingly routinized sense of national self and culture; women are for men the markers which maintain cultural distinctiveness.

The idealized good girl in Hindi film cannot, however, have no intercourse with the foreign; her very relation with a hero who articulates both local and European identity places her in a position of negotiation. In *Maine Pyār Kiyā*, the heroine must be taught to say willingly the English words 'I love you', a phrase for which there is no close translation in Hindi; the film title is itself an attempt at translation. In another film shown in Bombay several months earlier, *Bivī Ho To Aise*, the actress Rekha plays the heroine, a village girl fighting for the hearts of her husband's Westernized family against more 'mod' rivals. In the last scene the village belle reveals a dramatic secret, 'I am an Oxford graduate.' This fact, uncovered after the hero has proven his commitment to her homespun virtues, is offered not as essential to her local identity but as part of the armamentarium needed to defend it against the claims of the mod. These days, the film reveals, you've got to be an Oxford grad to survive as an authentic villager, which renders identity an almost impossible problem.

In his ICTAM lecture, Kothari attempts to offer himself as the village belle, forced into modern guise to preserve what is authentic and powerful about traditional Asian medicine. Audience reaction was mixed. Kothari's demonstration that what is most emblematic of the West, its sexual licence, was originally Indian, was a *tour de force*

---

[19]   P. Chatterjee, 'Colonialism, Nationalism, and Colonialized Women: The Contest in India', *American Ethnologist*, 16 (1989), 622–33.
[20]   A.L. Stoler, 'Carnal Knowledge and Imperial Power: Gender, Race, and Morality in Colonial Asia', Micaela di Leonardo (ed.), *Gender at the Crossroads of Knowledge: Feminist Anthropology in the Postmodern Era* (Berkeley, 1991), pp. 51–101.

obliterating any space of allopathic primacy or uniqueness. Yet, as in *Bīvī Ho To Aise*, the viewer of Kothari's slide show was left not with a sense of primacy but destabilization. These days, you've got to be pornographic to survive as local and authentic. Epistemology becomes vulgar mimesis.

Most panels were less visual. Slides were shown, but of data and flow charts. I attended a session on Rasāyana, given my research. The first panellist, Dr Bhave,[21] began with the emphatic declaration, 'The concept of Rasāyana is in no other system in the world. Maybe, now, it is beginning to emerge elsewhere.' Despite the uniqueness of Rasāyana, he focused his presentation not on Rasāyana itself but on the 'maybe, now', that is, on twentieth-century developments in physics and biomedicine. First addressed were 'the molecular concept' and 'particle wave dualism', both of which were for Bhave *approaching* the elegant truths of Rasāyana.

The legitimation of Āyurvedic practice through the invocation of indeterminacy metaphors from theoretical physics has become a routinized strategy, one which opened many of the papers of the Big Room sessions. Fritjof Capra, whose *Tao of Physics* and *Turning Point* elaborate the connections between (what he reads as) modern theoretical physics' rejection of a Cartesian universe and non-Cartesian 'Eastern' knowledges,[22] has become a charismatic icon within such presentations. In 1983, I attended the annual Dhanvantari Pūjā at the Institute of Medical Sciences in Varanasi, honouring both Dhanvantari, the god of medicine, and *Suśruta*, the classical exponent of Āyurveda and a local Varanasi boy made good. Yet far more frequent than the many invocations to *Suśruta* or Dhanvantari at the Pūjā were those to Fritjof Capra, who had achieved not only a hagiographic but a ritual status at the Institute, surpassing, it almost seemed, *Suśruta* himself.

Bhave followed his discussion of Rasāyana and the particle-wave

---

[21]   Names of most conference participants here and hereafter are fictional, my admittedly weak moral response to the meanness of subverting commonplace personal intention to a satirical reading of disciplinary intentionality. At the reading of an earlier draft of this paper, in Montreal in 1992, thoughtful objections to the inadvisability and possible racism of humour deployed from a privileged vantage point were raised. I struggle with the problems of representing the comic irony of a highly contingent and dialogically politicized epistemology against the frequently tragic epistemology of Laboratory Space and its constructed hermeticism. On the one hand, writing this way careens down a slippery slope towards the minstrel show or Shakespeare's Bottom, the subaltern as pretender and ass. Yet to ignore the tragicomedy of IASTAM is to ignore its goals of healing and understanding; such avoidance maintains an ongoing and far more profound dehumanization.

[22]   F. Capra, *The Tao of Physics: An Exploration of the Parallels between Modern Physics and Eastern Mysticism* (Berkeley, 1975), and *The Turning Point: Science, Society, and the Rising Culture* (New York, 1982).

duality with references to fermions and bosons, to 'systems theory', to the electron carrier NADH, to the structure of myelopeptides, to exostimuli and hormone cascades, to neurotension and fibroblasts, and to the specificity of polypeptides in the limbic system. He cited this material to demonstrate the scientific profundity of the textual claim that *ojas*, the quintessential substance behind the scheme of seven bodily tissues or *dhatus*, is derived from *surya*, the sun.

Skilfully weaving together frequent textual citations in Sanskrit with wildly eclectic references to cosmopolitan science and technology, Bhave accomplishes something quite interesting. Like the frequent references to endorphins, physics, and cybernetic holism which opened similar presentations a decade earlier, he legitimates Āyurveda through layered references to 'the West'. He has taken the art of the contemporary synthesis to a new degree of complexity. Against the tired references to neuropeptides of less cutting-edge colleagues, he offers myelopeptides; against Einstein's theory of relativity, he offers bosons; against holism, we are given systems theory. All fit together in a Rube Goldberg fantasy machine: the fermion hits the ancient text into the myelopeptide, which drops it onto NADH, which pushes into a hormone cascade, and so forth. Physiological progress is achieved without reference to bodies, to affliction, or to the clinic.

Narratively, Bhave achieves something more. He does not legitimate Rasāyana through physics and biomedicine; he rather legitimates new developments in these fields through Rasāyana. Like Kothari's dildos, Rasāyana is always already there. This counter-hegemonic ideology of contemporary Āyurveda as part of a discourse of national identity – beating 'the West' at its own game by claiming the game itself – has been a well-described theme of the sociology of Indian medicine for several decades, particularly in the work of Charles Leslie.[23] Zimmermann has pointed out the radical revisioning of Āyurveda which occurs when, to differentiate it from allopathy and modernity, its holism and gentleness are stressed.[24] Traditions of radical purgation and emesis, central not only to Rasāyana but to much of Āyurvedic therapeutics, are erased in such Capra-esque accounts.

The panel chairperson responded to the first minute of Bhave's talk,

[23]   C. Leslie, 'The Ambiguities of Medical Revivalism in Modern India', in C. Leslie (ed.), *Asian Medical Systems: A Comparative Study* (Berkeley, 1976), pp. 356–67, and 'Interpretations of Illness: Syncretism in Modern Āyurveda', in C. Leslie and A. Young (eds.), *Pathways to Asian Medical Knowledge* (Berkeley, 1992), pp. 177—208; see also P.R. Brass, 'The Politics of Āyurvedic Education', in S.H. Rudolph and L.I. Rudolph (eds.), *Education and Politics in India* (Cambridge, Mass., 1972), pp. 342–71.
[24]   F. Zimmermann, 'Gentle Purge: The Flower Power of Āyurveda', in C. Leslie and A. Young (note 23), pp. 209–23.

reiterating its opening statement on the originality and historical primacy of Rasāyana. None of the putatively substantive points were addressed, nor were they taken up by the audience. Audience questions in general during the panel did not engage the syntagmatic causal specifics of these myriad legitimating bits of science but rather their paradigmatic placement. A young man demanded to know if a 'high-protein diet as advocated by sports medicine' was in fact a better fit for one of the pieces of the Rube Goldberg machine than that which the author offered. He went on to ask if such a diet might not replace Rasāyana. The essential in these debates was a conscious and contestable poetics of placement.

The sports medicine question is itself intriguing, playing as it does on one of the great themes in tropical medicine and in Indian colonial discourse on the body, the debilitating effects of the Hindu diet. Young men who took ginseng in Varanasi were often concerned about their protein intake; late at night they might be found at one of the numerous omelette stands which constituted a dietary demi-monde near the Banaras Hindu University gate.

Eggs are meat, inappropriate and sometimes polluting for many high-status young men in complicated ways not at all adequately glossed by the usual purity–pollution sorts of distinctions in the field of Indian studies. Bohemian eggs are seductively displayed in vertically placed egg crates behind the counter of these small stalls. Like bottles in a liquor bar, the attraction is of multiple packets of dangerous but powerful stuff, here heightened by the erotic red of tomatoes which the egg shop vendor might substitute for some of the eggs to make enticing patterns of red and white. Male university students spoke to me of two contradictory strategies for maintaining the strong and inviolate body: purifying blood and muscle through the moral hygiene of restrained living (parallel to envisioning Āyurveda as holism) versus augmenting them through powerful but questionably clean substances like eggs (parallel to Āyurveda as radical therapy).

Ashis Nandy has drawn attention, in *The Intimate Enemy*, to the continued internalization by Indian élite men, several decades after Independence, of an infantilized and emasculated caricature of the 'Indian self' generated by a British colonial gaze.[25] Eggs and high-protein diets remain powerful signifiers of the powerful meat-fed body of the internalized other that one can never quite become. The sports medicine question suggests that more was at stake in the room than projects of institutional or professional legitimation, that the powerful

[25] Nandy (note 14), pp. 29–55.

body which Rasāyana holds forth points to important questions of the differences *between* bodies. Physiology, in the ICTAM Big Rooms, was always comparative, engaging not a generic but a national, contingent body, defined by what it was not.

Another panellist, a pharmacologist at a large allopathic hospital in Bombay, offered a paper on Rasāyana and the life-span. He began by noting that 'the concept of *kāla* in Āyurveda goes far beyond the concept of time today'. The point of the paper was that scientific research has demonstrated that ageing is correlated with the loss of body water, a fact evident in the shifting humoral balance across the life-course in Āyurvedic *tridoṣa* physiology. Rasāyana, he suggested, replenishes the moisture of the dhatus or bodily tissues.

The format and questions paralleled that of the earlier presentations, until a debate arose over whether Rasāyana was useful in the old. The debate, as we saw in the case of Chyawanprash, is not new, but given the heightened marketing of Rasāyana with both old and young models proclaiming their virtues, it had taken on new salience. One audience member suggested that, in avoiding the context of radical purgative therapies by which the giving of the Rasāyana drug must be preceded, these papers were ignoring a critical component of the bodily transformations of the field. Others responded that their old patients had been rejuvenated by the drug in itself, or that they had read a report to this effect. Against a critique that the commodification of the tonic in the age of Zandu was reducing Āyurveda from medicine to pharmacy, they insisted on the power of the drug in itself as fundamental to Āyurvedic legitimacy.

My own paper addressed some of these issues. It was also booked into a Big Room, one of the few papers not by a practitioner of real or nominal Āyurveda. I was later told the booking was a mistake. 'They thought you were from India.' Unlike the majority of my North American and European colleagues, I thus had the benefits of a disputation where a hegemonic agenda did not obliterate all dialogue. The paper discussed jhandū Chyawanprash and ginseng, the embodied meanings of weakness across class, and the commodification of Āyurveda.

In addition to ginseng, I addressed a second compound which has been labelled Āyurvedic with considerable controversy, Vick's Vapo-Rub. A competitive cold-balm manufacturer had sued Proctor and Gamble, the manufacturers of Vick's, for falsely claiming Vick's was Āyurvedic. In both cases, I was interested in the marketability of labelling a product Āyurvedic. After the panel, a flurry of questions arose. Several young Āyurvedic physicians surrounded me. 'Is ginseng

Āyurvedic or not?' They were under pressure to prescribe it, they said, given a powerful advertising campaign by several pharmaceutical houses, but were uneasy at its claims to be Āyurvedic. Ginseng is not technically in the mainstream Āyurvedic pharmacopoeia, and mine was one of the few papers to take up its authenticity, an important question for these young doctors. An older man took me aside, and confided:

I am from a dynasty of vaidyas, three generations on my father's and on my mother's side. I would like to talk with you about ginseng. It is a very important issue. I agree that we cannot call ginseng Āyurvedic, especially as we do not know its *dosic* [humoral] properties. But as for Vick's Vapo-Rub, I am the consultant to Proctor and Gamble in their defence. Their case as to whether Vick's is Āyurveda or not is now before the Supreme Court. I am showing that it is.

He detailed at length why Vapo-Rub was indeed Āyurvedic: its ingredients, its holistic potential and lack of side-effects, its humoral properties, and so forth. He had the zeal of a salesman. I looked around me for support, but saw only more young men queuing to ask me about ginseng. Was this dialogue? The Proctor and Gamble vaidya finally summed up his proof of the Āyurvedic-ness of Vick's. And then he paused, a long pause, followed by a stage whisper, 'Personally, let me tell you, it *isn't!*'

Bombay: the Small Rooms

The rest of the conference participants were packed into the two Small Rooms, which not surprisingly were overflowing and overheated. These rooms were themselves further segmented. One divide was between medical anthropology papers presented by North Americans and those presented by West Germans, with what constituted legitimate ethnography and theory clearly disputed along national lines. There were other splits. Against the interpretive stance of the anthropologists was the pragmatic 'How do we translate traditional belief into biomedically sound practice?' stance of the psychiatric and public health contingents. Against practice-oriented approaches where one had little sense of historical process were textual approaches which tended to ignore all non-canonical silences in their construction of a hermeneutic. The air was thick with colliding assumptions and bad tempers.

One panel included several transcultural psychiatrists from South and East Asia who had received some formal or informal training in ethnographic methods from American anthropologists. Their papers did not flow as smoothly as those of the vaidyas or the social scientists. The psychiatrists struggled with the difficulties of integrating their psychiatric and epidemiological training with interpretive paradigms, and often English, the language of struggle, was not their own. Unlike the Big Rooms, where Sanskrit, Hindi, and Marathi were called upon with some regularity, the 'international' climate of the Small Rooms precluded any heteroglot readings. There was silence during these papers, and few questions. The discussant – a North American anthropologist – arose, and began to lambast the panel for what he saw as a uniform poverty of analysis. It seemed a set-up, and indeed the flow of authority in the Small Rooms was continually from foreign expert to local physician or healer. A message was being offered: the locals just don't get it.

The message is not limited to the conference, however, but permeates other fora where 'TAM' is discussed in Small Room settings. *Pathways to Asian Medical Knowledge* is a collection of cutting-edge articles in the study of traditional Asian medicine.[26] In its introduction, editors Charles Leslie and Allan Young review the state of the art since Leslie's last and now classic anthology, *Asian Medical Systems*.[27] In discussing social science developments in Āyurveda, they include two Indian scholars, the prominent translator P.V. Sharma and the psychoanalyst and cultural theorist Sudhir Kakar. But they conclude that 'the prevailing tendency among Indian ethnologists and sociologists has been to neglect research on Āyurveda, Unāni, and other forms of indigenous medicine, in favour of biomedical institutions'.[28]

An unfortunate fact, if true, and one which legitimates the racial divides of Small Room politics. But it is not true – that is, there are many critical historians, sociologists, and cultural theorists in contemporary India who are interested in Āyurveda, Unāni, and other forms of indigenous medicine and who have been working between the publication of these two books. They need no apologist, but if the politics of knowledge of IASTAM are to shift, their inclusion is merited here. Some I will refer to only briefly: Shiv Visvanathan and Ashis Nandy are at the core of a group of critics at the Centre for the Study of Developing Societies who have turned to Āyurveda as a central part of a more general engagement with post-colonial ideologies of nationalism and the sociology of science. The social anthropologist J.P.S. Uberoi has been leading critical reading groups of *Suśruta* at the Delhi School of Economics.

Debiprasad Chattopadhyaya was a Marxist historian and philosopher of science in Calcutta once influential throughout India. He was one of a group of historians working with Sanskrit texts to further a complex

[26]   C. Leslie and A. Young (note 23).
[27]   C. Leslie (note 23).
[28]   C. Leslie and A. Young (note 23), pp. 11–12.

project, the use of dialectical materialism to guide the reading of a text while simultaneously using the text to construct an Indic vision of what a critical materialism might be. His early work focused on the study of heterodox Lokāyata materialism.[29] In the late 1970s, Chattopadhyaya looked more closely at Āyurveda. His argument in *Science and Society in Ancient India* is that early pre-Gupta Āyurveda was a heterodox and materialist tradition often allied with Buddhism which challenged Brahmanic ideology and power. With the re-establishment of Brahmanic hegemony by the Gupta period Āyurveda was reconstructed as a far less threatening, more theistic, and 'superstitious' system mystifying and naturalizing the caste-linked origins of human affliction.[30]

To make his argument, Chattopadhyaya subjects the language of the text to an archaeological analysis, looking for interpolations based on philological evidence. I mentioned him to some European and American Āyurvedic scholars at ICTAM-III, but they dismissed his work as of marginal scholarship. When I protested, they unleashed the ultimate weapon, 'If you knew Sanskrit . . .' *Nolo contendere*. And yet my excitement in reading Chattopadhyaya was not based on a naïve assessment of the accuracy of his claims. There is much in his analysis to distress a medical historian or anthropologist. The aggressive opposition of science and superstition central to Chattopadhyaya's analysis makes multiple unwarranted assumptions about both and about the nature and scope of rationality and healing. His Marxism is crude, and must awkwardly assume the consistent subordinacy of doctors and their identification with the most marginalized.

But what Chattopadhyaya offers is an analysis of a text and a tradition of practice rooted in a complex and hierarchical social world in which epistemology is forever the site of contest. At a time when Indian scholars are represented as doing little more than translating texts so that their foreign colleagues can read them, Chattopadhyaya offered an ambitious programme of critique and reinterpretation, less the final word on the subject than the outlines of a critical medical anthropology of Āyurveda. It is a path to medical knowledge, one of many absent from ICTAM-III. Like World Wrestling Foundation bouts, intellectual engagements at ICTAM-III lacked the feel of real action. Enormous lacunae in the roster of local contributors were interpreted through the narrative space of the conference as a dearth of local theory and knowledge and critique. Not so.

---

[29] D. Chattopadhyaya, *Lokāyata: A Study in Ancient Indian Materialism* (New Delhi, 1959).
[30] D. Chattopadhyaya, *Science and Society in Ancient India* (Calcutta, 1977), pp. 7–19, 363–426.

Whither and whence

In reviewing a passage on Āyurvedic philosophy from the historian R.C. Majumdar, one which traces the philosophic referents of Āyurveda in Sāmkhya, Nyāya, and Vedānta, Chattopadhyaya comments:

> This looks like a queer junk-shop in which dismantled parts of various metaphysical models – sometimes with random labels stuck to these – are sought to be joined to each other, uninhibited by any consideration of their mutual coherence and, what is worse for our present discussion, with a total disregard for the question of their possible relevance to the theoretical requirements of medical practice.[31]

The junk-shop, for Chattopadhyaya, marks the battle site of ideological struggle between the materialist roots of clinical practice and later superimpositions of Brahmanical authority. He reads the text's contradictions dialectically, and separates the poles of the dialectic in time, positing after Engels an antediluvian period of proto-Communism and its decline.

The reading is vulgar and simplistic, but the analysis of the text through its contradictions critical. A key problem for Chattopadhyaya is his assumption that contradiction must be explained through superimpositions over time as opposed to contradictions inherent in the practice and complex social location of the physician-redactor. The redactors of *Suśruta* and of *Caraka* might be less simplistically reconstructed, not as early proto-Marxist heroes versus later mystifying reactionaries with no commitment to patient care, but as authors with variable access to state patronage, i.e., with conflicting allegiances and cultural identities given this patronage, and yet, at the same time, a possible involvement in the embodied life of marginal communities. At least part of the palimpsest Chattopadhyaya sees in the texts might indeed be the result not of contradictory addenda over time but of the contradictions – within economies of capital, power, and knowledge – of medical practice itself.

The junk-shop of course is an uncanny depiction of the Big Room bricolage at ICTAM-III, with Rasāyana and fermions and cybernetics and sports medicine welded together into routinized heteroglossia. The similarity is instructive, and denies what was the most common, modernist reading of the IASTAM chaos I heard from European and American participants, that what was going on down the hall was but the sad politics of contemporary Āyurveda, the residual, in Dumont's sense, and not the structural. But perhaps the Big Room contribution to

[31] Ibid., p. 11.

carnival meant more, perhaps it reflected the embodied contradictions of affliction in a certain time and place, and perhaps such contradictory epistemologies are themselves a tradition in Āyurveda, a structured and structuring response to the local and global politics and physiologies of bodies. Like Mr Casaubon's endless search, in *Middlemarch*, for the Key to all Mythologies, the drive for a coherent Āyurvedic – or any other – epistemology of medicine may bear stunted fruit and ultimately be less about the object of the search than other projects of mastery.

In listening to Small Room participants complain – continually – about the others at the conference, I felt much as I had when I spent some time with North American Hare Krishnas in the Indian temple town of Brindavin. Krishna, for his devotees from Long Island and Toronto, was of course the supreme personality of Godhead. But Hindus, they sadly observed, had forgotten how to worship him properly. India without Indians: it is an old, and still quite alarming, Orientalist theme. Scholarship as neutron bomb.

Nothing in Bombay was as it appeared. Discussions on holism and Āyurvedic attention to diet were sandwiched between rich banquets of five-star cuisine. Anthropologists and historians involved in the laboured hermeneutics of understanding the other did not interact with the hundreds of Āyurvedic doctors down the hall. Foreign scholars did join vaidyas in criticizing biomedical hegemony, but wouldn't have much interaction with other foreigners who took up Āyurveda professionally: medical pluralism became museological repression. And yet, despite these myriad disjunctions within discourses and between them, the stability of Āyurveda as conceptual category and of system and epistemology as royal roads to unlocking disciplinary intentionality and practice went unchallenged. Both Big Room and Small Room academics at the Oberoi maintained a sense of systematic coherence and boundary which their own practice as well as the conference itself continually belied.

What was at stake in Bombay? I had a sense, throughout the conference, of a profound pessimism at both ends of the hall. Āyurveda was jhandū, the all-but-unattainable after the fact, for more than just its most marginal low caste interlocutors. The body laid out for discussion was neither the body of the foreign scholar, which had little at stake in Āyurvedic practice, nor of the vaidya, for whom the more powerful presence of the international body cut off local sensation. Presentations in the Big Rooms engaged substantive issues, but these issues and the research undertaken were erased within the meta-discourse organizing the sessions. The only paper which was seriously criticized by the chairperson during the Rasāyana session was that of Dr Kapur, a researcher who demonstrated the suppression of stress-induced cortisol in rats with several Rasāyana plants. Like the other papers, she integrated Rasāyana with biomedical modelling. But she did not use biomedicine iconically, as exploded pieces of discourse to legitimate a theoretical argument in Rasāyana, but rather indexically, as a translation of Rasāyana into cosmopolitan and biomedical terms. She was hit with a flurry of questions. Is your methodology itself epistemologically appropriate? Did you purge and oil and sweat the rats before giving them the medicine? Kapur countered defensively, 'I am trying to make these drugs available to many, by simplifying their grouping into systems.' The audience was unimpressed, and continued to attack her aggressively.

Others in the session had used biomedicine in similar ways, but were not attacked. Kapur failed to preface her talk with the requisite originality and uniqueness of Rasāyana. Others reversed the direction of narrative legitimation: Rasāyana proved modern science and not vice versa. Most avoided detailed discussions of therapy for abstract discussions of 'basic principles'. Kapur's presentation challenged the integrity of Rasāyana and of Āyurveda by assuming it, rather than performatively rehearsing and reconstituting it. It was not characterized by what Roland Barthes has called 'enumerative obsession' in his discussion of de Sade, the elaborate and excessive production of a signifier to fill an unsignifiable void.[32] The elaboration of system, in the Big Rooms, was an obsessive response to the anxiety that such a void existed.

Is this anxiety a response to the colonial delegitimation of Āyurveda and the larger loss of self chronicled by Nandy? Or does it respond to other vacancies, those summed up in jhandū medicine and the sick body of marginal class and caste and gender, an inscription of difference more evident in Āyurveda than in biomedicine's unyielding corpus, which is more clotted with capillary power? Questions at least worth further consideration.

In the Small Rooms, the sense of vacancy was all the more urgent: bodies, in at least one powerful sense, were not there. Packed together lifeboat-style by the vaidyas' takeover of ICTAM-III, the rest of the conference participants confronted each other at close quarters. All that united them was not being in the Big Rooms, not being, that is, practitioners of 'TAM'. The authenticity of Āyurveda here had little to do with its resemblances to more hegemonic canons, little to do, that is, with the need to reinvent a totalizing systematicity in the face of multiple dislocations. For many Small Room scholars, Āyurveda did not have to

[32] R. Barthes, Sade, Fourier, Loyola (Paris, 1971).

map onto lived daily experience nor to reflect post-colonial, or other, quandaries of embodiment. One could establish an affectively moving relationship with a practitioner or a community or a text and then go safely home, to a world where the local and the global appear happily to coincide and five-star space isn't confined to the lobby.

Authenticity has little relationship to the world beyond the text, or the carefully delineated forum of practice, when one's own embodied experience is not at stake. Epistemology can remain a clean realm; IASTAM–ICTAM–III is Āyurveda. A stage whisper, again: 'Personally, let me tell you, it *isn't*!'

Part 4

Commentaries

16   Commentary

Amos Funkenstein

Someone spoke of our endeavour as building a house in which the foundation is solid. But perhaps it's more like repairing a ship while at sea, where the foundation is not all solid but somehow it floats. And indeed, the whole foundation of what we tried to do, namely, to compare cultures, to compare bodies of knowledge, is, I would say, very flimsy, very unsafe, very uncertain both from a philosophical vantage point but also from a historian's vantage point.

First, there is the perennial problem that, when we compare two bodies of knowledge – say Indian, Chinese, Western medicine or within the Western tradition, medieval, early modern, Greek, Arabic – what is it precisely that we compare? Furthermore – and this is a philosophical question – is comparison logically possible? How do we safeguard the objectivity or vantage point for such a comparison? And do we have to give up the claim for truth if we relativize radically?

Now this logical problem of comparison is that if you compare the theories of science, or the periods of science, and even more so if you compare the very disparate bodies of knowledge, there is the question of commensurability. How do you translate a term, an observation, any item of one theory to the other? How do you translate from one language into another, from one system or concept to another? Is such a translation at all possible? Can one look for similarities?

These are questions of principle and you may argue that such translations are *a priori* impossible. You may argue, as some historians of science do, that there is no point in comparing, say, the notion of impetus developed in the Middle Ages and the principle of inertia as underlying the physics of the seventeenth century; that there can be no one-to-one correspondence between the terms of one theory and the terms of the theory which replace it, let alone the terms of a totally disparate theory. So this is the question of logical possibility. But comparisons somehow do take place. I believe they have some value.

Then there is the question of objectivity, that is, of choosing a vantage point for such a comparison, because after all we ourselves are captive in our point of view in what Gadamer calls our *Verstehenshorizont* from which there is no escaping. In other words, we are always, as historians, captive in a kind of hermeneutical circle. We construct the context from the text and we give meaning to the text from the context, be the context the immediate surrounding of the artefact we want to explain or be the surrounding our own surrounding which can be influenced by those artefacts.

Lastly, there is the question of radical relativization and the plane of truth. Now, when we compare, say, two cultures, two kinds of medicine, two kinds of science, do we have to give up all claim for truth or validity of the claims of the one as against the claims of the other? The answer, of course, is 'not at all', because it is a wrong perception that radical relativization deprives itself of reason, that the proposition 'all propositions are relative', because it includes itself, generates a paradox. It does not. The proposition 'all propositions are false' (which implies that 'this proposition is also false') does indeed generate a paradox – it is true only if it is false and false only if it is true. But the proposition 'all propositions are relatively true' (or 'this proposition is relatively true') can also be relative, that is, temporarily true or true until replaced by another or infinitely regressing; but it is not, because of that, paradoxical.

Nevertheless, even though being radically relativistic is not a self-defying position, the most relativizing or externalist interpretation of science or truth will still not base its attempt to persuade us of its validity by appealing to relative circumstances such as our health, or economic conditions, but will still try to make an argument. So we have to live, so to say, within contradictory perceptions of rationality. Rationality is context-dependent on the one hand but nonetheless it can appeal only to itself when it argues. That is, science in this sense differs from rain-making or play-acting. It still argues even if it is, as it always has been, aware of the fragility of its own assumptions and structure.

So these are questions, perennial questions of principle. Now let me sum up some of my discomforts about comparing the body of ancient Greek and medieval European medicine and science with the Indian and Chinese varieties. What I aim to do is to underline somewhat, and to systematize somewhat more, some of the matters which I became aware of during the course of our discussions.

Now the question for me, lacking much knowledge about Indian and Chinese affairs, is: what is specific or maybe unique in the development of science in the Greek, Arabic and medieval European traditions, as against these others? And one thing which came to my mind very early was that, at least since the fourth century BC, every Greek science was engaged with the question, 'What is it that makes it into a distinct body of science?' What is it that makes science a science, which establishes its independence, or at least its relative independence, from other bodies of knowledge? What is it that makes physics different from mathematics? What is it that makes physics different from medicine and so forth?

It's a question of the criteria of knowledge and of the validity of a body of knowledge and it is a question, I think, at least from all I heard, first asked by the Greeks and not asked in the other cultures. In this context, I and others referred to the Aristotelian attempt to secure the intentions and criteria of one science as against the other. Aristotle asked this question, 'What is it that distinguishes physics, say, from mathematics, or physics from metaphysics?' What kinds of principles are involved?

And I think it is of cardinal importance that it is also Aristotle who, for the first time, issued this curious injunction that one should refrain from employing the methods and forms of argument of one discipline in another (which is not subaltern to it). It was Professor Hankinson, I think, who mentioned in this context, as I also did in another, that this is in close proximity to Aristotle's very firm belief that a specific difference will never occur in more than one genus. Aristotle was certain that if being a rational animal or having the power of deliberation is the specific difference between some kind of higher mammals and us, then this kind of specific difference will never appear among minerals or among different members of any other genera.

And this Aristotle knew, not *a posteriori* because he never happened to have met a thinking stone or a mineral with social inclinations, but he knew it *a priori*. This kind of ontological commitment allowed him to claim that the ordering of nature is not arbitrary, because if a specific difference were to appear in more than one genus then why shouldn't we, if we so wished, take those instances of that specific difference and make them into a genus and make the genus out of that specific difference?

There must be something in nature itself which guarantees that our ordering into genera and species is objective, is part of nature itself. This is, I think, the deeper reason for Aristotle's certainty that a specific difference will not occur in more than one genus. It is as if he had read Mary Douglas and knew the rules of purity and danger and that one shouldn't mix categories because nature usually doesn't mix categories. Such a mixture is a monstrosity against nature. And it is, I think, the same impulse which led him also to keep the disciplines clean, in a period of scientific investigation which was just coming into its own and becoming aware of the peculiarity of this kind of an enterprise.

And he was indeed very strict. Mathematics dealt only with intelligible matter, or matter without motion. And even in mathematics one should not, without very careful devices, compare, say, curves to straight lines. They don't have a common measure. They are incommensurable. One can compare proportions of the one, or relations of the one to relations of the other. But one cannot straightforwardly compare between two kinds of magnitude.

For example, for a Greek mathematician, at least of Aristotle's guild, one could never write a very simple, innocuous equation as we have done since the seventeenth century that says 'distance equals velocity times time'. This, to Aristotle, was mixing different categories like cabbages and tomatoes. It is a meaningless expression. You can compare proportions of velocity to proportions of time but you cannot straightforwardly put time, velocity and distance in one expression. This is mixing the categories. Mixing categories is a bad thing both in nature and in theories. This injunction was to be repeated time and again in the Middle Ages, at least in the Western tradition as I know it, except that it became less and less binding. In fact, it became more and more a lip service the more one got towards the later Middle Ages – certainly after the Nominalist Revolution of the fourteenth century.

To put it differently, Aristotle claimed that there are some sciences in which there is an eclecticism of methods and which do not have first principles of their own and he calls them '*scientia media*', middle sciences. In its original Greek, it is an Aristotelian expression. And medicine was first such an eclectic science. In the Middle Ages more and more sciences, in fact almost all of them, became 'scientiae mediae'.

Together with this development the ideal of science or scientific proof also became very different toward the end of the Middle Ages. Rather than asking for demonstrative proofs of the nature of mathematical proofs in all disciplines, the criteria had become much more lax for scientific proof. I remember Albert of Saxony saying about some proofs in optics, 'this is sufficient for physics'. In physics this kind of proof is sufficient; you don't need mathematical certainty. We can't reach that degree of certainty.

So the criteria of proof in science became more relaxed. Mixing disciplines, taking methods, say, from mathematics and transporting them into theology became an everyday habit amongst the Mertonians in Oxford in the fourteenth century. Eventually, in the seventeenth century, the Aristotelian injunction was not only violated, but what Aristotle decried as a vice became for Descartes a clear virtue, namely taking the method of one science and trying to apply it to all. From this came the birth of the ideal of a universal method or a '*mathesis universalis*' which, if possible, will unlock the secrets of everything including medicine, once it too becomes 'mechanized'.

But, side by side with the relaxation of this injunction against *metabasis*, against mixing categories, against transporting methods from one discipline to another, emerged an ever-growing professionalization in the social domain of the sciences. That is, there was an increasing insistence on the social or academic independence of the discipline. If you were a philosopher you used to sit in one faculty and have privileges and obligations which were different from those of a theologian or a lawyer or a man of medicine and so forth. So it is not as if a growing cross-fertilization of disciplines brought also greater sociability amongst the practitioners.

And so I would say that one mark of the Western traditions I know, and this would be true of the Greek, the medieval, and also the modern, is the perennial question, 'What makes a discipline into a discipline?' What distinguishes it from other bodies of knowledge? Should these distinctions be relativized? How firm are they? How fruitful would it be to overcome them? These are reflexive questions which I don't find either in the social development nor in the theoretical development of other traditions, but of course I may be totally wrong there.

Let me add one more word about this separation of disciplines and the status of medicine, at least in the Middle Ages, as a 'scientia media', which I would say is a status which medicine has not lost, even today. The comparison was made by Professor Zimmermann between Indian scholasticism and Western scholasticism and we discussed at length what Western scholasticism looked like. That is, we considered whether there was in India a kind of *disputatio* as we find in, say, medieval universities in the philosophical or theological faculty, and whether Indian commentaries are at all comparable to, say, commentaries like those of fourteenth-century schoolmen which were made up of debates with earlier and present authorities. And it crossed my mind that perhaps our comparison was on the wrong object, because, curiously enough, medical instruction in the Middle Ages did not proceed in this same scholastic manner of *quaestiones disputatae* or at least not in so strict a form. It was much more the learning and reciting of a body of knowledge than was the case with any other discipline, certainly more than with theology or Aristotelian physics.

When you heard a lecture or when you studied Aristotle's physics you really did pose a question, a thesis and an anti-thesis, along with all kinds of corollary propositions which you developed and answered in a very intricate way until you evolved a very complex answer. And the answer becomes more and more complex as we move to the later Middle Ages. But none of this was true of the body of medical knowledge that was taught in the medical faculties. It was not so scholastic a form of instruction as was the case in the other faculties. It was perhaps much closer to the Indian model, say. And this is because medicine was, in their sense as in ours, a 'scientia media'.

The other feature which caught my attention as being so peculiar is that, apart from the constant awareness of the kind of theory one builds and what makes a science into a science, in other words, apart from this constant posture of reflexivity in Western science, be it ancient, medieval or early modern, there was also a readiness, sometimes stronger, sometimes weaker, to accept that which doesn't fit, to accept the singular, the unique, the not-as-yet-explained. Now this was certainly true even in the bodies of science which were regarded as very firm, such as astronomy and physics. But this was all the more true in medicine which simply, almost from its onset as a discipline, lived from case-histories, case-histories which were *narrated* in the singular. There is such and such a case which takes preponderance over its explanation and aetiology. Admittedly, the language of case-histories was still highly theoretical and people still believed when they saw what they were preconditioned to see. But there was a willingness to accept that which is unique, that which is not explained.

Take, for example, the history of ancient and medieval astronomy. It is the history of perhaps the most successful discipline, at least in the sense of prediction. Nonetheless, it was also admitted that it was not capable of a physical interpretation. The physics to which these early scientists were committed, namely Aristotelian physics, could not be harmonized with Ptolemaic astronomy. Now, whether they then said that the postulate of an equant or of an epicycle merely 'saves the phenomena' or what it means 'to save the phenomena' we can set aside. But there was this fundamental recognition that a theory is basically, intrinsically incomplete because it has no physical interpretation and the physics to which we are committed is not sufficient to generate astrophysics.

And that which was true of mathematics and physics was all the more true, I would say, of the lesser disciplines such as medicine which were regarded as less firm. In other words, perhaps we don't have the theories but we can accumulate what is called observation. This posture was true for the Middle Ages, and it was true for early modern science. Even though humoral pathology and other such theories were used, even though they were sometimes cited, and even though, for many, they were almost a dogma, nonetheless, an ancient or medieval methodologist would always say, upon reflection, that he was willing to abandon them for better models, if and when they were found.

As Professor Kuriyama has argued in his paper, it is indeed true that the Greeks perceived differently, that they saw differently from, say, the Chinese. But eventually the Greeks were always willing to exchange one model of interpretation for another, or to try on for size different models of interpretation. They were of course not always aware of their own practices. That is why they were willing, on the one hand, to debate whether or not the earth stands at the centre of the universe, and yet never debated the possibility that the celestial orbits are not circular. This remained an unchallenged premiss until Kepler, a premiss not even challenged by Copernicus. This obsession with circularity was so ingrained that an alternative was never really seriously developed.

But still, in principle, I would say, the Greek sciences were willing to look at the models they were operating with, to try to articulate them, and to endeavour at times to size up alternative models. Eventually, with a growing degree of self-consciousness, they asked, as we of that same tradition also ask, 'What is a model?' What are the forms of perception of which we are captive? These are questions that are heir to the very same willingness to entertain alternative models of explanation. I don't know that any of the other bodies of science, Indian or Chinese, were willing to entertain such possibilities.

I shall finish with a sociological observation or remark. Together with a friend of mine I once published, in Hebrew, in a lighter vein, a small booklet which we called 'The Sociology of Ignorance'. The gist of it was that, in very few societies (and they are the exception rather than the rule), a new ideal, not a reality but an ideal emerged, that of open science – science or knowledge which is accessible to everyone. Now this does not mean only the difference between accessibility and inaccessibility. It is not only that the items of knowledge are open or closed in such societies, in contrast to other societies in which knowledge is the property of a guild, of a group, of a class, or even of a community as a whole, sometimes with injunctions of secrecy. Nor is it the fact of accessibility alone that marks the new ideal. Rather, it is that the very criteria of what constitutes knowledge are inarticulate, opaque, in most societies, whereas they are meant to be accessible, transparent, open for debate in those cultures which entertain an ideal of open knowledge.

That the reality is, of course, very different, that knowledge, even today, is in fact accessible only to a few chosen by class, economic conditions, or state law, may be true. Nonetheless, even in the medical profession, we regard an item of knowledge as secure and as valid only if it has been published, i.e., only if it has withstood open debate. This doesn't mean the medical profession is open for everyone to practise or even that access to medical knowledge is really open to everyone. But it does mean that, in theory, it is open to everyone because the journals are out there for everyone to read. The ideal of open knowledge was articulated in the Greek, Jewish, Christian and modern European traditions. And perhaps it does not characterize other cultures to the same degree.

This, I think, covers what crossed my mind as matters worth discussing when comparing cultures of science, which of course I cannot do by myself. I know nothing about Indian or Chinese medicine or any other discipline enough to compare, and it is natural that, when visiting alien territory, I should look for those features of the landscape either strongly resembling or strongly differing from my own.

17   Commentary

Allan Young

My work as an anthropologist has been divided between two medical traditions: traditional Ethiopian (Amhara) medical beliefs and practices and psychiatric medicine in North America. Ethiopian medicine includes a textual tradition, derived from Graeco-Arabic sources, but my knowledge of texts extends only to recipe books and divinatory texts – humble stuff compared to the traditions discussed at this workshop. On the other hand, while psychiatric medicine has a rich textual tradition, it is also rather far removed from the humoral traditions represented here. So I can claim no expertise in any of the scholarly discourses represented among the workshop's participants.

Because my own research has focused on clinical settings, I am disposed to see these textual traditions in a similar context. Throughout the workshop, I have been asking myself these two questions. What is or was the relation between these various texts and the medical practices that each encodes? What is or was the relation of the texts cum practices to sickness in these societies? I recognize that in many instances, we have only the texts and there is no plausible way to reconstruct the clinical realities. In my comments, I want to suggest that the questions are worth asking anyway, as a tentative step to contextualizing these literate traditions.

What I require at this point is a textual tradition to which I can claim equal access and expertise with the workshop's other participants. Fortunately for me, Dr Kuriyama has introduced just the thing. You may have missed it, since his (chance) remark flashed by before the start of his splendid paper on visual knowledge in classical Chinese medicine. I am referring to Dr Kuriyama's comment on Sherlock Holmes and his legendary mastery of logical inference. What! Mixing Conan Doyle's detective stories with learned medical treatises! Please, give me a few minutes and I think that I can show that these stories have something useful to tell us.

Perhaps I should say a few words about the connection between Sherlock Holmes and medicine before I proceed. Conan Doyle was a practising physician. While studying medicine at Edinburgh, he was a student of the great surgeon, Joseph Bell, a man whose powers of observation and skills in diagnosing were famous throughout the British medical community. According to one of his students, Bell could

diagnose people as they came in, before they had opened their mouths. He would tell them their symptoms, he would give them details of their lives, and he would hardly ever make a mistake. 'Gentlemen', he would say to us students standing around, 'I am not quite sure whether this man is a cork-cutter or a slater. I observe a slight callus ... on one side of the forefinger, and little thickening on the outside of his thumb, and that is a sure sign he is either one or the other.'[1]

The set pieces in which Holmes makes his remarkable inferences are modelled on Joseph Bell's demonstrations of his virtuosity in medical semiotics. Indeed, many of the Sherlock Holmes stories can be read as metaphorical accounts of medical diagnoses, in which the great detective reconstructs the past symptomatically.

'It is an old maxim of mine, that when you have excluded the impossible, whatever remains, however improbable, may be the truth', Holmes tells Watson in *The Beryl Coronet*. Although Holmes claims to proceed in this manner, he actually does not. His much vaunted deductive method is more a 'mythod' than a method, relying more on intuition than logic.[2] Holmes's greatest asset is not his superior intellect, but rather Conan Doyle, who never fails to provide the detective with a radically pared-down environment and a small set of unusual signifiers (clues). The stories work not so much because Holmes gradually excludes the impossible, but rather because Conan Doyle has success-fully excluded so much of the possible, even before Holmes arrives. (Is it possible that Bell provided himself with similar advantages when he selected his patients for his clinical demonstrations?) The overall effect is that Holmes's action and thinking, as well as the reader's attention, are channelled into a single stream. *The Speckled Band* is typical of these stories. A murdered man is discovered in a bedroom whose door and windows are locked from the inside. The remaining point of entry is a ventilator over the bed, too tiny for a human to squeeze through. This becomes the focus of Holmes's attention. He develops a hypothesis, via an intuitive leap, involving a poisonous snake that might have descended down the rope that regulates the ventilator. His idea is that the snake bites the sleeping occupant and then slithers out under the door where it

---

[1]   R. Blathwayt, 'A Talk with Dr Conan Doyle', *Bookman*, 2 (1892), 50. Quoted in Michael Shepherd, *Sherlock Holmes and the Case of Dr Freud* (London: Tavistock, 1985), pp. 11–12.

[2]   Shepherd, ibid., p. 20.

is collected by its handler. Holmes then tests his hypothesis. It is confirmed and he nabs the murderer.

Of course it is altogether preposterous, from beginning to end. But why are we so gullible as to accept Holmes's claims about his style of reasoning? Part of the explanation has to do with our sense of time. If we examine these texts from a real time perspective – that is, tracing Holmes's mental steps from the point of his arrival at the scene of the crime up to the story's denouement – the role played by intuition and contingency becomes obvious. This is not how the text (Watson) relates the events, however. First, it is Holmes's conclusions or observations rather than his reasoning processes that Watson provides; second, he narrates them *backwards* (in the concluding pages of the story), starting with the discovery of the murder. In this way, Conan Doyle produces a retrospective chain of sufficient causes and (nearly) inevitable effects that we are eager to mistake for Sherlock Holmes's style of reasoning.

There are obvious parallels with medical texts. To make my point, I will use the example of biomedicine. There is a growing literature dedicated to the rhetoric of scientific writing. A favourite argument of these authors is that, when scientists write journal articles, they erase the boundary between real time (contingent, undetermined) and narrative time (logical, causal). The erasure is achieved through rhetorical conventions, such as the use of the passive voice ('results were obtained') and the absence of any reference to human agency (no personal pronouns). My impression is that, despite these devices, competent readers of scientific journals can tacitly recognize the co-existence of the two kinds of time – real/contingent and narrative/determined – in the work they read. On the other hand, in popular science magazines, erasure is attempted through other means: original reports are aggre-gated, renarrated, and oriented to a shared telos (a notable scientific 'discovery'). Non-scientist readers of these magazines are analogous to the readers of Watson's accounts, in that they seem inclined to mistake narrative time for real time.

My point is the obvious one that it would be a mistake to confuse the styles of reasoning that are realized in clinical practice with the ones that are encoded in medical and scholarly texts. I can take the point a step further with the help of Sherlock Holmes. One of the features that seems to disqualify Holmes as someone to be taken seriously is that he is a fictional character, and his mode of operation is not even remotely related to how real detectives work. Holmes himself made this last point, but as a way of disparaging the mental acuity of policemen. Now I want to argue that these differences are worth examining because they illuminate the relation of medical texts to their subject, sickness.

Medical practitioners, in contrast to medical texts, are more like real-life detectives than they are like Sherlock Holmes.

1. As I have indicated, Watson's claims concerning Holmes's deductive powers must be examined in the context of a pared-down reality. Each of their cases has been reduced to a small set of extraordinary features and each feature (clue) permits only a very limited number of interpretations. On the other hand, real detectives are usually dealing in situations that are open-ended, and that engender almost limitless possibilities. In contrast to what happens in *The Speckled Band*, the real detective's case is likely to involve a murdered man who is discovered in a room with an unlocked door and an open window. He can rule out snakes and ventilators but not much else. In these circumstances, he does what the rest of us would do. He reasons analogically rather than deductively, and bases his inferences on his background knowledge of precedents and probabilities.

According to Sherlock Holmes, the goal of detection is the discovery of a *particular truth*, the identity of the individual who is responsible for the particular crime under investigation. Real detectives sometimes work this way, but it would be more precise to say that their goal is an *indictable suspect* – someone who plausibly fits into a category or matches some precedent – rather than a particular truth.

2. Holmes is interacting mainly with objects rather than (human) subjects. He constructs an edifice of facts, within which he eventually encloses the guilty party and the reader. Holmes's intervention leads to closure, usually involving an explicit or implicit confession of guilt. Holmes is never dragged into court to be cross-examined by some clever attorney, and never obliged to explain and defend his inferences before a jury. It is a curiously desocialized world, in which Holmes's main contact with the legal apparatus is through an occasional police inspector. Holmes is beholden to nothing and no one – only to the truth. Everything is quite different for the real-life detective. A good (ethical) detective may serve justice, he may be an agent of justice, but he does not determine justice (guilt). He is never sufficient unto himself, but is part of a *system* of knowledge and practice.

The same two qualities are reflected in the narrative perspective of Conan Doyle's stories. Each story is centred in the consciousness of the composite figure Holmes/Watson; all of the events are filtered through his mind. Most of the medical texts discussed at the workshop are also centred. Although not necessarily located in the consciousness of an identifiable individual (author), the texts are each rooted in a single perspective, a particular view looking out from a particular expert tradition. If we are interested simply in texts and traditions, then the mono-perspective might be enough, I suppose. On the other hand, if we are interested in the relation of textual traditions to *sickness* – that is, to events and processes that affect people and their families, rather than to the disembodied concepts and accounts represented in texts – it is necessary to think beyond the mono-perspective. I suppose the analogy would be to ask Conan Doyle to rewrite *The Speckled Band* in the style of Kurosawa's *Rashomon*.

Each of the textual traditions we have considered at this workshop is the product of a complex social formation. Given what we have learned about medical beliefs and practices in the contemporary world, it seems safe to assume that, wherever people live in complex societies, they also utilize multiple medical traditions. To see the significance of this point for understanding the relationship between our texts and sickness, it will be useful if we make a distinction between 'medical traditions' and 'medical systems'.

A medical *tradition* is equivalent to sets of practices and technologies organized around historically situated ideas about aetiology, sympto-matology, and treatment. Biomedicine, Āyurveda, classical Chinese medicine are examples of medical traditions. But not all medical traditions are textual traditions nor does the presence of one textual tradition preclude the presence of one or more others. A medical *system*, on the other hand, is equivalent to the collection of traditions and sectors that are available to people living in a particular community.

Medical beliefs and practices are useful to patients and their families because they know how to incorporate them into *patterns of resort*. These are the paths that people create in the course of actual sickness episodes, as they navigate their way from one medical sector to another, picking and choosing among their options. The ethnographic literature suggests two main patterns of resort.

In the first, a pattern is created when the patient or a surrogate *simultaneously* consults alternative traditions. People have various motives for following this strategy. In some cases patients believe the effects of multiple interventions are cumulative, in other cases they are unsure which, if any, of the available traditions will provide an effective cure. In some communities, the simultaneous pattern of resort reflects a therapeutic division of labour. In South Asia today, biomedicine is prized for its quick effects against causal agents, such as 'microbes', and its ability to treat symptoms such as high fevers. Āyurveda is valued for its ability to counter the perceived iatrogenic side-effects of biomedicines, especially antibiotics, and for its ability to restore an equilibrium among the body's organs and humours. The alternative strategy consists of a *sequential* pattern of resort, in which the individual's strategy is to exhaust the resources of a given tradition or sector before moving on to an alternative tradition in the medical system.

For perfectly good reasons, the workshop's participants have concentrated on texts and mono-perspectives. At the same time, it is useful to remember that, within any society, people and sicknesses are likely to traverse traditions.

Index

364   Index

Greek medicine (*cont.*)
  social strictures and, 48–9
  testimony by women, 15, 41n, 45–7,
    48–9, 53–7
  traditional remedies, 47
  understanding of bodies by doctors,
    15, 41–59
  written works
    diffusion and transformation, 7–12
    epistemological debate, 25–39
  see also Galenism
Gregory of Tours, 121
Guṇāpāṭha ('The Recitation of the Virtues
  [of Simples]'), 316–17
gynaecology
  Chinese, 236n, 238n
  Greek, 42
  see also women's health

Hart, James, 162
Henri de Mondeville, 147
Herophilus, 63–4
Hinduism, 281–2
  see also Āyurvedic medicine
Hippocrates, 8
  On Affections, 32
  On Ancient Medicine, 26–8, 31, 33, 35–6
  On the Art, 28–9, 33–4
  De aëris, aquis et locis (*Airs, Waters,
    Places*), 115, 166
  De mulierum affectibus, 116, 117
  De salubri dieta, 115
  De victus ratione, 115–16
  On Diseases, 31–2, 45
  On Diseases of Women, 45, 47, 48, 49–50,
    53, 54, 55, 56
  early medieval texts ascribed to, 113–17,
    118
  Fractures, 45, 226
  On the Nature of the Child, 46
  On the Nature of Man, 33–4
  On the Places in Man, 32
  Prognosticon, 114–15
  On Regimen in Acute Disease, 28, 31,
    35–6
  On the Seven-month Child, 46
  On Sterile Women, 46, 53–5
  works in medieval medicine, 138
Holmes, Sherlock, 355–8
Hortus Indicus Malabaricus, 317–18
Hua Shou: illustration of human body,
  205, 206
Hua Tuo, 222
Huangdi bashiyi nanjing, see Inner Canon of
  the Yellow Lord: Canon of Eighty-
  one Problems

Huang Di Nei Jing; *Huangdi neijing zhangju
  suoyin, see* Inner Canon of the
  Yellow Lord
Huang-ti chia i ching ('A–B' Canon of the
  Yellow Lord), 192
  knowledge lineage, 187
Huang-ti nei ching, see Inner Canon of the
  Yellow Lord
Huang-ti nei ching ling shu, see Inner Canon
  of the Yellow Lord: Divine Pivot
Huang-ti nei ching su wen, see Inner Canon
  of the Yellow Lord: Basic Questions
Huang-ti pa-shih-i nan ching, see Inner
  Canon of the Yellow Lord: Canon
  of Eighty-one Problems

IASTAM, *see* International Association for
  the Study of Traditional Asian
  Medicine
Ibn Buṭlān, al-Mukhtār, 84–100
Ibn Riḍwān, ᶜAlī, 84–100
Ibn Sīnā, *see* Avicenna
India, 281
  caste system (*jati*), 293–5, 326–7
  Dharmashastra texts, 282, 293–5
  diet, Hindu, 335
  IASTAM: conference, 1990, 322–43
  marketing of Chyawanprash tonic, 326
  non-text-based knowledge, 296
  Sanskrit, 295, 300
  scholars, Indian, 338–9
  sexual mores, 330–2
  see also Āyurvedic medicine
indicative sign-inference, 65, 66, 74–5
Inner Canon of the Yellow Lord: Basic
  Questions (*Huang-ti nei ching su
  wen*), 237n
  facial colours, 210–11
  knowledge lineage, 186, 190
  se concept, 228, 229
  sexual maturation, 236–7
Inner Canon of the Yellow Lord: Divine
  Pivot (*Huang-ti nei ching ling shu*),
  237n
  anatomy, 224
  botanical analogies, 228
  colours, body, 210–11, 219, 223
  enlightened gaze, 209
  oral teachings, 186
Inner Canon of the Yellow Lord (*Huang-ti
  nei ching*), 190, 191, 192, 237n, 287,
  288, 291
  Canon of Eighty-one Problems (*Huang-
  ti pa-shih-i nan ching*), 192, 209,
  213, 228
  divergent medical practices, 29–30

natural philosophy, Greek
contrasted with medicine, 33–5
medical training and, 127–9
in role of physician, 141–2, 145–6, 148
Near East, *see* Arab-Islamic medicine
Neijing, see Inner Canon of the Yellow
Lord
neo-Confucianism, 190–1
Nidānasthāna (Book of Aetiology), 311

Oribasius, 110
Outer Canon of the Yellow Lord, 191, 192

Paths of Renowned Senior Chinese
Doctors (*Ming Laozhongyi zhi Lu*),
252–3, 253n, 257
People's Republic of China, *see* China
person-based knowing, 19–20
Chinese traditional medicine, 19–20,
272, 273–4
Petrus Alfonsi, 130
Petrus Hispanus, 134
Phayre, Thomas, 167
physicians
Chinese hereditary, 183, 195, 199
see also laozhongyi; learned physicians
Plato, 34–5
Gorgias, 34–5, 225
Timaeus, 225–6
pseudo-Apuleius, 110
Pulse Books of the Yellow Lord and Pien
Ch'ueh (*Huang-ti Pien Ch'ueh mo
shu*), 179
pulse examination, 51, 51n, 213, 246–7,
247n, 273n
Pyrrhonism, 65
Empiricism and, 76–8

Quintus Serenus, 108

radical relativization, 348
Rationalists, *see* Dogmatism
'Recitation of the Virtues [of Simples]'
(*Guṇapāṭha*), 316–17
revelatory texts, 12–13, 192–3, 194

Samkhya-karika, 294
Sanskrit, 295, 300
Sapentia artis medicinae, 111, 113n, 121–2
scholarly medicine, 23
scholarly physicians, *see* learned physicians
scientia, 133, 141–2, 146, 348–53
se concept, *see* Chinese visual knowledge
Securis, John, 168–9
Sextus Empiricus, 61, 65–7, 77, 79
Sextus Placitus, 108

sexual differences: Chinese traditional
medicine compared to Greek,
235–7
sexual mores: India, 330–2
Shanghan lun, 209
Shangshu zhengyi (Shujing), 217
Sheng chi ching (Canon of Sagely
Benefaction), 193
Shi Ji (Shih chi/Shiji) of Sima Qian, 177–8,
179–80, 208–9, 212, 218
Ch'un-yü I, 177–8
diagnosis, 30, 183–4
disciples, 181–2
medical studies, 179–82
Shujing, see Shangshu zhengyi
Sigerist, Henry, 101, 124–5
Sima Qian, 30, 218
see also Shi Ji
Skepticism, 60–1, 61n, 77
Empiricism and, 60–83
Pyrrhonism, 65, 76–8, 82
slave trade, 131
Soranus, 46
Sowerby, Leonard, 159–60
Springs and Autumns of Lü Pu-wei (*Lü
shih ch'un-ch'iu*), 188
Sun Ssu-mo, 189–90
Susruta-Samhita, 286

text editing
classical methodology, 102–4, 106–7
florilegia (anthologies), 10, 104, 105–7,
110–11, 125–6
manuscript books compared with
printed books, 104–5
traditions, *see* medical traditions
transition to the similar, 65, 71–3
Tung Chung-shu, 190

Vaughn, William, 159
Venner, Tobias, 156–8
Vesalius, Andreas: illustration of human
body, 205, 207
Vincent de Beauvais, 135, 136
Vindicianus Afer, 108, 116, 121
Visvanathan, Shiv, 338
Vivarium (monastery), 114

Wang Chong, 29, 217–18
Wang Mang, 223–4
Wang Shu-ho, Mo ching (Canon of the
Pulse), 192
Weber, Max, 4
'Western' medicine, 359
China and, 254, 259, 260, 261–2, 262n,
267

Lightning Source UK Ltd.
Milton Keynes UK
UKHW042206170919
349987UK00013BA/155/P

9 780521 480710